Cellular Physiology

Cellular Physiology

Mordecai P. Blaustein, M.D.
Professor, Departments of Physiology and Medicine
Director, Maryland Center for Heart, Hypertension and Kidney Disease
University of Maryland School of Medicine
Baltimore, Maryland

Joseph P.Y. Kao, Ph.D.
Professor
Medical Biotechnology Center
University of Maryland Biotechnology Institute
and
Department of Physiology
University of Maryland School of Medicine
Baltimore, Maryland

Donald R. Matteson, Ph.D.
Associate Professor
Department of Physiology
University of Maryland School of Medicine
Baltimore, Maryland

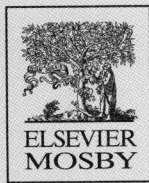

ELSEVIER
MOSBY

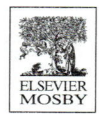

The Curtis Center
Independence Square West
Philadelphia, Pennsylvania 19106

CELLULAR PHYSIOLOGY   ISBN 0-323-01341-4
Copyright © 2004, Elsevier, Inc. All rights reserved.

Cartoon in Chapter 1 reproduced with the permission of *The New Yorker*.

No part of this publication may be reproduced, stored in a retrieval system, or transmitted in any form or by any means, electronic, mechanical, photocopying, recording, or otherwise, without prior permission of the publisher.

Permissions may be sought directly from Elsevier's Health Sciences Rights Department in Philadelphia, USA: phone: (+1)215-238-7869, fax: (+1)215-238-2239, email: healthpermissions@elsevier.com. You may also complete your request on-line via the Elsevier Science homepage (http://www.elsevier.com), by selecting 'Customer Support' and then 'Obtaining Permissions'.

NOTICE

Medicine is an ever-changing field. Standard safety precautions must be followed, but as new research and clinical experience broaden our knowledge, changes in treatment and drug therapy may become necessary or appropriate. Readers are advised to check the most current product information provided by the manufacturer of each drug to be administered to verify the recommended dose, the method and duration of administration, and contraindications. It is the responsibility of the licensed prescriber, relying on experience and knowledge of the patient, to determine dosages and the best treatment for each individual patient. Neither the publisher nor the editor assumes any liability for any injury and/or damage to persons or property arising from this publication.

Library of Congress Cataloging-in-Publication Data
Blaustein, Mordecai P.
 Cellular physiology/Mordecai P. Blaustein, Joseph P.Y. Kao, and Donald R. Matteson.
   p. cm.
 Inludes bibliographical references and index.
 ISBN 0-323-01341-4
   1. Cell physiology.   I. Kao, Joseph P.Y. II. Matteson, Donald R. III. Title.

QH631 .B556 2002
571.6–dc21   2002029562

Acquisitions Editor: William Schmitt
Developmental Editor: Kevin Kochanski
Publishing Services Manager: Patricia Tannian
Book Design Manager: Gail Morey Hudson

Printed in United States of America

Last digit is the print number: 9 8 7 6 5 4 3 2

Preface

Knowledge of cellular and molecular physiology is fundamental to understanding tissue and organ function as well as integrative systems physiology. Pathological mechanisms and the actions of therapeutic agents can best be appreciated at the molecular and cellular level. Moreover, a solid grasp of the scientific basis of modern molecular medicine and functional genomics clearly requires an education with this level of sophistication.

The explicit objective of *Cellular Physiology* is to help medical and graduate students bridge the divide between basic biochemistry and molecular and cell biology, on the one hand, and organ and systems physiology, on the other. The emphasis throughout is on the functional relevance of the concepts to physiology. Our aim at every stage is to provide an intuitive approach to quantitative thinking. The essential mathematical derivations are presented in boxes for those who wish to verify the more intuitive descriptions presented in the body of the text. Physical and chemical concepts are introduced wherever necessary to assist students with the learning process, to demonstrate the importance of the principles, and to validate their ties to clinical medicine. Applications of many of the fundamental concepts are illustrated with examples from systems physiology, pharmacology, and pathophysiology.

The book is organized into four major sections, each of which is divided into several chapters. Each chapter begins with a list of learning objectives and ends with a set of study problems. Many of these problems are designed to integrate concepts from two or more chapters or sections; the answers are presented in Appendix D. Throughout the book, key concepts and new terms are highlighted. A set of multiple-choice review questions and answers is contained in Appendix E. A review of basic mathematical techniques and a summary of elementary circuit theory, which are useful for understanding the material in the text, are included in Appendixes A and C, respectively.

We thank our many students and our teaching colleagues who, by their critical questions and insightful comments over the years, have helped us to refine and improve the presentation of this fundamental and fascinating material. Nothing pleases a teacher more than a student whose expression indicates that the teacher's explanation has clarified a difficult concept that, just a few moments earlier, was completely obscure.

Mordecai P. Blaustein
Joseph P.Y. Kao
Donald R. Matteson

Acknowledgments

We thank Professor Clara Franzini-Armstrong for providing original electron micrographs, as well as Professors Luis Reuss and Martin F. Schneider for their very helpful comments and suggestions on preliminary versions of, respectively, Chapters 10 and 11 and Chapters 12 to 14. We also thank Professors David M. Warshaw and Toby C. Chai for valuable help with Chapter 14.

Contents

SECTION I
Fundamental Physicochemical Concepts

1 Introduction: Homeostasis and Cellular Physiology, 1
- Homeostasis enables the body to survive in diverse environments, 1
- The body is an ensemble of functionally and spatially distinct compartments, 2
  - The biological membranes that surround cells and subcellular organelles are lipid bilayers, 3
  - Biomembranes are formed primarily from phospholipids but may also contain cholesterol and sphingolipids, 3
  - Biomembranes are not uniform structures, 3
- Transport processes are essential to physiological function, 4
- Cellular physiology focuses on membrane-mediated processes and on muscle function, 5
- Summary, 5
- Key words and concepts, 6

2 Diffusion and Permeability, 7
- Diffusion is the migration of molecules down a concentration gradient, 7
- Fick's First Law of Diffusion summarizes our intuitive understanding of diffusion, 7
- Essential aspects of diffusion are revealed by quantitive examination of random, microscopic movements of molecules, 9
  - Random movements result in meandering, 9
  - The root-mean-squared (RMS) displacement is a good measure of the progress of diffusion, 10
  - Square-root-of-time dependence makes diffusion ineffective for transporting molecules over large distances, 11
  - Diffusion constrains cell biology and physiology, 11
- Fick's First Law can be used to describe diffusion across a membrane barrier, 12
  - The net flux through a membrane is the result of balancing influx against efflux, 15
  - The permeability determines how rapidly a solute can be transported through a membrane, 17
- Summary, 20
- Key words and concepts, 20
- Study problems, 20

3 Osmotic Pressure and Water Movement, 21

- Osmosis is the transport of *solvent* driven by a difference in *solute* concentration across a membrane that is impermeable to solute, 21
- Water transport during osmosis leads to changes in volume, 22
- Osmotic pressure drives the net transport of water during osmosis, 22
- Osmotic pressure and hydrostatic pressure are functionally equivalent in their ability to drive water movement through a membrane, 25
  - The direction of fluid flow through the capillary wall is determined by the balance of hydrostatic and osmotic pressures, as described by the Starling equation, 26
- Only impermeant solutes can have permanent osmotic effects, 30
  - *Transient* changes in cell volume occur in response to changes in the extracellular concentration of *permeant* solutes, 30
  - *Persistent* changes in cell volume occur in response to changes in the extracellular concentration of *impermeant* solutes, 31
  - The amount of *impermeant* solute inside the cell determines the cell volume, 32
- Summary, 32
- Key words and concepts, 35
- Study problems, 35

4 Electrical Consequences of Ionic Gradients, 37

- Ions are typically present at different concentrations on opposite sides of a biomembrane, 37
- Selective ionic permeability through membranes has electrical consequences: the Nernst equation, 37
- The stable resting membrane potential in a living cell is established by balancing multiple ionic fluxes, 42
  - Cell membranes are permeable to multiple ions, 42
  - The resting membrane potential can be quantitatively estimated by use of the Goldman-Hodgkin-Katz equation, 45
  - A permeant ion already in electro-chemical equilibrium does not need to be included in the GHK equation, 47
  - The Nernst equation may be viewed as a special case of the GHK equation, 47
- The cell can change its membrane potential by selectively changing membrane permeability to certain ions, 48
- The Donnan effect is an osmotic threat to living cells, 48
- Summary, 49
- Key words and concepts, 52
- Study problems, 52

SECTION II
Ion Channels and Excitable Membranes

5 Ion Channels, 53

- Ion channels are critical determinants of the electrical behavior of membranes, 53
- Distinct types of ion channels have several common properties, 54
  - Ion channels increase the permeability of the membrane to ions, 54
  - Ion channels are integral membrane proteins that form gated pores, 55
  - Ion channels exhibit ionic selectivity, 55
- Ion channels share structural similarities and can be grouped into gene families, 56
  - Channel structure is studied with biochemical and molecular biological techniques, 56

Contents

- ○ Structural details of a K⁺ channel are revealed by x-ray crystallography, 58
- Summary, 59
- Key words and concepts, 61
- Study problems, 61

6 Passive Electrical Properties of Membranes, 63

- The time course and spread of membrane potential changes are predicted by the passive electrical properties of the membrane, 63
- The equivalent circuit of an excitable membrane has a resistor in parallel with a capacitor, 64
  - ○ Membrane conductance is established by open ion channels, 64
  - ○ Capacitance reflects the ability of the membrane to separate charge, 65
- Passive membrane properties produce linear current-voltage relationships, 65
- Membrane capacitance affects the time course of voltage changes, 65
  - ○ Ionic and capacitive currents flow when a channel opens, 65
  - ○ The exponential time course of the membrane potential can be understood in terms of the passive properties of the membrane, 67
- Membrane and axoplasmic resistances affect the passive spread of subthreshold electrical signals, 69
  - ○ The decay of subthreshold potentials with distance can be understood in terms of the passive properties of the membrane, 70
  - ○ The length constant is a measure of how far away from a stimulus site a membrane potential change will be detectable, 73
- Summary, 73
- Key words and concepts, 73
- Study problems, 74

7 Generation and Propagation of the Action Potential, 75

- The action potential is a rapid and transient depolarization of the membrane potential in electrically excitable cells, 75
  - ○ The properties of the action potential can be studied with intracellular microelectrodes, 75
- Ion channel function is studied with a voltage clamp, 77
  - ○ Ionic currents are measured at a constant membrane potential with a voltage clamp, 77
  - ○ Ionic currents are dependent on voltage and time, 79
  - ○ Voltage-gated channels exhibit voltage-dependent conductances, 81
- Individual ion channels have two conductance levels, 83
- Sodium channels inactivate during maintained depolarization, 84
- The action potential is generated by voltage-gated Na⁺ and K⁺ channels, 86
  - ○ The equivalent circuit of a patch of membrane can be used to describe action potential generation, 86
  - ○ The action potential is a cyclical process of channel opening and closing, 87
  - ○ Both Na⁺ channel inactivation and open voltage-gated K⁺ channels contribute to the refractory period, 87
  - ○ Pharmacological agents that block Na⁺ or K⁺ channels, or interfere with Na⁺ channel inactivation, alter the shape of the action potential, 89
- Action potential propagation occurs as a result of local circuit currents, 89
  - ○ In nonmyelinated axons an action potential propagates as a continuous wave of excitation away from the initiation site, 89
  - ○ Conduction velocity is influenced by τ, by λ, and by I_{Na} amplitude and kinetics, 91

- ○ Myelination increases action potential conduction velocity, 93
- Summary, 96
- Key words and concepts, 96
- Study problems, 97

8 Ion Channel Diversity, 99

- Various types of ion channels help to regulate cellular processes, 99
- Voltage-gated Ca^{2+} channels contribute to electrical activity and mediate Ca^{2+} entry into cells, 99
  - ○ Calcium currents can be recorded with a voltage clamp, 101
  - ○ Ca^{2+} channel blockers are useful therapeutic agents, 104
- Potassium-selective channels are the most diverse type of channel, 104
  - ○ Neuronal K^+ channel diversity contributes to the regulation of action potential firing patterns, 105
  - ○ Rapidly inactivating voltage-gated K^+ channels cause delays in action potential generation, 107
  - ○ Ca^{2+}-activated K^+ channels are opened by intracellular Ca^{2+}, 109
  - ○ ATP-sensitive K^+ channels are involved in glucose-induced insulin secretion from pancreatic β-cells, 109
- Ligand-gated channels are gated by agonist binding, 111
  - ○ Acetylcholine opens channels at the neuromuscular junction, 112
- Ion channel activity can be regulated by second-messenger pathways, 113
  - ○ β-Adrenergic receptor activation modulates L-type Ca^{2+} channels in cardiac muscle, 113
- Summary, 115
- Key words and concepts, 115
- Study problems, 116

SECTION III
Solute Transport

9 Electrochemical Potential Energy and Transport Processes, 117

- Electrochemical potential energy drives all transport processes, 117
  - ○ The relationship between potential energy and force is revealed by an examination of gravity, 117
  - ○ A gradient in chemical potential energy gives rise to a chemical force that drives the movement of molecules, 118
  - ○ An ion can have both electrical and chemical potential energy, 118
  - ○ The Nernst equation is a simple manifestation of the electrochemical potential energy, 120
  - ○ How to use the electrochemical potential energy to analyze transport processes, 121
- Summary, 126
- Key words and concepts, 126
- Study problems, 126

10 Passive Solute Transport, 127

- Diffusion across biological membranes is limited by lipid solubility, 127
- Channel, carrier, and pump proteins mediate transport across biological membranes, 128
  - ○ Transport through channels is relatively fast, 129
  - ○ Permeability through channels depends on the density of channels in the membrane, 129
  - ○ The rate of transport through open channels depends on the net driving force, 130
  - ○ Transport of substances through some channels is controlled by "gating" the opening and closing of the channels, 130

Contents

- Carriers are integral membrane proteins that open to only one side of the membrane at a time, 130
  - Carriers facilitate transport through membranes, 130
  - Transport by carriers exhibits kinetic properties similar to those of enzyme catalysis, 132
- Coupling the transport of one solute to the "downhill" transport of another solute enables carriers to move the cotransported or countertransported solute "uphill" against an electrochemical gradient, 134
  - Sodium/proton exchange is an example of Na^+-coupled countertransport, 134
- Sodium is cotransported with a variety of solutes such as glucose and amino acids, 136
  - How does the electrochemical gradient for one solute affect the gradient for a cotransported solute? 137
  - Glucose uptake efficiency can be increased by a change in the Na^+-glucose coupling ratio, 139
- Net transport of some solutes across epithelia is effected by coupling two transport processes in series, 139
  - A variety of inherited defects of glucose transport have been identified, 140
- Sodium is exchanged for solutes such as calcium and protons by countertransport mechanisms, 141
  - Na^+/Ca^{2+} exchange is an example of coupled countertransport, 141
  - Na^+/Ca^{2+} exchange is influenced by changes in the membrane potential, 143
  - Na^+/Ca^{2+} exchange is regulated by several different mechanisms, 143
  - Intracellular Ca^{2+} plays many important physiological roles, 143
- Multiple transport systems can be functionally coupled, 144
  - Tertiary active transport, 145
- Summary, 146
- Key words and concepts, 147
- Study problems, 147

11 Active Transport, 149

- Primary active transport converts the chemical energy from ATP into electrochemical potential energy stored in solute gradients, 149
  - Three broad classes of ATPases are involved in active ion transport, 150
- The plasma membrane Na^+ pump (Na,K-ATPase) maintains the low Na^+ and high K^+ concentrations in the cytosol, 150
  - Nearly all animal cells normally maintain a high intracellular K^+ concentration ($[K^+]_i$) and a low intracellular Na^+ concentration ($[Na^+]_i$), 150
  - The Na^+ pump hydrolyzes ATP while transporting Na^+ out of the cell and K^+ into the cell, 150
  - The Na^+ pump is "electrogenic," 152
  - The Na^+ pump is the receptor for cardiotonic steroids such as ouabain and digoxin, 152
- Intracellular Ca^{2+} signaling is universal and is closely tied to Ca^{2+} homeostasis, 154
- Ca^{2+} storage in the sarcoplasmic/endoplasmic reticulum is mediated by a Ca^{2+}-ATPase, 157
  - SERCA has three isoforms, 158
- The plasma membrane of most cells also has an ATP-driven Ca^{2+} pump, 158
  - The relative roles of the several Na^+ and Ca^{2+} transporters differ in different cell types, 159
  - Different functions account for the different distribution of the Na^+/Ca^{2+} exchanger and PMCA in the same plasma membrane, 159

- Transport systems may be functionally coupled in parallel or in series, 160
- Several other plasma membrane transport ATPases also play important physiological roles, 160
  - An H^+,K^+-ATPase mediates gastric acid secretion, 160
  - Two copper-transporting ATPases play essential physiological roles, 162
  - ATP-binding cassette (ABC) transporters are a superfamily of P-type ATPases, 163
- Net transport across epithelial cells depends on the coupling of apical and basolateral membrane transport systems, 165
  - Epithelia are continuous sheets of cells, 165
  - Epithelia exhibit great functional diversity, 167
  - What are the sources of Na^+ for apical membrane Na^+-solute cotransport? 168
  - Absorption of Cl^- occurs by several different mechanisms, 169
  - Substances can also be secreted by epithelia, 170
  - Net water flow is coupled to net solute flow across epithelia, 172
- Summary, 174
- Key words and concepts, 175
- Study problems, 175

SECTION IV
Molecular Motors and Muscle Contraction

12 Molecular Motors and the Mechanisms of Muscle Contraction, 177

- Molecular motors produce motility by converting chemical energy into kinetic energy, 177
  - The three types of molecular motors are myosin, kinesin, and dynein, 177
- Single skeletal muscle fibers are composed of many myofibrils, 178
- The sarcomere is the basic unit of contraction in skeletal muscle, 178
  - The sarcomere consists of interdigitating thin and thick filaments, 178
  - Thick filaments are composed mostly of myosin, 182
  - Thin filaments in skeletal muscle are composed of four major proteins: actin, tropomyosin, troponin, and nebulin, 182
- According to the "sliding filament" mechanism, muscle contraction results from thin and thick filaments sliding past each other, 182
- The cross-bridge cycle powers muscle contraction, 184
- In skeletal and cardiac muscles, Ca^{2+} activates contraction by binding to the regulatory protein troponin C, 188
- The structure and function of cardiac muscle and smooth muscle are distinctly different from those of skeletal muscle, 188
  - Cardiac muscle is striated, 188
  - Cardiac muscle cells require a continuous supply of energy, 190
  - To act as a pump, the muscle cells that make up each chamber of the heart must contract synchronously, 190
  - Smooth muscles do not exhibit the striations observed in other muscle types, 190
  - In smooth muscle, elevation of the cytosolic Ca^{2+} concentration activates contraction by promoting the phosphorylation of the myosin regulatory light chain, 191
- Summary, 196
- Key words and concepts, 196
- Study problems, 197

13 Excitation-Contraction Coupling in Muscle, 199

- Skeletal muscle contraction is initiated by a depolarization of the surface membrane, 199
    - In skeletal muscle, depolarization initiates contraction, 199
    - Skeletal muscle has a high resting Cl⁻ permeability, 200
    - A twitch is a transient contraction that results from a single action potential, 201
    - How does depolarization increase $[Ca^{2+}]_i$ in skeletal muscle? 202
- Direct mechanical interaction between sarcolemmal and sarcoplasmic reticulum membrane proteins may mediate excitation-contraction coupling in skeletal muscle, 202
    - In skeletal muscle, depolarization of the T-tubule membrane is required for excitation-contraction coupling, 202
    - In skeletal muscle, extracellular Ca^{2+} is *not* required to activate contraction, 202
    - In skeletal muscle, the sarcoplasmic reticulum stores all of the Ca^{2+} needed for contraction, 203
    - The triad is the structure that mediates excitation-contraction coupling in skeletal muscle, 205
    - In skeletal muscle, excitation-contraction coupling is believed to be mechanical, 205
    - Skeletal muscle relaxes when Ca^{2+} is returned to the sarcoplasmic reticulum by the sarcoplasmic reticulum Ca^{2+} pump, 207
- Ca^{2+}-induced Ca^{2+} release is central to excitation-contraction coupling in cardiac muscle, 208
    - In cardiac muscle, communication between the SR and sarcolemmal membrane occurs at dyads and peripheral couplings, 209
    - In cardiac muscle, excitation-contraction coupling requires extracellular Ca^{2+} and Ca^{2+} entry through L-type Ca^{2+} channels, 210
    - The Ca^{2+} that enters the cell during the cardiac action potential must be removed to maintain a steady state, 211
    - Cardiac contraction can be regulated by an alteration in $[Ca^{2+}]_i$, 211
- Activation of smooth muscle differs in fundamental ways from excitation-contraction coupling in skeletal and cardiac muscles, 211
    - Smooth muscles are highly diversified, 211
    - The density of innervation varies greatly among different types of smooth muscles, 214
    - Some smooth muscles are normally activated by depolarization, 215
    - Some smooth muscles are normally activated by agents that induce little or no depolarization, 215
    - Inositol-1,4,5-trisphosphate activates the release of Ca^{2+} from smooth muscle sarcoplasmic reticulum, 218
    - Long-term Ca^{2+} balance is maintained by Ca^{2+} extrusion mechanisms that compensate for the Ca^{2+} entry during smooth muscle activation, 218
- Summary, 221
- Key words and concepts, 222
- Study problems, 222

14 Mechanics of Muscle Contraction, 225

- The total force generated by a skeletal muscle can be varied by several mechanisms, 225
    - Whole muscle force can be increased by recruitment of motor units, 225
    - A single action potential produces a twitch contraction, 226
    - Repetitive stimulation produces fused contractions, 228

- Skeletal muscle mechanics is characterized by two fundamental relationships, 229
  - The relationship between initial muscle length and force can be understood in terms of the sliding filament mechanism, 230
  - The velocity of shortening decreases as force increases in isotonic contractions, 231
- There are three main types of phasic skeletal muscle motor units, 232
- The force generated by cardiac muscle is regulated by various mechanisms that control $[Ca^{2+}]_i$, 234
  - Cardiac muscle generates long-duration contractions, 234
  - The total force developed by cardiac muscle is related to the level of $[Ca^{2+}]_i$ attained during activation, 235
- The mechanical properties of cardiac and skeletal muscle are similar, but there are significant quantitative differences, 235
  - Isolated cardiac muscle and skeletal muscle have similar length-tension relationships, 235
  - The force of contraction of the intact heart varies as a function of its initial (end-diastolic) volume, 237
  - The velocity of shortening in cardiac muscle is slower than in skeletal muscle, 238
- The dynamic properties of smooth muscle contraction differ markedly from those of skeletal and cardiac muscle, 238
  - Three key relationships can be used to define the kinetic properties of smooth muscle function, 238
  - The length-tension relationship in smooth muscles is consistent with the sliding filament mechanism of contraction, 238
  - The velocity of shortening is much lower in smooth muscle than in skeletal muscle, 239
- Some properties of specific types of smooth muscles can be resolved by a study of individual myosin motors, 241
  - Analysis of single actin and myosin molecule interactions has resolved the question of how smooth and skeletal muscles generate the same amount of stress despite very different shortening velocities, 241
  - The kinetic properties of the cross-bridge cycle depend largely on the myosin isoforms expressed in the cells, 242
  - Myosin light chain phosphorylation determines the velocity of smooth muscle shortening and the amount of stress generated, 242
- The relationship among $[Ca^{2+}]_i$, myosin light chain phosphorylation, and force in smooth muscles is complex, 242
  - Tonic smooth muscles can maintain tension with little consumption of ATP, 243
  - Perspective: smooth muscles are functionally diverse, 246
- Summary, 246
- Key words and concepts, 249
- Study problems, 249

Epilogue, 251

Appendixes

A A Mathematical Refresher, 255
- Exponents, 255
  - Definition of exponentiation, 255
  - Multiplication of exponentials, 255
  - Meaning of the number 0 as exponent, 256
  - Negative numbers as exponents, 256
  - Division of exponentials, 256
  - Exponentials of exponentials, 256
  - Fractions as exponents, 256

Contents

- Logarithms, 257
  - Definition of the logarithm, 257
  - Logarithm of a product, 257
  - Logarithm of an exponential, 257
  - Changing the base of a logarithm, 258
- Solving quadratic equations, 258
- Differentiation and derivatives, 258
  - The slope of a graph and the derivative, 258
  - Derivative of a constant number, 260
  - Differentiating the sum or difference of functions, 260
  - Differentiating composite functions: the chain rule, 261
  - Derivative of the natural logarithm function, 262
- Integration: the antiderivative and the definite integral, 263
  - Indefinite integral (also known as the antiderivative), 263
  - Definite integral, 263
- Differential equations, 264
  - First-order equations with separable variables, 264
  - Exponential decay, 264
  - First-order linear differential equations, 265

B Root-Mean-Squared Displacement of Diffusing Molecules, 267

C Summary of Elementary Circuit Theory, 271
- Cell membranes are modeled with electrical circuits, 271
- Definitions of electrical parameters, 271
  - Electrical potential and potential difference, 271
  - Current, 272
  - Resistance and conductance, 272
  - Capacitance, 273
- Current flow in simple circuits, 273
  - A battery and resistor in parallel, 273
  - A resistor and capacitor in parallel, 274

D Answers to Study Problems, 281

E Review Examination, 295
- Answers to review examination, 309

Cellular Physiology

CHAPTER 1

SECTION I Fundamental Physicochemical Concepts

Introduction: Homeostasis and Cellular Physiology

Objectives:

1. Understand the need to maintain the constancy of the internal environment of the body and the concept of homeostasis.
2. Understand the hierarchical view of the body as an ensemble of distinct compartments.
3. Understand the composition and structure of the lipid bilayer membranes that encompass cells and organelles.
4. Understand why the protein-mediated transport processes that regulate the flow of water and solutes across biomembranes are essential to all physiological functions.

■ HOMEOSTASIS ENABLES THE BODY TO SURVIVE IN DIVERSE ENVIRONMENTS

Humans are independent, free-living animals who can move about and survive in vastly diverse physical environments. Thus we find humans inhabiting habitats ranging from the frozen tundra of Siberia and the mountains of Nepal* to the jungles of the Amazon and the deserts of the Middle East. Nevertheless, the elemental constituents of the body are cells, whose survival and function are possible only within a narrow range of physical and chemical conditions, such as temperature, oxygen concentration, osmolarity, and pH. Therefore the whole body can survive under diverse external conditions only by maintaining the conditions around its constituent cells within narrow limits. In this sense the body has an **internal environment,** which is maintained constant to ensure survival and proper biological functioning of the body's cellular constituents. The process whereby the body maintains constancy of this internal environment is referred

---

*The adaptability of humans can be surprising: humans can survive on Mount Everest, which, at 29,028 feet above sea level, is at the cruising altitude of jet airplanes. At the summit the temperature is about −40° Celsius (same as −40° Fahrenheit), the thin atmosphere supplies only about one third of the oxygen at sea level, and the relative humidity is zero.

1

to as **homeostasis**.* When homeostatic mechanisms are severely impaired, as in a patient in an intensive care unit, artificial life support systems become necessary for maintaining the internal environment.

Achieving homeostasis requires various component physiological systems in the body to function coordinately. The musculoskeletal system enables the body to be motile and to acquire food and water. The gastrointestinal system extracts nutrients (both sources of chemical energy, such as sugars, and essential minerals, such as sodium, potassium, and calcium) from food. The respiratory (pulmonary) system absorbs oxygen, which is required in oxidative metabolic processes that "burn" food to release energy. The circulatory system transports nutrients and oxygen to cells, while carrying metabolic waste away from cells. Metabolic waste products are eliminated from the body by the renal and respiratory systems. The complex operations of all the component systems of the body are coordinated and regulated through **biochemical signals** released by the endocrine system and disseminated by the circulation, as well as through electrical signals generated by the nervous system.

■ THE BODY IS AN ENSEMBLE OF FUNCTIONALLY AND SPATIALLY DISTINCT COMPARTMENTS

The organization of the body may be viewed hierarchically (Figure 1-1). The various systems

---

*The concept of the internal environment was first advanced by the 19th-century French pioneer of physiology Claude Bernard, who discussed it in his book, *Introduction à l'étude de la médecine expérimentale* in 1865. Bernard's often-quoted dictum is: "The constancy of the internal environment is the pre-requisite for a free life." ("*La fixeté du milieu intérieur est la condition de la vie libre,*" from *Leçons sur les phénomènes de la vie communs aux animaux et aux végétaux*, 1878). The term "homeostasis" was introduced by the American physiologist Walter B. Cannon in his physiology text, *The Wisdom of the Body* (1932).

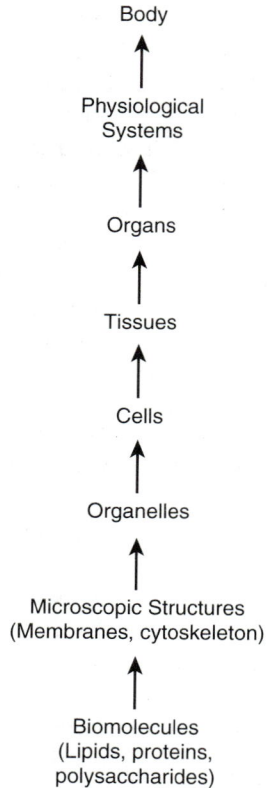

Figure 1-1 ■ **Hierarchical view of the organization of the body.** (Modified from Eckert R, Randall D: *Animal physiology*, ed 2, San Francisco, 1983, WH Freeman.)

of the body not only constitute functionally distinct entities, but also comprise spatially and structurally distinct compartments. Thus the lungs, the kidneys, the various endocrine glands, the blood, and so on are distinct compartments within the body. Each compartment has its own local environment that is maintained homeostatically to permit optimal performance of different physiological functions.

Compartmentation is an organizing principle that applies not just to macroscopic structures in the body, but to the constituent cells as well. Each cell is a compartment distinct from the extracellular environment and separated from that environment by a membrane (the *plasma membrane*). The intracellular space of each cell is further divided into subcellular compartments (cytosol, mitochondria, endoplasmic reticulum, etc.). Each of these subcellular compartments is encompassed within its own membrane, and each has a different microscopic internal environment to allow different cellular functions to be carried out optimally (e.g., protein synthesis in the cytosol and oxidative metabolism in mitochondria).

The Biological Membranes That Surround Cells and Subcellular Organelles Are Lipid Bilayers

As noted previously, cells and subcellular compartments are separated from the surrounding environment by biomembranes. Certain specific membrane proteins are inserted into these **lipid bilayer membranes.** Many of these proteins are **transmembrane proteins** that mediate the transport of various solutes or water across the bilayers. Ion channels and ion pumps are examples of such transport proteins. Other transmembrane proteins have signaling functions and transmit information from one side of the membrane to the other. Receptors for peptide hormones and growth factors are examples of signaling proteins.

Biomembranes Are Formed Primarily from Phospholipids but May Also Contain Cholesterol and Sphingolipids

The majority of the lipids that make up biomembranes are *phospholipids*. These **amphiphilic (or amphipathic) phospholipids** consist of a **hydrophilic** (water-loving), or **polar,** phosphate-containing head group attached to two **hydrophobic** (water-fearing), or **nonpolar,** fatty acid chains. The phospholipids assemble into a sheet or *leaflet*. The polar head groups pack together to form the hydrophilic surface of the leaflet, and the nonpolar hydrocarbon fatty acid chains pack together to form the hydrophobic surface of the leaflet. Two leaflets combine at their hydrophobic surfaces to form a bilayer membrane.

The bilayer presents its two hydrophilic surfaces to the aqueous environment, while the hydrophobic fatty acid chains remain sequestered within the interior of the membrane (Figure 1-2). The individual lipid molecules within the bilayer are free to move and are not rigidly packed. Therefore the lipid bilayer membrane behaves in part like a two-dimensional fluid and is frequently referred to as a **fluid mosaic.**

Biomembranes typically also contain other lipids such as cholesterol and sphingolipids. For example, in animals, biomembranes usually contain significant amounts of cholesterol, a nonphospholipid whose presence alters the fluidity of the membrane.

Biomembranes Are Not Uniform Structures

Different biomembranes vary in their lipid composition. For example, the plasma membrane is rich in cholesterol but contains almost no cardiolipin (a structurally complex phospholipid); the reverse is true for the mitochondrial membranes. Even the lipid compositions of the two leaflets constituting a single bilayer membrane can differ. For example, whereas phosphatidyl choline is most abundant in the outer leaflet of the plasma membrane, phosphatidyl serine is found almost exclusively in the inner leaflet. Such asymmetry can be maintained because flip-flop of lipid molecules from one leaflet to the other occurs naturally at an extremely slow rate.

Some cytoskeletal proteins bind to membrane proteins. These interactions enable the cytoskeleton to confer structural integrity on the membrane. Just as important, such interactions, by grouping and "tethering" membrane proteins, also organize membrane proteins into functional

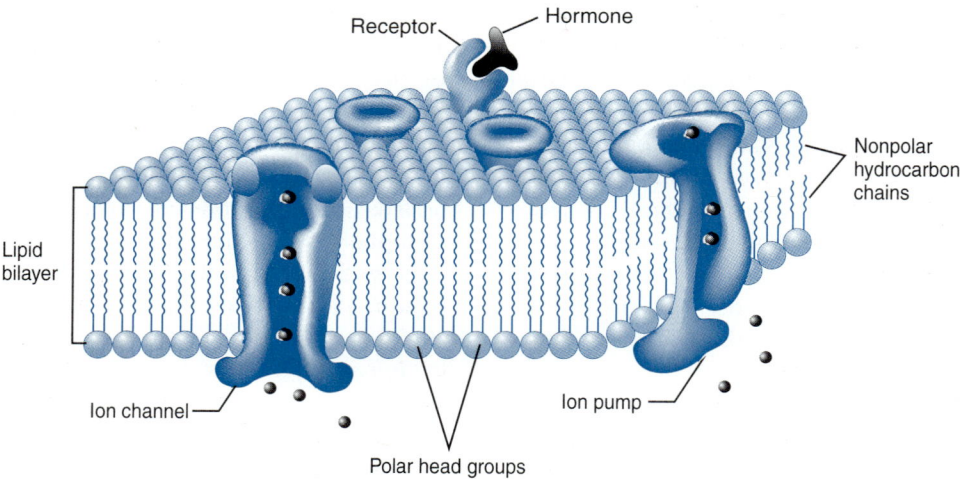

Figure 1-2 ■ Lipid bilayer of the plasma membrane, with various membrane proteins that serve transport and signaling functions. The locations of the polar head groups and nonpolar hydrocarbon chains of the phospholipids in the bilayer are shown. Also represented are a hormone receptor, an ion channel, and an ion pump.

membrane **microdomains.** Such microdomains are compositionally and functionally different from other regions of the membrane. Thus it should be apparent that most biomembranes are not uniform either in composition or in architecture but are highly organized structures with different microdomains serving different functions.

■ TRANSPORT PROCESSES ARE ESSENTIAL TO PHYSIOLOGICAL FUNCTION

Each compartment within the body, whether microscopic or macroscopic, has the optimal biochemical composition to enable a different set of physiological processes to take place. But those very physiological processes tend to alter the composition within the compartments. In this light, homeostasis within each compartment implies that transport processes must operate continuously to adjust and maintain the internal environment of each compartment, including microscopic compartments such as those within subcellular organelles. Therefore transport mechanisms are central to homeostasis. Moreover, coordinated regulation of the physiological functions that occur in distinct compartments implies communication, that is, the transmission and reception of signals, between different compartments. At the subcellular level this is achieved through the generation and movement of biochemical signals, including **second messengers** such as inositol trisphosphate (IP_3), cyclic adenosine monophosphate (cAMP), or calcium ions (Ca^{2+}). As noted earlier, extracellular (or intercellular) communication is mediated by biochemical signals as well as electrical signals. The biochemical signals (e.g., hormones and growth factors) are secreted by specialized cells and disseminated through the circulation. The electrical signals are generated and propagated through the transport of certain ions across the membranes of "excitable" cells (see Chapters 5 to 7). By their nature, the signaling mechanisms themselves alter the composition of the cells from which they originate. Thus the composition of those cells, too, must be continually restored. Therefore transport processes are also fundamental to the coordinated regulation of physiological processes in the body. Indeed, when membrane transport processes go awry, as may occur with mutations in transport proteins, homeostatic mechanisms are disrupted and physiology is adversely affected (this is referred to as **pathophysiology**). Examples of pathophysiological mechanisms are presented throughout this book.

■ CELLULAR PHYSIOLOGY FOCUSES ON MEMBRANE-MEDIATED PROCESSES AND ON MUSCLE FUNCTION

The foregoing description implies that homeostasis and its regulation depend on transport and signaling processes that occur at or through biological membranes. For this reason such **membrane-mediated processes** are essential to physiology and are a central theme of this text (Chapters 2 to 11). Of these membrane-mediated processes, passive diffusion and osmosis are fundamental physical processes that can occur *directly* through any lipid bilayer membrane and are the topics of Chapters 2 and 3, respectively. The vast majority of the membrane-mediated processes can occur only through the agency of diverse protein machinery (e.g., ion channels, solute transporters, and transport ATPases or "pumps") residing in cellular membranes. These membrane protein-dependent processes are the subject of Chapters 4 to 11. A schematic representation of a cellular (plasma) membrane and some of the transport and signaling processes it mediates is shown in Figure 1-2.

Although processes mediated by cellular membranes are fundamental to physiological function, they take place on a microscopic scale. The maintenance of life also requires action on a macroscopic scale. Thus acquisition of food and water requires body mobility; nutrient extraction requires maceration of food and its passage through the gastrointestinal tract; intake of oxygen and expulsion of carbon dioxide require expansion and contraction of air sacs in the lungs; and distribution of nutrients and dissemination of endocrine signals to various tissues require rapid transport of material through the circulation. All of these processes require movement on a macroscopic scale. The evolutionary solution to the problem of large-scale movements is *muscle*. For this reason the cellular mechanisms underlying muscle function constitute the other major theme of this text (see Chapters 12 to 14). The subject of cellular physiology comprises the two major themes described above.

■ SUMMARY

1. To survive under extremely diverse conditions, the body must be able to maintain a constant internal environment. This process is referred to as *homeostasis*.
2. Homeostasis requires the coordination and regulation of numerous complex activities in all the component systems of the body.
3. The body can be viewed in terms of a hierarchical organization in which compartmentation is a major organizing principle.
4. Cells and subcellular organelles are compartments that are encompassed within biomembranes, which are essentially lipid bilayer membranes.
5. Biomembranes are composed primarily of phospholipids and integral membrane proteins; the membranes may also contain other lipids such as cholesterol and sphingolipids.
6. Most of the integral membrane proteins span the membrane (i.e., they are transmembrane proteins) and are involved in signaling or in

the transport of water and solutes across the membrane. These processes are essential for homeostasis.
7. Biomembranes are usually nonuniform structures: the inner and outer leaflets often have different composition. Many integral membrane proteins bind to elements of the cytoskeleton and may be organized into microdomains with specialized functions.
8. The transport processes mediated by integral membrane proteins such as channels, carriers, and pumps in cell and organelle membranes are essential for physiological function.
9. The maintenance of life also depends on movement on a macroscopic scale. Such movements are mediated by muscle.

■ KEY WORDS AND CONCEPTS

- Internal environment
- Homeostasis
- Biochemical signals
- Compartmentation
- Lipid bilayer membranes
- Transmembrane proteins
- Amphiphilic (or amphipathic) phospholipids
- Hydrophilic (polar)
- Hydrophobic (nonpolar)
- Fluid mosaic
- Membrane microdomains
- Second messengers
- Pathophysiology
- Membrane-mediated processes

■ BIBLIOGRAPHY

Alberts B, Johnson A, Lewis J, et al: *Molecular biology of the cell*, ed 4, New York, 2002, Garland Science.

Bernard C: *An introduction to the study of experimental medicine* (translated by H.C. Greene, from the French: *Introduction à l'étude de la médecine expérimentale*, Paris, 1865, JB Baillière), New York, 1957, Dover.

Bernard C: *Leçons sur les phénomènes de la vie communs aux animaux et aux végétaux, Tome 1*, Paris, 1878, JB Baillière.

Cannon WB: *The wisdom of the body*, New York, 1932, WW Norton.

Eckert R, Randall D: *Animal physiology*, ed 2, San Francisco, 1983, WH Freeman.

Gennis RB: *Biomembranes*, New York, 1989, Springer-Verlag.

Vance DE, Vance JE: *Biochemistry of lipids and membranes*, Menlo Park, Calif, 1985, Benjamin/Cummings.

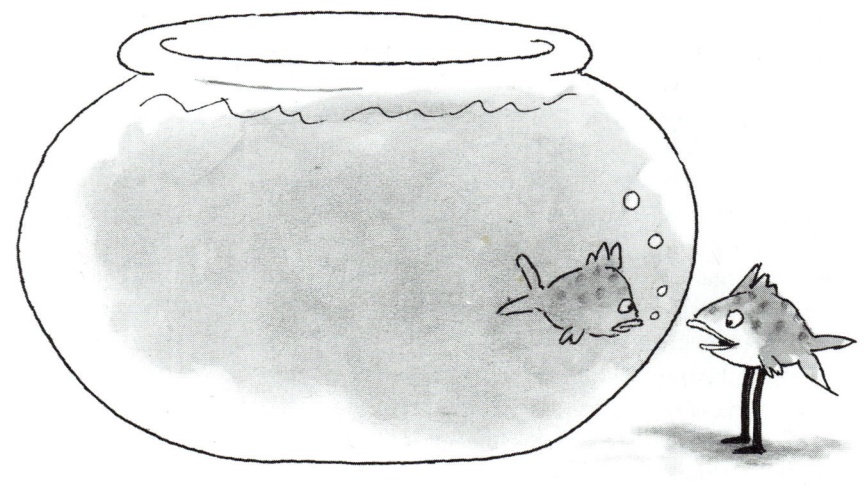

"In order to be free I had to make certain adjustments."

CHAPTER 2

Diffusion and Permeability

Objectives:

1. Understand that diffusion is the migration of molecules *down* a concentration gradient.
2. Understand that diffusion is the result of the purely *random* movement of molecules.
3. Define the concepts of *flux* and membrane *permeability* and the relationship between them.

■ DIFFUSION IS THE MIGRATION OF MOLECULES DOWN A CONCENTRATION GRADIENT

Experience tells us that molecules always move spontaneously from a region where they are more concentrated to a region where they are less concentrated. As a result, concentration differences between regions become gradually reduced as the movement proceeds. **Diffusion** always transports molecules from a region of high concentration to a region of low concentration because the underlying molecular movements are completely *random*. That is, any given molecule has no preference for moving in any particular direction. The effect is easy to illustrate. Imagine two adjacent regions of comparable volume in a solution (Figure 2-1). There are 5200 molecules in the left-hand region and 5000 molecules in the right-hand region. For simplicity, assume that the molecules may move only left or right. Because the movements are random, at any given moment approximately half of all molecules would move to the right and approximately half would move to the left. This means that, on average, roughly 2600 would leave the left side and enter the right side, while 2500 would leave the right and enter the left. Therefore a *net* movement of about 100 molecules would occur across the boundary going from left to right. Note that this net transfer of molecules caused by **random movements** is indeed from a region of higher concentration into a region of lower concentration.

■ FICK'S FIRST LAW OF DIFFUSION SUMMARIZES OUR INTUITIVE UNDERSTANDING OF DIFFUSION

The preceding discussion indicates that the larger the difference in the number of molecules between adjacent compartments, the greater the

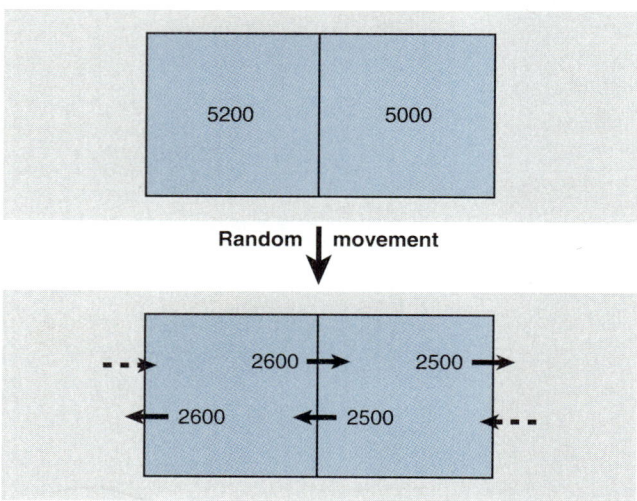

Figure 2-1 ■ Two adjacent compartments of comparable volume in a solution. The left compartment contains 5200 molecules, and the right compartment contains 5000 molecules. If the molecules can only move randomly to the left or to the right, approximately half of all molecules would move to the right and approximately half would move to the left. This means that, on average, roughly 2600 would leave the left side and enter the right side, while 2500 would leave the right and enter the left.

net movement of molecules from one compartment into the next. In other words, the *rate* at which molecules move from one region to the next depends on the concentration difference between the two regions. The following definitions can be used to obtain a more explicit and quantitative representation of this observation:
1. **Concentration gradient** is the change of concentration, ΔC, with distance, Δx (i.e., $\Delta C/\Delta x$).
2. **Flux** (symbol J) is the amount of material passing through a certain cross-sectional area in a certain amount of time.

With these definitions, the earlier observation can be simply restated as "flux is proportional to concentration gradient," or

$$J \propto \frac{\Delta C}{\Delta x} \qquad [1]$$

By inserting a proportionality constant, D, we can write the above expression as an equation:

$$J = -D\frac{\Delta C}{\Delta x} \qquad [2]$$

The proportionality constant, D, is referred to as the **diffusion coefficient** or **diffusion constant**. The minus sign accounts for the fact that the diffusional flux, or movement of molecules, is always *down* the concentration gradient (i.e., flux is from a region of high concentration to a region of low concentration). The graphs in Figure 2-2 illustrate this sign convention.

Equation [2] applies to the case in which the concentration gradient is linear, that is, a change in concentration, ΔC, for a given change in distance, Δx. For cases in which the concentration gradient may not be linear, the equation can be generalized by replacing the linear concentration gradient, $\Delta C/\Delta x$, with the more general expression for concentration gradient, dC/dx (a derivative). The diffusion equation now takes the form

Diffusion and Permeability

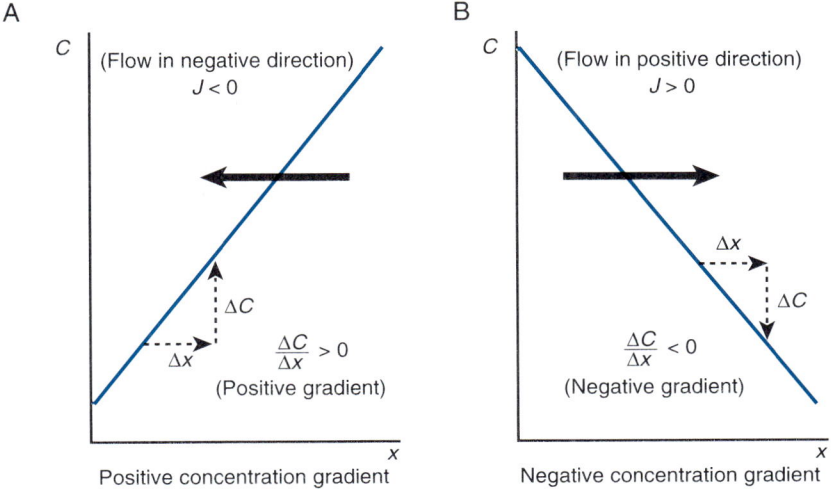

Figure 2-2 ■ The direction (sign) of the concentration gradients is opposite to the direction (sign) of the flux. A, A positive concentration gradient: the concentration increases as we move in the positive direction along the *x*-axis ($\Delta C/\Delta x > 0$). The flux being driven by this positive gradient is in the negative direction. The concentration increases from left to right, but the flux is going from right to left. B, A negative concentration gradient: the concentration decreases as we move in the positive direction along the *x*-axis ($\Delta C/\Delta x < 0$). The flux being driven by this negative gradient is in the positive direction. The concentration increases from right to left, but the flux is going from left to right.

$$J = -D\frac{dC}{dx} \qquad [3]$$

This equation is also known as **Fick's First Law of Diffusion**. It is named after Adolf Fick, a German physician who first analyzed this problem in 1855.

To complete the discussion of Fick's First Law, we should examine the dimensions (or units) associated with each parameter appearing in Equation [3]. Because flux, J, is the quantity of molecules passing through unit area per unit time, it has the dimensions of "moles per square centimeter per second" ($= (mol/cm^2)/s = mol \cdot cm^{-2} \cdot s^{-1}$). Similarly, the concentration gradient, dC/dx, being the rate of change of concentration with distance, has dimensions of "moles per cubic centimeter per centimeter" ($= (mol/cm^3)/cm = mol \cdot cm^{-4}$). For all the units to work out correctly in Equation [3], the diffusion coefficient, D, must have dimensions of cm^2/s ($= cm^2 \cdot s^{-1}$).

■ ESSENTIAL ASPECTS OF DIFFUSION ARE REVEALED BY QUANTITATIVE EXAMINATION OF RANDOM, MICROSCOPIC MOVEMENTS OF MOLECULES

Random Movements Result in Meandering

The most important characteristics of diffusion can be appreciated just by considering the simplest case of random molecular motion—that of a single molecule moving randomly along a single dimension. The situation is presented graphically in Figure 2-3.

The molecule is initially (at Time = 0) at some location that for convenience we simply refer to as 0 on the distance scale. During every

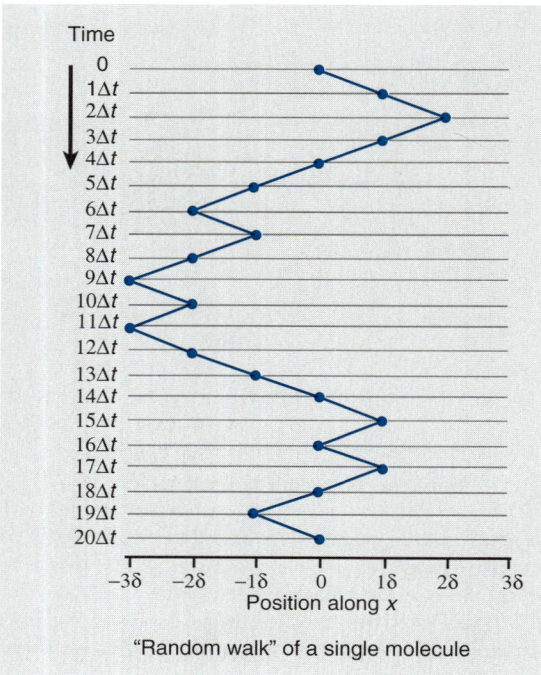

Figure 2-3 ■ "Random walk" of a single molecule. A molecule is initially at position $x = 0$. During each increment of time, Δt, the molecule can take a step of size δ, either to the left or to the right. The position occupied by the molecule after each time increment is marked by a dot. A typical series of 20 steps is shown.

time increment, Δt, the molecule can take a step of size δ either to the left or to the right. A typical series of 20 random steps is shown in Figure 2-3. Two features are immediately apparent from the figure. First, when a molecule is moving randomly, it does not make very good progress in any particular direction; it tends to meander back and forth aimlessly. Second, because the molecule meanders, its net movement away from its starting location is not rapid. These two features manifest themselves in important ways when we consider the aggregate behavior of a large number of molecules.

Figure 2-4 presents the results of a numerical simulation of diffusive spreading of 2000 molecules initially confined at $x = 0$ (Figure 2-4, *A*). At each time point, each molecule takes a random step (forward and backward steps are equally probable). After each molecule has taken 10 random steps (Figure 2-4, *B*), some molecules are seen to have moved away from the initial position and the number of molecules remaining at precisely $x = 0$ has dropped to ~250. After 100 steps have been taken (Figure 2-4, *C*), many molecules have moved farther afield, with a corresponding drop in the number remaining at $x = 0$ to ~100. The trend continues in Figure 2-4, *D* (after 1000 steps). Note the change in magnitude of the vertical axis in each panel to rescale the spatial distribution for visual clarity. Clearly, the spatial distribution of molecules is gradually broadened by diffusion.

One might ask what the average position of all the molecules is after diffusion has caused the spatial distribution to broaden. Figure 2-4 shows that as the molecules move randomly, they spread out progressively, but *symmetrically*, so that their average position is always centered on $x = 0$. This is reasonable: because moves to the right and left are equally probable, at any time, there should always be roughly equal numbers of molecules to the right and to the left of 0. The average position of such a distribution must be $x = 0$ at all times. This observation indicates that the average position is not an informative measure of the progress of diffusion.

The Root-Mean-Squared (RMS) Displacement Is a Good Measure of the Progress of Diffusion

We seek a quantitative description of the fact that, with time, the molecules will cluster less and will progressively spread out in space. The desired measure is the **root-mean-squared displacement,** d_{RMS} (see Appendix B). For diffusion in one dimension,

Diffusion and Permeability

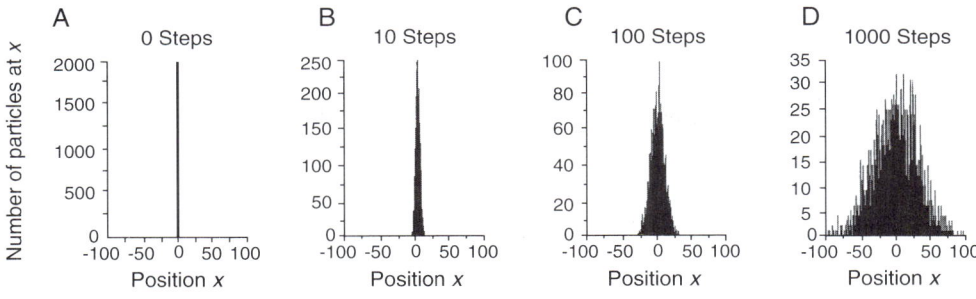

Figure 2-4 ■ Spreading of molecules in space by random movements. The "experiment" is exactly the same as shown in Figure 2-3, except that 2000 molecules are being monitored. Initially 2000 molecules are located at $x = 0$. For each step in time, each of the molecules may move 1 step to the left or to the right. The number of molecules found at each position along the x-axis is shown, A, at time = 0 and after each molecule had taken, B, 10 steps, C, 100 steps, and, D, 1000 steps. The result of each molecule's undergoing an independent random walk is to cause the entire ensemble of molecules to spread out in space.

$$d^{1-D}_{RMS} = \sqrt{2Dt} \qquad [4]$$

where D is the diffusion coefficient (as in Fick's First Law) and t is time. For diffusion in two and three dimensions, the RMS displacements are given by, respectively,

$$d^{2-D}_{RMS} = \sqrt{4Dt} \qquad [5]$$

and

$$d^{3-D}_{RMS} = \sqrt{6Dt} \qquad [6]$$

Square-Root-of-Time Dependence Makes Diffusion Ineffective for Transporting Molecules over Large Distances

The most important aspect of the RMS displacement is that it does not increase linearly with time. Rather, random molecular movement involves meandering and thus causes spreading that increases only with the *square root* of time. Figure 2-5 shows the difference between displacement that varies directly with time and displacement that varies with the square root of time. The thing to notice is that over long distances the square root function seems to "flatten out." This means that to diffuse just a little farther takes a lot more time. In fact, because of the square-root dependence on time of the RMS displacement, to go 2 times farther takes 4 times as long, 10 times farther takes 100 times as long, and so on. Therefore, for long distances, diffusion is an ineffective way to move molecules around.

Diffusion Constrains Cell Biology and Physiology

The practical significance of the fact that diffusion has a square-root dependence on time (Equations [4], [5], and [6]) can be shown by a simple calculation. Diffusion constants for biologically relevant small molecules (e.g., glucose, amino acids) in water are typically about 5×10^{-6} cm^2/s. For such molecules to diffuse a distance of 100 μm (0.01 cm) would take $(0.01)^2/6D = 3.3$ sec (use Equation [6] and solve for t). For the same molecules to diffuse a distance of

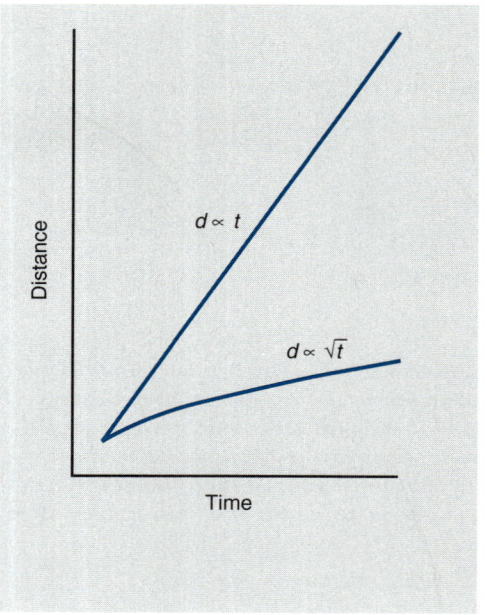

Figure 2-5 ■ Comparison of linear and square-root dependence of distance on time. With a linear time dependence, equal increments of time give equal increments of distance traveled. With a square-root time dependence, as the distance to be traveled becomes greater, the time required to cover the distance becomes disproportionately longer.

1 cm (slightly less than the width of a fingernail), however, would take $1^2/6D$ = 33,000 sec = 9.3 hours! These results show that diffusion is sufficiently fast for transporting molecules over microscopic distances but is extremely slow and ineffective over even moderate distances. Not surprisingly, therefore, most cells in the body are within 100 μm of a capillary and thus only seconds away from both a source of nutrient molecules and a sink for metabolic waste (Box 2-1). These calculations also demonstrate why even small insects (e.g., a mosquito) must have a circulatory system to transport nutrients into, and waste out of, the body.

■ FICK'S FIRST LAW CAN BE USED TO DESCRIBE DIFFUSION ACROSS A MEMBRANE BARRIER

A membrane typically separates two compartments in which the concentrations of some solutes can be different. We may designate the two compartments as i (inside) and o (outside), corresponding, for example, to the cytosol and extracellular fluid, respectively. The concentration difference between the two compartments, $\Delta C = C_i - C_o$, gives rise to a concentration gradient across the membrane, which has a certain thickness, say Δx. The concentration gradient, $\Delta C/\Delta x$, drives the diffusion of the solute across the membrane, thus leading to a flux of material, J, through the membrane. This description suggests that Fick's First Law in the form of Equation [2] would be well suited for analyzing such a situation:

$$J = -D\frac{\Delta C}{\Delta x} = -D\frac{C_i - C_o}{\Delta x} \qquad [7]$$

In this form the equation applies to a solute diffusing across a membrane of thickness Δx, provided that the solute dissolves as well in the membrane as it does in water (i.e., the concentration of the solute just inside the membrane matches the solute concentration in the adjacent aqueous solution; Figure 2-6, A).

In Figure 2-6, A, C_o^{mem} is the concentration of solute in the part of the membrane in immediate contact with the outside aqueous solution; C_i^{mem} is the concentration of solute in the part of the membrane in immediate contact with the inside aqueous solution. Realistically, because biological membranes are hydrophobic and nonpolar, while the aqueous solution is highly polar, solutes typically show different solubilities in the membrane relative to aqueous solution. To take such differential solubilities into account, we can define a quantity, β, the **partition coefficient**:

$$\beta = \frac{C^{mem}}{C^{aq}} \qquad [8]$$

BOX 2-1

The Density of Capillaries Is a Function of the Metabolic Rate of a Tissue

Oxygen diffuses passively from tissue capillaries to cells in the tissue. To provide adequate O_2 to meet cellular metabolic needs, capillaries must be spaced closely enough in tissue to ensure that that O_2 concentration does not fall below the level required for mitochondrial function. We would expect capillary density in a particular tissue to depend on the metabolic rate of that tissue. Thus, in slowly metabolizing tissue (e.g., subcutaneous), cells are typically separated by larger average distances from tissue capillaries. In contrast, in metabolically active tissues, cells are much closer to capillaries. In the cerebral cortex or the heart, for example, cells are typically only 10 to 20 μm from a capillary. In skeletal muscle the density of active capillaries depends strongly on the level of physical activity. At rest, skeletal muscle fibers are, on average, 40 μm from a functioning capillary. During strenuous exercise, many more capillaries are "recruited" and the average separation between muscle fibers and capillaries falls below 20 μm.

The necessity of capillaries in delivering oxygen to cells can be exploited clinically. Solid tumors require an adequate supply of O_2 for growth. Angiogenesis (growth of new blood vessels) is therefore essential for tumor growth. As a result of the pioneering research of Dr. Judah Folkman, new therapeutic regimens, involving drugs that inhibit angiogenesis, are being developed to promote the destruction of solid tumors.

---

where C^{aq} is the solute concentration in aqueous solution and C^{mem} is the solute concentration just inside the membrane. With the use of the partition coefficient, the solute concentrations just inside either face of the membrane can be written:

$$C_i^{mem} = \beta \times C_i \quad \text{and} \quad C_o^{mem} = \beta \times C_o$$

The diffusion equation can now be cast in the following form:

$$J = -D\left[\frac{\Delta C}{\Delta x}\right]_{\text{Across membrane}} = -D\frac{C_i^{mem} - C_o^{mem}}{\Delta x} \quad [9]$$

$$= -D\frac{\beta C_i - \beta C_o}{\Delta x} = -D\beta\frac{C_i - C_o}{\Delta x}$$

This form of the equation shows that the partition coefficient serves to modulate the solute concentration gradient within the membrane: When $\beta > 1$ (solute dissolves better in the membrane than in aqueous solution), the concentration gradient in the membrane is enhanced and flux is proportionally increased (Figure 2-6, B). Conversely, when $\beta < 1$ (solute dissolves better in aqueous solution than in the membrane), the concentration gradient in the membrane is diminished and flux is proportionally decreased (Figure 2-6, C).

Equation [9] also predicts that when $\beta = 0$, the flux, J, through the membrane would also be zero. In other words, if a substance is completely insoluble in the membrane, its flux through the membrane would be zero; that is, the membrane is completely *impermeable* to a substance that is not soluble in the membrane. This suggests that Equation [9] can also be used to describe **membrane permeability.** Indeed, we can rearrange Equation [9] to yield the following form:

$$J = -\left(\frac{D\beta}{\Delta x}\right)(C_i - C_o) = -P(C_i - C_o) \quad [10]$$

where $P (= D\beta/\Delta x)$ is the **permeability** (or **permeability coefficient**) of the membrane for passage of a solute.* The dimensions of P are

---

*Equation [10] describes the diffusion of a substance across a membrane barrier. As such, it is applicable to many physiological situations, including gas exchange in the lung between the air space of an alveolus and the blood in a capillary (see Box 2-2).

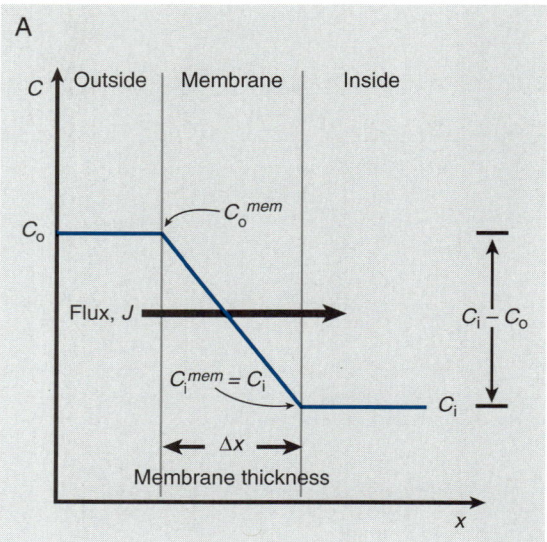

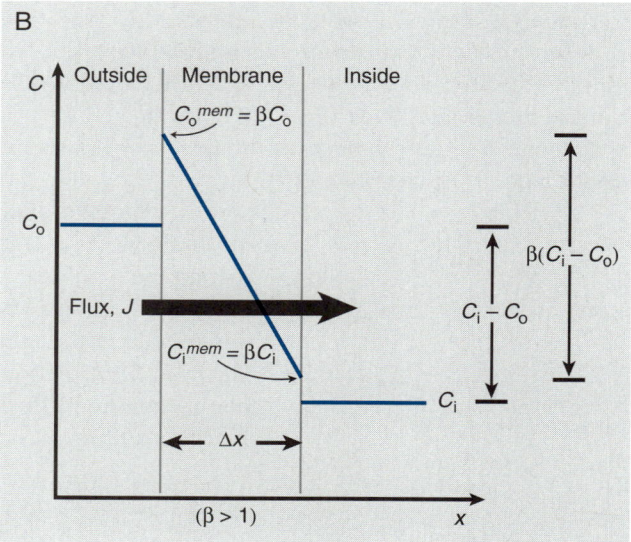

Figure 2-6 ■ Diffusion of a solute across a membrane is driven by the solute concentration gradient in the membrane. A solute is present in the outside solution at concentration C_o, and in the inside solution at concentration C_i. C_o^{mem} and C_i^{mem} are the solute concentrations in the part of the membrane immediately adjacent to the outside and inside solutions, respectively. The partition coefficient, β, is the ratio of the solute concentration in the membrane to the solute concentration in the aqueous solution in contact with the membrane ($\beta = C_o^{mem}/C_o = C_i^{mem}/C_i$). A, A solute that dissolves equally well in the membrane and in aqueous solution is characterized by $\beta = 1$. B, A solute that preferentially dissolves in the membrane has $\beta > 1$.

Diffusion and Permeability

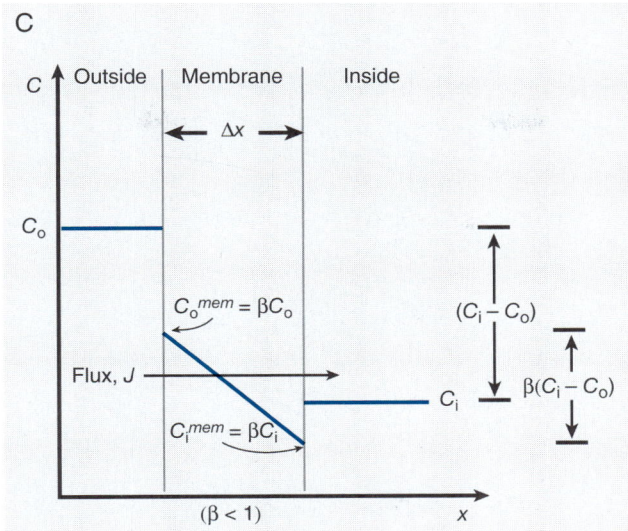

Figure 2-6, cont'd ■ **C**, A solute that dissolves better in aqueous solution than in the membrane has $\beta < 1$. In B, a larger β makes the solute concentration gradient steeper in the membrane and leads to a larger flux of the solute through the membrane. Conversely, in C, a smaller β makes the solute concentration gradient shallower in the membrane and leads to a smaller flux of the solute through the membrane.

cm/s (i.e., a velocity), so that when P is multiplied by the concentration difference (with units of mol/cm³), the result is (mol/cm²)/s — the appropriate units for flux. In the mathematical description above, P is seen to contain microscopic properties such as D, the diffusion coefficient of solute inside the lipid membrane; β, the partition coefficient of the solute; and Δx, the thickness of the membrane. In actuality, the permeability coefficient can be determined empirically for each solute, without the need to measure the microscopic parameters described above.

The Net Flux Through a Membrane Is the Result of Balancing Influx Against Efflux

An alternative way of looking at fluxes and permeabilities is suggested by Equation [10]:

$$J = -P(C_i - C_o) = PC_o - PC_i = J_{out \to in} - J_{in \to out} \quad [11]$$

In other words, the **net flux** of a solute, J, is the result of balancing the inward flux (**influx**),

$$J_{out \to in} = P \times C_o \quad [12]$$

against the outward flux (**efflux**),

$$J_{in \to out} = P \times C_i \quad [13]$$

The two individual fluxes are *unidirectional* fluxes. Influx can thus be viewed as the inward flux being driven by the presence of solute on the outside at concentration, C_o, while efflux can be viewed as the outward flux being driven by the presence of solute on the inside at concentration, C_i. Mathematically, it is useful to note that multiplying a permeability and a concentration yields a unidirectional flux. It is also important

BOX 2-2

Fick's First Law of Diffusion Is Used to Describe Gas Transport in the Lung

Ventilation delivers O_2 to, and removes CO_2 from, the lungs. Exchange of O_2 and CO_2 between the lung and pulmonary blood occurs through a thin (~0.3 µm) membranous barrier separating the alveolar air space from the blood inside capillaries apposed to the outer surface of the alveolus (see Figure B-1 in this box).

The concentration (or partial pressure) of a physiologically important gas typically differs between the alveolar space and the blood. This concentration (or partial pressure) difference drives the diffusion of the gas between the two compartments. Pulmonologists use a variant form of Fick's First Law to describe gas exchange across the alveolocapillary barrier:

$$\dot{V}_{gas} = A \times \left[\frac{-D \cdot \beta_m}{t} (p_B - p_A) \right] \quad [B1]$$

where $\dot{V}_{gas}$ is the volume of a gas transported per unit time across a membrane barrier of area, A, and thickness, t; D is the diffusion coefficient, and β_m the solubility, of the gas in the membrane barrier; and p_B and p_A are the partial pressures of the gas in the blood and in the alveolus, respectively. Comparison of Equation [B1] with Equation [10] in the text immediately shows their similarity of form (i.e., the amount of substance transported is driven by a concentration difference). All of the proportionality factors in Equation [B1] can be grouped together as the *diffusing capacity of the lung* (D_L) for a particular gas. Equation [B1] then takes the very simple form

$$\dot{V}_{gas} = D_L (p_A - p_B) \quad [B2]$$

We note that this equation has the same form as the equation for flux in the text (Equation [10]). Inspection of Equation [B1] shows how various physiological or environmental changes could alter the amount of oxygen transported into the body. For example, if edema (accumulation of fluid) occurs to some extent in the alveoli, thus increasing the total thickness (t) of the alveolocapillary barrier, $\dot{V}_{O_2}$ would decrease. Similarly, destruction of alveoli by disease would reduce the total surface area (A) across which gas exchange may take place, and thus lower $\dot{V}_{O_2}$. Finally, at high altitudes, where the partial pressure of oxygen is diminished, p_A of O_2 is correspondingly lower, leading also to decreased $\dot{V}_{O_2}$.

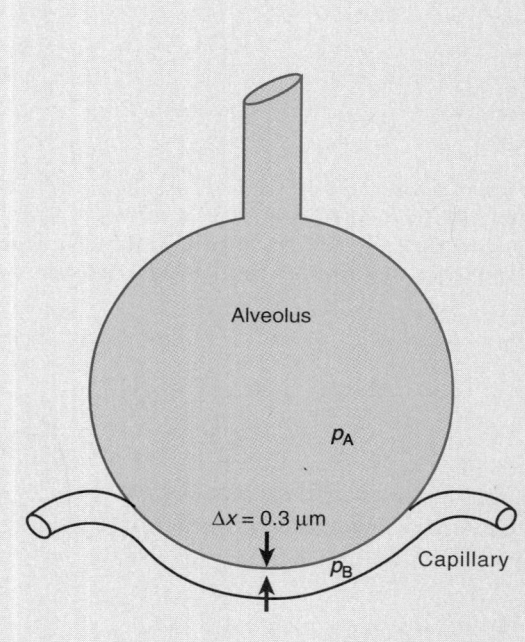

Figure B-1 ■ Schematic representation of a capillary apposed to an alveolus. The oxygen partial pressures in the alveolar air space and the capillary blood are symbolized by p_A and p_B, respectively. The diffusion barrier between the air space and the blood is typically ~0.3 µm.

Diffusion and Permeability

TABLE 2-1

Permeability of plain lipid bilayer membrane to solutes

Solute	P [cm/s]	τ^*
Water	10^{-4}-$10^{-3\dagger}$	0.5-5 sec
Urea	10^{-6}	~8 min
Glucose, amino acids	10^{-7}	~14 hr
Cl$^-$	10^{-11}	~1.6 yr
K$^+$, Na$^+$	10^{-13}	~160 yr
CO$_2$	.16 cm^2/sec ≈	10^7 cm/sec

*Calculated for a spherical cell with diameter = 20 μm (see Box 2-3). τ is the time constant that indicates how rapidly a solute concentration difference across the membrane can be dissipated by diffusion.

$\dagger$Plain phospholipid bilayers are relatively permeable to water, but water permeability is reduced by the presence of cholesterol, which is found in all animal cell membranes.

to notice that, given the way Equations [10] and [11] are defined, a net flux that brings solute *into* a cell is a positive quantity.

The Permeability Determines How Rapidly a Solute Can Be Transported Through a Membrane

Membrane permeability coefficients for several biologically relevant molecules are shown in Table 2-1. The permeability coefficients give a fairly good idea of the relative permeability of a membrane to different solutes. In general, small neutral molecules (e.g., water, O$_2$, and CO$_2$, with MW 18, 32, and 48, respectively) permeate the membrane readily. Larger, highly hydrophilic organic molecules (e.g., glucose, MW 180) barely permeate. Inorganic ions (e.g., Na$^+$, K$^+$, Cl$^-$, Ca^{2+}) are essentially impermeant.

An approximate description of how fast a solute concentration difference across a membrane is abolished as solute molecules diffuse through the membrane is given by Equation [B8] in Box 2-3:

$$\Delta C(t) = \Delta C^0 e^{-\frac{t}{\tau}}$$

where $\tau = 1/(P \times$ surface-to-volume ratio) is a *time constant* that describes the time scale on which concentration differences change. With the aid of Equation [B8] from Box 2-3 and the permeabilities in Table 2-1, we can calculate corresponding values of the time constant and immediately get a sense of how fast concentration differences for a given substance across the cell membrane would be evened out. For a spherical cell that is 20 μm in diameter, the surface area is $A_{cell} = 2.83 \times 10^{-5}$ cm^2, and the volume is $V_{cell} = 1.41 \times 10^{-8}$ cm^3, giving a surface-to-volume ratio of 2000 cm^{-1}. The τ values corresponding to the various P values are given in Table 2-1. Now the permeability properties of lipid bilayer membranes are easier to grasp. Small neutral molecules such as water, O$_2$, and CO$_2$ permeate readily and *fast*—on the order of seconds. Common nutrients such as glucose and amino acids take well over 10 hours to permeate, which means that in any real biological context, they might as well be considered impermeant. Ions such as Cl$^-$, Na$^+$, K$^+$, and Ca^{2+} are so impermeant that years to centuries are required for them to permeate through a simple lipid bilayer membrane. Although measurements have never been made, we can infer that proteins, being very large molecules and often carrying multiple ionic charges, are also essentially impermeant.

The main point of this discussion is that, except simple, small, neutral molecules, essentially everything that is biologically relevant and important cannot readily pass through a simple lipid bilayer membrane. For this reason a diversity of special mechanisms has evolved to transport a broad spectrum of biologically important species across cellular membranes. Ion pumps and channels permit influx and efflux of Na$^+$, K$^+$, Ca^{2+}, and Cl$^-$. A range of carrier proteins allows movement of sugars and amino

BOX 2-3

How Rapidly Can Diffusion Abolish Concentration Differences Across a Membrane?

With a little bit of mathematics, we can improve our understanding of relative permeabilities and better appreciate what is meant when something is called permeant or impermeant. Recall that the permeability coefficient, P, has dimensions of cm/sec. That is, the concept of *time* (and thus *rate*) is somehow embodied in the description of permeability presented in the text. We now make this connection explicit.

Text Equation [10] stated that the flux (J) of molecules across a cell membrane is driven by the concentration difference of that molecule between the inside and the outside:

$$J = -P(C_i - C_o) = -P\Delta C \quad \text{[B1]}$$

When the membrane is permeable to a particular species, for that species, any concentration difference between inside and outside cannot persist. As molecules start to permeate the membrane from one side to the other, any concentration difference between inside and outside will gradually diminish. To determine how the concentration difference is gradually abolished, we need only to figure out how the concentration inside the cell is changed by the flux of molecules. Given that flux (J) is in units of *moles per cm^2 per second* (amount of molecules passing through a unit area of membrane in unit time), the number of moles of molecules entering the cell through its entire surface area (A_{cell}) in unit time must be

$$J \times A_{cell} \quad \text{with units of moles/sec}$$

These moles of molecules are added to the total internal volume of the cell (V_{cell}). The resulting concentration change in the cell must be

$$(J \times A_{cell})/V_{cell} \quad \text{with units of (moles/cm}^3\text{)/sec}$$

Merging this with Equation [B1] above, we can write the rate of change of the concentration difference as

$$\frac{\Delta[\Delta C]}{\Delta t} = J \times \frac{A_{cell}}{V_{cell}} = -P\frac{A_{cell}}{V_{cell}}\Delta C \quad \text{[B2]}$$

The ratio A_{cell}/V_{cell} is the *surface-to-volume ratio* of the cell. If we redefine the product of the permeability coefficient and the surface-to-volume ratio as k, Equation [B2] can be written more compactly as

$$\frac{\Delta[\Delta C]}{\Delta t} = -k\Delta C \quad \text{[B3]}$$

or, with derivative notation, as

$$\frac{d[\Delta C]}{dt} = -k\Delta C \quad \text{[B4]}$$

Equation [B4] can be rearranged and integrated:

$$\int_{t=0}^{t} \frac{1}{\Delta C}\frac{d[\Delta C]}{dt}dt = \int_{t=0}^{t} -k\,dt \quad \text{[B5]}$$

The result of integration is

$$\ln\frac{\Delta C(t)}{\Delta C^0} = -kt \quad \text{[B6]}$$

In terms of exponentials, Equation [B6] is

$$\frac{\Delta C(t)}{\Delta C^0} = e^{-kt} \quad \text{or} \quad \Delta C(t) = \Delta C^0 e^{-kt} \quad \text{[B7]}$$

Equation [B7] describes how the concentration difference across a cell membrane (initially at ΔC^0) will change with time if the membrane is permeable: the concentration difference will decrease exponentially with time. The time course of such a change is shown in Figure B-1.

The constant k is called a *rate constant*, and its magnitude governs how fast the concentration difference is abolished (large k means rapid abolition of concentration difference between inside and outside). If we recall that

$$k = P \times \text{(surface-to-volume ratio)}$$

this makes sense: the higher the permeability of the membrane, the faster molecules will be able to

Diffusion and Permeability

BOX 2-3

How Rapidly Can Diffusion Abolish Concentration Differences Across a Membrane?—Cont'd

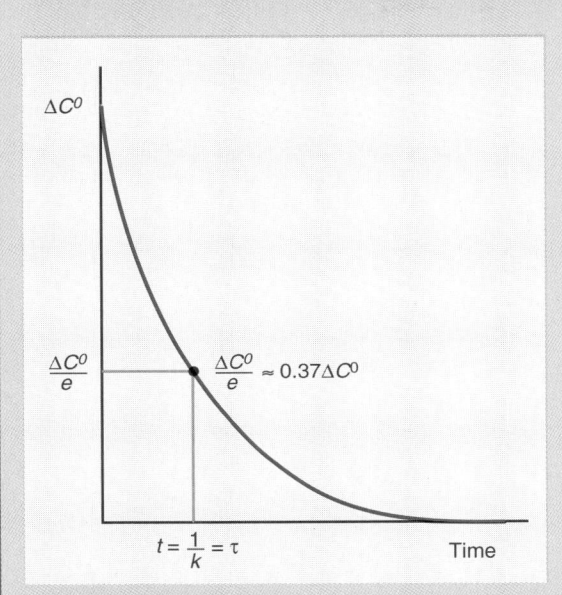

Figure B-1 ■ Exponential decay of a solute concentration difference across a cell membrane. Initially ($t = 0$), the concentration difference, ΔC, is at initial value, ΔC^0. With time, ΔC diminishes and asymptotically approaches 0. The time constant, τ (which is equal to the inverse of the rate constant, k), is the time at which ΔC has dropped to $1/e$ (or ~37%) of its initial value.

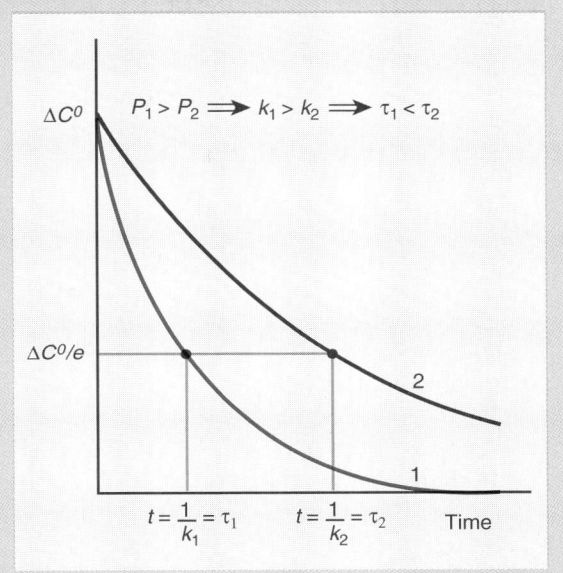

Figure B-2 ■ The higher the membrane permeability, the faster the disappearance of a solute concentration gradient across the cell membrane. For two solutes (1 and 2) with the same initial concentration difference (ΔC^0) across the membrane, if the membrane is more permeable to solute 1 than to solute 2 ($P_1 > P_2$), the concentration difference of solute 1 will decrease faster than that of solute 2. This is equivalent to saying that the rate constants and time constants for the two solutes have the following relationships: $k_1 > k_2$ and $\tau_1 < \tau_2$.

move through the membrane, and the more rapidly the concentration difference across the membrane will be abolished. The reciprocal of the rate constant is called the *time constant* and is given the symbol τ (Greek letter "tau"):

$$\tau = 1/k$$

τ is the time it takes for the concentration difference to drop to $1/e$ (~37%) of its initial value.

Put another way, when $t = \tau$, $\Delta C = 0.37\ \Delta C^0$. A solute that has higher permeability has a shorter τ, whereas one with lower permeability has a longer τ. These relationships are illustrated in Figure B-2.

Because τ is just the reciprocal of k, Equation [B7] can also be written as

$$\Delta C(t) = \Delta C^0 e^{-\frac{t}{\tau}} \qquad [B8]$$

acids across membranes. Elaborate and highly regulated machinery governs endocytosis and exocytosis to bring large molecules like proteins into and out of cells. Endocytosis and exocytosis lie in the realm of cell biology and are not discussed in detail in this text. Ion channels, pumps, and carriers are basic to cellular functions that underlie physiology and neuroscience and are discussed in later chapters.

■ SUMMARY

1. Diffusion causes the movement of molecules from a region where their concentration is high to a region where their concentration is low; that is, molecules tend to diffuse down their concentration gradient.
2. Fick's First Law describes diffusion in quantitative terms: the flux of molecules is directly proportional to the concentration gradient of those molecules.
3. Diffusion results entirely from the random movement of molecules.
4. The distance that molecules diffuse is proportional to the square root of time.
5. Because of the square-root dependence on time, diffusion is effective in transporting molecules and ions over short distances that are on the order of cellular dimensions (i.e., micrometers). Diffusion is extremely ineffective over macroscopic distances (i.e., a millimeter or greater).
6. The net flux of molecules diffusing across a cell membrane may be viewed as the net balance between an inward flux (influx) and an outward flux (efflux).
7. The ease with which a species may diffuse through a membrane barrier is characterized by the membrane permeability, P. Higher permeability permits a larger flux.
8. The product of a permeability and a concentration is a flux. For example, $P_{Na} \times [Na^+]_o$ represents a flux of Na^+ into the cell (an influx), whereas $P_{Cl} \times [Cl^-]_i$ represents a flux of Cl^- out of the cell (an efflux).
9. With the exception of small neutral molecules such as oxygen, carbon dioxide, water, and ethanol, essentially no biologically important molecules and ions can spontaneously diffuse across biological membranes.

■ KEY WORDS AND CONCEPTS

- Diffusion
- Random movement
- Concentration gradient
- Flux
- Diffusion coefficient (or diffusion constant)
- Fick's First Law of Diffusion
- Root-mean-squared (RMS) displacement
- Partition coefficient
- Membrane permeability
- Permeability or permeability coefficient
- Net flux
- Influx
- Efflux

STUDY PROBLEMS

1. If a collection of molecules diffuses 5 μm in 1 second, how long will it take for the molecules to diffuse 10 μm?
2. The permeability of the plasma membrane to K^+ is given the symbol P_K. If the intracellular and extracellular K^+ concentrations are $[K^+]_i$ and $[K^+]_o$, write the expressions representing influx (J_{inward}) and efflux ($J_{outward}$) of K^+. What is the expression for the net flux of K^+?

■ BIBLIOGRAPHY

Feynman RP: *Feynman lectures on physics*, New York, 1970, Addison-Wesley.
Ferreira HG, Marshall MW: *The biophysical basis of excitability*, Cambridge, Eng, 1985, Cambridge University Press.

CHAPTER 3

Osmotic Pressure and Water Movement

Objectives:

1. Understand the nature of osmosis.
2. Define osmotic pressure in terms of solute concentration through van't Hoff's Law.
3. Define the driving forces that control water movement across membranes.
4. Understand that fluid movement across a capillary wall is determined by a balance of hydrostatic and osmotic pressures.
5. Know how cell volume changes in response to changing concentrations of permeant and impermeant solutes in the extracellular fluid.

■ OSMOSIS IS THE TRANSPORT OF *SOLVENT* DRIVEN BY A DIFFERENCE IN *SOLUTE* CONCENTRATION ACROSS A MEMBRANE THAT IS IMPERMEABLE TO SOLUTE

Because of diffusion, a net movement of molecules occurs *down* concentration gradients, and substances tend to move in a way that abolishes concentration differences in different regions of a solution. Alternatively, it could be said that diffusion results in *mixing*. We now examine the consequences when a solute is prevented from diffusing down its concentration gradient. Figure 3-1, *A*, shows two aqueous compartments, 1 and 2, separated by a semipermeable membrane. Initially compartment 1 contains pure water and compartment 2 contains a solute dissolved in water. The membrane is permeable to water but impermeable to the solute. Because the solute concentration differs between the two compartments (higher in 2 than in 1), normally a net flux of solute molecules from 2 into 1 would occur. Because the membrane is impermeable to the solute, however, such a flux cannot take place; that is, the solute molecules cannot move from 2 into 1 to abolish the concentration difference between the two compartments.

The situation can be viewed from another perspective. When a solute is dissolved in water to form an aqueous solution, as the concentration of solute in the solution is increased, the concentration of *water* in the same solution must correspondingly decrease. In the two compartments shown in Figure 3-1, *A*, whereas the solute concentration is higher in 2 than in 1,

21

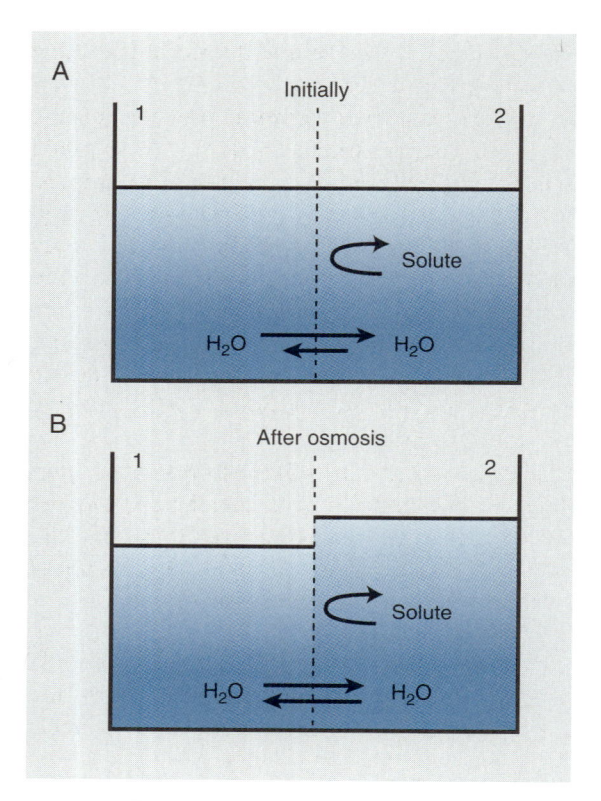

Figure 3-1 ■ Two aqueous compartments separated by a semipermeable membrane that allows passage of water but not solute. Compartment 1 contains pure water; compartment 2 contains a solute dissolved in water. **A,** Before any osmosis has taken place. **B,** After osmosis has occurred.

the water concentration is higher in 1 than in 2. Therefore, although the membrane does not permit the solute to move across from 2 into 1, it does allow water to move from 1 into 2. The presence of the water concentration difference allows us to predict, correctly, that a net flux of water will occur from 1 into 2. This movement of water through a semipermeable membrane, from a region of higher water concentration to a region of lower water concentration, is called **osmosis.**

■ WATER TRANSPORT DURING OSMOSIS LEADS TO CHANGES IN VOLUME

In light of the foregoing, we can think about simple diffusion again. Because an increase in solute concentration dictates a corresponding decrease in water concentration, when a solute concentration gradient exists, a water concentration gradient running in the opposite direction must also be present. We can therefore view simple diffusion as a net flux of solute molecules down their concentration gradient occurring *simultaneously* with a net flux of water molecules down the water concentration gradient.

In osmosis, the membrane does not permit solute movement, so the only flux is that of water. Because the net flux of water in one direction is not balanced by a flux of solute in the opposite direction, the net movement of water would be expected to contribute to a change in volume: as water moves from compartment 1 to compartment 2, the volume of solution in 2 should increase, as shown in Figure 3-1, *B*.

■ OSMOTIC PRESSURE DRIVES THE NET TRANSPORT OF WATER DURING OSMOSIS

In the two-compartment situation depicted in Figure 3-1, as osmosis proceeds, the solution volume in 2 will increase and a "head" of solution will build up (Figure 3-1, *B*). The head of solution will exert a **hydrostatic pressure,** which will tend to "push" the water across the membrane back to compartment 1, thus reducing the net flux of water from 1 into 2. As the solution volume in 2 increases, a point will be reached when the hydrostatic pressure from the solution head is sufficient to exactly counteract the net flow of water from 1 into 2.

This view suggests that we could also think of osmotic flow of water as being driven by some "pressure" that forces water to flow from 1 into 2. This pressure, arising from unequal solute concentrations across a semipermeable membrane, is termed **osmotic pressure**. From the earlier discussion, we expect that the larger the solute concentration difference between two solutions separated by a semipermeable membrane, the larger the osmotic pressure difference driving water transport. Therefore the osmotic pressure of a solution should be proportional to the concentration of solute. Indeed, for any solution, the osmotic pressure can be described fairly accurately by **van't Hoff's Law***:

$$\pi = RTC_{solute} \qquad [1]$$

where π is the osmotic pressure, C_{solute} is the concentration of the **impermeant solute**, T is the absolute temperature (T = Celsius temperature + 273.15, in absolute temperature units, i.e., Kelvins), and R is the universal gas constant (0.08205 liter·atmosphere/mole·Kelvin). The various units of measurement used in the study of osmosis are described in Box 3-1.

In Figure 3-1 the osmotic pressure of the solution in compartment 1 is 0 ($C_{solute} = 0$), while the osmotic pressure of the solution in compartment 2 is equal to RTC_{solute}. In practice, the magnitude of the osmotic pressure is equal to the amount of pressure that must be applied to the compartment with the higher solute concentration in order to stop the net flux of water into that compartment. The magnitude of osmotic pressures encountered in physiology is typically very high (Box 3-2).

When impermeant solute is present on both sides of a semipermeable membrane, the net osmotic pressure driving water across the membrane will depend on the net imbalance of solute concentrations across the membrane:

$$\Delta\pi = RT\Delta C_{solute} \qquad [2]$$

where $\Delta\pi$ is the osmotic pressure across the membrane, ΔC_{solute} is the difference in concen-

---

*Derived by the Dutch scientist Jacobus Henricus van't Hoff, who received the Nobel Prize in Chemistry in 1901.

BOX 3-1

Units of Measurement Used in the Study of Osmosis

Osmotic pressure is proportional to the total concentration of dissolved particles. Each mole of osmotically active particles is referred to as an osmole. One mole of glucose is equivalent to 1 osmole, because each molecule of glucose stays as an intact molecular particle when in solution. One mole of NaCl is equivalent to 2 osmoles, because when in solution, each mole of NaCl dissociates into 1 mole of Na$^+$ ions and 1 mole of Cl$^-$ ions, both of which are osmotically active.

One osmole in 1 liter of solution gives a 1 *osmolar* solution. Alternatively, one osmole in 1 kilogram of solution gives a 1 *osmolal* solution. Because *osmolarity* is defined in terms of solution volume, whereas *osmolality* is defined in terms of the weight of solution, osmolarity changes with temperature, whereas osmolality is independent of temperature. For simplicity, in this chapter all concentrations of osmotically active solutes are given in units of molar (M = mole/liter) or millimolar (mM = 10^{-3} mole/liter).

With commonly used factors, van't Hoff's Law (Equation [1] in text) gives the osmotic pressure in units of atmospheres. Physiological pressures are typically given in units of millimeters of mercury (mm Hg). The conversion factor is 1 atmosphere = 760 mm Hg.

> **BOX 3-2**
>
> ### *Physiologically Relevant Osmotic Pressures Are High*
>
> All fluid compartments in the body contain dissolved solutes. Extracellular fluid is high in Na$^+$ and Cl$^-$ and low in K$^+$, whereas intracellular fluid is high in K$^+$ and phosphate in various forms and low in Na$^+$ and Cl$^-$. For cells in the body to maintain constant volume, the osmotic pressure arising from solutes inside cells must be equal to the osmotic pressure arising from solutes in the extracellular fluid. The total solute concentration in the fluids is typically close to 300 mM. The osmotic pressure resulting from this solute concentration at 37° C (310.15 Kelvin) can be estimated with van't Hoff's Law:
>
> $$\pi = RTC = 0.08205 \, \frac{l \cdot atm}{mol \cdot K} \times 310.15K \times 300 \times 10^{-3} \, \frac{mol}{l} = 7.63 \, atm$$
>
> At 7.63 atmospheres, the osmotic pressure of intracellular and extracellular fluids is quite high, especially in light of the fact that air pressure at sea level is just 1 atmosphere. This is why red blood cells, which are much more permeable to water than to solutes, will swell very rapidly and burst (lyse) when they are placed into water or dilute solutions.
>
> A note about units of measurement: 1 atmosphere is equivalent to 760 mm of mercury (Hg).

trations of the impermeant solute across the semipermeable membrane, and R and T are as defined for Equation [1].

In real life, membranes are never completely impermeable to solute. What happens when the membrane is only partially impermeable to solute? We can deduce the answer by considering the two extreme cases we already know: (1) If the membrane allows the solute molecules to pass through as freely as water molecules can, the flux of water is counterbalanced by the flux of solute in the opposite direction and the situation is no different from free diffusion; therefore no osmotic pressure would be present. (2) If the membrane is completely impermeable to solute molecules but completely permeable to water molecules, the maximum osmotic pressure that can be achieved is given by Equation [2]. The behavior of real-life membranes must lie somewhere between these two extremes. Because the relative permeability of the membrane to solute and water determines the actual behavior, we can define a parameter, called the **reflection coefficient**, represented by the symbol σ:

$$\sigma = 1 - \frac{P_{solute}}{P_{water}} \quad [3]$$

When the membrane permeability to solute, P_{solute}, has the value of 0, the reflection coefficient takes on the value of 1. In this case the membrane "reflects" all solute molecules and does not allow them to pass through, and full osmotic pressure should be achieved. When the solute molecules permeate the membrane as readily as do water molecules ($P_{solute}/P_{water} = 1$), the reflection coefficient takes on the value of 0. In this case the membrane allows free passage of both water and solute, and the osmotic pressure should be 0. By incorporating the reflection coefficient into the osmotic pressure equation, we can more accurately describe real-life behavior:

$$\Delta\pi = \sigma RT \Delta C_{solute} \quad [4]$$

where $\Delta\pi$ is the effective osmotic pressure difference across a membrane.

The fact that, even at the same concentration, solutes with different reflection coefficients can generate different osmotic pressures gives rise

Osmotic Pressure and Water Movement

> ### BOX 3-3
>
> ### *Tonicity and Osmolarity*
>
> Each mole of dissolved solute particles contributes 1 osmole to the solution; therefore any dissolved solute contributes to the osmolarity of a solution. With regard to the ability to drive water flow by osmosis, not all solutes are equal. Solutes with low membrane permeability (σ close to 1) have far greater osmotic effect than those with high membrane permeability (σ close to 0). Therefore two solutions of equal osmolarity can have different osmotic effects on cells. As an example, take a cell initially equilibrated with extracellular fluid (ECF). When a solute is added to the ECF, the ECF becomes *hyperosmolar* with respect to the intracellular fluid (ICF). If the added solute has $\sigma = 1$ (is impermeant), the cell will lose water and shrink; the ECF is then said to be *hypertonic* with respect to the cell. If the added solute has $\sigma = 0$ (is completely membrane permeant), the osmotic pressure of the ECF will not change and neither will the cell volume. In this case the ECF is said to be *isotonic* with respect to the cell. Similarly, a solution that causes the cell to gain water and swell is said to be *hypotonic*.

to a distinction between **osmolarity** and **tonicity**, which is explained in Box 3-3.

■ OSMOTIC PRESSURE AND HYDROSTATIC PRESSURE ARE FUNCTIONALLY EQUIVALENT IN THEIR ABILITY TO DRIVE WATER MOVEMENT THROUGH A MEMBRANE

In the previous section we noted that hydrostatic pressure can counteract water movement driven by osmotic pressure. This suggests that as far as water movement through a membrane is concerned, hydrostatic and osmotic pressures act equivalently—both are capable of driving water movement through a membrane. When water movement is described, it is customary to consider the *volume* of water that passes through a unit area of membrane per unit time. **Volume flow** through a membrane, given the symbol J_v, is quantitatively described by the following equation (sometimes called the **Starling equation***):

$$J_v = L_p(\Delta\pi - \Delta P) = L_p(\sigma RT\Delta C_{solute} - \Delta P) \quad [5]$$

wherein ΔP is the hydrostatic pressure difference across the membrane and L_p is a proportionality constant called the **hydraulic conductivity** (a measure of the ease with which a membrane allows water to pass through). Another name for the proportionality constant L_p is the **filtration constant**, symbolized as K_f. Equation [5] emphasizes the equivalence of hydrostatic and osmotic pressures in driving water volume flow through membranes. Furthermore, it indicates that the direction of water volume flow across a membrane is determined by the *balance* of hydrostatic and osmotic pressures across the membrane.*

---

*Named after Ernest Starling, a 19th-century British physiologist who first investigated fluid movement driven by osmotic and hydrostatic forces.

*That the balance of hydrostatic and osmotic forces determines the direction of water movement across a membrane is the basis for a water purification process called reverse osmosis. By application of high pressure to salty water on one side of a semipermeable membrane, water can be made to flow by "reverse osmosis" from the side of high salt concentration to become water with low salinity on the other side. Reverse osmosis is used on an industrial scale to generate fresh water from seawater in some parts of the world where fresh water is in short supply.

Once again, it is instructive to check the dimensions of the various quantities in Equation [5]. The pressure terms (hydrostatic and osmotic), naturally, have units of pressure (often in the form of force per unit area, e.g., dyne/cm^2). L_p, then, has units of cm^3/dyne·s. We can figure out that J_v must have units of cm/s—seemingly bizarre units for *volume* flow! However, if we recognize that cm/s is exactly equivalent to cm^3 per cm^2 per second, we see that J_v does indeed have the right physical meaning of *volume* of water flowing through unit *area* of membrane per unit *time*.

The Direction of Fluid Flow Through the Capillary Wall Is Determined by the Balance of Hydrostatic and Osmotic Pressures, as Described by the Starling Equation

In analyzing fluid movement across capillary walls, Starling recognized the importance of hydrostatic and osmotic forces. The Starling equation (Equation [5]) succinctly summarizes how net fluid movement is determined by hydrostatic and osmotic pressures. Figure 3-2 shows the four pressures that are in play; the direction of water movement driven by each pressure component is indicated by an arrow associated with that pressure. The capillary hydrostatic pressure (blood pressure) is P_c; the hydrostatic pressure in the interstitium is P_i. The principal contributors to osmotic pressure are dissolved proteins, which are too large to pass through the capillary walls. The osmotic pressure of the capillary is termed the capillary **colloid osmotic pressure**, or the capillary **oncotic pressure**, and is symbolized as π_c. The osmotic pressure resulting from dissolved proteins in the interstitial fluid is called the interstitial colloid osmotic pressure, or the interstitial oncotic pressure, and is symbolized as π_i. The capillary hydrostatic pressure tends to push water out of the capillary, whereas any inter-stitial hydrostatic pressure tends to push water into the capillary. The osmotic components operate in just the opposite way. The capillary osmotic pressure is due to impermeant solutes inside the capillary and would tend to retain water inside the capillary (or "pull" water from the interstitium into the capillary). Similarly, the interstitial osmotic pressure tends to retain water in the insterstitium (or "pull" water out of the capillary into the interstitium). As blood passes through a capillary, whether net movement of water occurs into or out of the capillary is determined by the balance of the four pressure components. The net movement of fluid out of the capillary is called filtration, and the net movement of fluid into the capillary is called absorption.

If we consider the net movement of fluid out of the capillary (filtration) as a positive quantity,

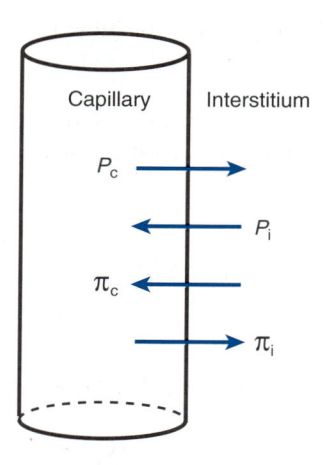

Figure 3-2 ■ Pressures that determine fluid movement between the interstitium and the lumen of a capillary. Capillary hydrostatic pressure, P_c, and interstitial oncotic (colloid osmotic) pressure, π_i, drive fluid movement from the capillary into the interstitium (filtration). Capillary oncotic pressure, π_c, and interstitial hydrostatic pressure, P_i, drive fluid movement from the interstitium into the capillary (absorption).

Osmotic Pressure and Water Movement

the meaning of the Starling equation can be summarized as follows:

Fluid movement ∝ (Pressures that drive fluid out) − (Pressures that drive fluid in)

but

(Pressures that drive fluid out) = $P_c + \pi_i$

and

(Pressures that drive fluid in) = $P_i + \pi_c$

If we use the filtration constant (K_f), which is the same as the hydraulic conductivity (L_p), the Starling equation (Equation [5]) can be written as:

Fluid movement = $J_v = K_f([P_c + \pi_i] - [P_i + \pi_c])$ [6]

Analysis of the situation in Figure 3-3, A, illustrates the principles involved in applying the Starling equation. Typical pressure values are shown in Figure 3-3. The arteriolar and venular hydrostatic pressures are 32 and 15 mm Hg, respectively. The interstitial hydrostatic pressure is typically ~0. The capillary and interstitial oncotic pressures are π_c = 25 mm Hg and π_i = 2 mm Hg, respectively (Box 3-4).

We wish to determine whether fluid moves into or out of the capillary at two key points along the capillary, the arteriolar and venular ends of the capillary. Two observations are useful: (1) At the point where the capillary is connected to the arteriole, the capillary hydrostatic pressure should be essentially identical to the blood pressure in the arteriole, that is, P_c = 35 mm Hg. (2) At the point where the capillary is connected to the venule, the capillary hydrostatic pressure should be essentially the same as the blood pressure in the venule, that is, P_c = 15 mm Hg. All other pressure components (P_i, π_c, and π_i) do not vary with location. Determination of the

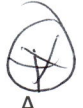

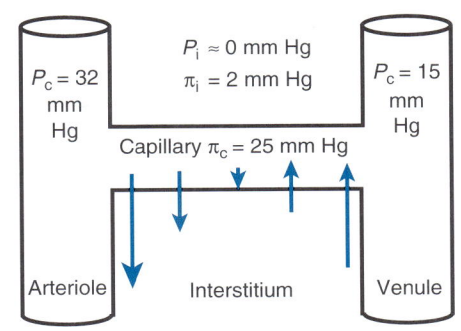

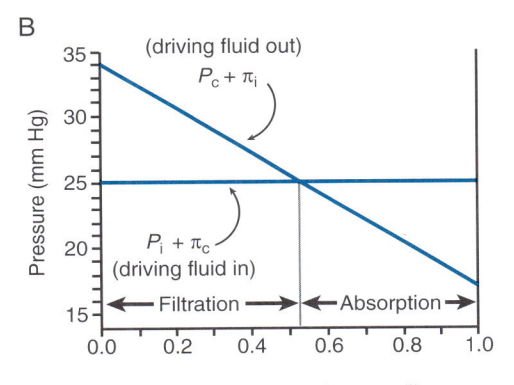

Figure 3-3 ■ **A**, Capillary connecting an arteriole and a venule. The magnitudes of all hydrostatic and osmotic pressures are marked. Arrows indicate the direction (in or out) and magnitude of the fluid movement at various distances along the capillary. **B**, Plot showing how the driving force ($P_c + \pi_i$) for outward fluid flow, as well as the driving force ($P_i + \pi_c$) for inward fluid flow, vary along the length of the capillary. The portions along the capillary length where filtration (net outward fluid flow) and absorption (net inward fluid flow) occur are indicated.

net effect of the various pressure components is now a straightforward calculation. At the arteriolar end,

$(P_c + \pi_i) - (P_i + \pi_c) = (32 + 2) - (0 + 25) = +9$ mm Hg

BOX 3-4

Dissolved Proteins Give Rise to the Colloid Osmotic (Oncotic) Pressure in the Plasma and the Interstitium

By far the most abundant solutes in blood plasma are low-molecular weight ions and molecules (e.g., Na^+, Cl^-). The total concentration of such small solutes is close to 300 mM. If a membrane barrier were completely impermeable to these solutes, an osmotic pressure close to 6000 mm Hg (i.e., ~7.6 atm; see Box 3-1) would develop. In reality, the wall of a typical capillary is quite permeable to small solutes (reflection coefficient, $\sigma \approx 0$). Thus, with respect to small solutes, the interstitial fluid has approximately the same composition as plasma, with the consequence that small solutes exert very little net osmotic effect across the capillary wall. Incidentally, it is reasonable that the walls of most capillaries are quite permeable to low molecular weight solutes, because the circulating blood brings small nutrient molecules (e.g., glucose, amino acids) that must leave the capillaries to nourish the cells in tissue, which cells, in turn, generate metabolic waste (e.g., carbon dioxide) that must enter the capillaries and be borne away by the blood.

Two types of proteins are found in significant amounts in the plasma. Albumin, with MW $\approx$ 69,000, is present at ~4.5 g/dl (grams/deciliter, same as grams/100 milliliters), or ~0.65 mM. Globulins, with MW $\approx$ 150,000, are present at ~2.5 g/dl, or ~ 0.17 mM. These proteins, being macromolecules, do not readily pass through the capillary wall ($\sigma \gtrsim 0.9$); therefore the plasma is protein rich whereas the interstititial fluid is low in proteins. Since the total protein concentration in plasma is close to 0.82 mM, we expect the maximum osmotic pressure contributed by the proteins to be

$$\pi_c = \sigma RTC = 0.9 \times 0.08205 \frac{l \cdot atm}{mol \cdot K} \times 310.15K \times 0.82 \times 10^{-3} \frac{mol}{l} = 0.0216 \text{ atm}$$

or 15.8 mm Hg. This number is still quite a bit less than the π_c = 25 mm Hg that is typically measured. This suggests that each protein molecule exists in solution not as a single particle, but rather as an ionic macromolecule with some associated small ions. Because the proteins cannot leave the capillary, the population of small "counter-ions" that are associated with them must also remain within the capillary, thereby increasing the total amount of effectively impermeant solute. In other words, if we ignore the fact that proteins can dissociate into more than one ionic particle, we underestimate the osmotic contribution of proteins.

The most important point is that proteins, because they do not readily pass through the capillary wall, are the predominant contributor to osmotic forces across the capillary wall.

This means that a net positive pressure is driving fluid out of the capillary near the arteriolar end. At the venular end,

$$(P_c + \pi_i) - (P_i + \pi_c) = (15 + 2) - (0 + 25) = -8 \text{ mm Hg}$$

This means that a net negative pressure is driving fluid out, which is the same as saying that the net pressure effect is to drive fluid back into the capillary near the venular end. In this capillary, filtration occurs toward the arteriolar end and absorption takes place toward the venular end. It is worth emphasizing that because P_i, π_c, and π_i tend to be relatively constant, the capillary hydrostatic pressure, P_c, being the only variable, becomes the primary determinant of whether filtration or absorption occurs.

If the capillary hydrostatic pressure decreases linearly from the arteriolar to the venular end, we can estimate the magnitude of the Starling forces along the entire length of the capillary. The result is shown in Figure 3-3, *B*. At the arteriolar end, where the capillary hydrostatic pressure is high, the forces driving fluid out override the forces driving fluid in and the result is filtration of fluid out of the capillary. Advancing along the capillary, capillary hydrostatic pressure wanes and fluid filtration correspondingly decreases. Eventually the capillary hydrostatic pressure declines to the point where the forces driving fluid in overtake the forces driving fluid out and the result is absorption of fluid back into the capillary. In the example shown in Figure 3-3, filtration occurs over a little more than the first half of the length of the capillary and absorption takes place over the remainder. The end result is that over the length of the capillary, there is a slight excess of filtration over absorption, with a net flow of a small amount of fluid into the interstitium. The fluid that "leaks" into the interstitium is gathered by the lymphatic system and eventually returned into circulation. During inactivity, lymph production in humans amounts to 3 to 4 liters over a 24-hour period. Since blood circulates at the rate of about 5 liters per minute, over a 24-hour period more than 1400 liters of blood passes through the capillaries. This shows that capillary filtration and fluid reabsorption typically are finely balanced. Under certain circumstances the relative balance of filtration and absorption is disrupted, leading to **edema,** or excess accumulation of fluid in tissue (Box 3-5).

BOX 3-5

Edema: Excess Accumulation of Fluid

The Starling equation (Equation [6] in main text) shows that whether fluid leaves or enters the capillary is determined by the balance of capillary and interstitial hydrostatic and osmotic pressures. Altered pressure balance leads to altered fluid flow. When venous blood pressure is raised as a result of venous blood clots or congestive heart failure, the result is elevated hydrostatic pressure (P_c) in the capillary, which leads to more fluid filtration. Liver disease and severe starvation can both lead to greatly reduced albumin production by the liver. Since albumin is the predominant contributor to plasma colloid osmotic pressure (π_c), loss of albumin drastically lowers the retention of fluid in the capillaries. Finally, some factors in insect venom (e.g., mellitin from bees), as well as endogenous biochemical agents secreted during the allergic response (e.g., histamine released from mast cells), markedly increase the permeability of capillary walls. Plasma proteins that are normally impermeant can then leave the capillary and enter the interstitium, which lowers π_c and raises π_i. All of the processes described above lead to increased movement of fluid from the capillaries into the interstitium and give rise to edema.

Accumulation of fluid in the brain (cerebral edema) is dangerous. The brain is encased by the cranium; therefore enlargement of the brain resulting from edema can give rise to excessive intracranial pressure, which can lead to abnormal neurological symptoms. In contrast to capillaries in the peripheral circulation, cerebral capillaries have exceedingly low permeability to most solutes, including even small molecules such as glucose (MW 180). This blood-brain barrier makes it possible to reduce brain edema by introducing a small solute such as mannitol (MW 182) into the circulation. Because mannitol cannot cross the blood-brain barrier, it increases the osmotic pressure of blood plasma relative to the cerebrospinal fluid. Water is thus drawn out of the brain into the circulatory system, with a corresponding reduction in brain volume. Neurosurgeons routinely use this technique to treat brain edema or to reduce brain volume during neurosurgery.

ONLY IMPERMEANT SOLUTES CAN HAVE PERMANENT OSMOTIC EFFECTS

Transient Changes in Cell Volume Occur in Response to Changes in the Extracellular Concentration of *Permeant* Solutes

The discussion on solute permeability in Chapter 2 shows that equilibration of a **permeant solute** across a membrane is only a matter of time. As long as the membrane has some finite permeability for a solute, that is, $P_{solute} \neq 0$, or equivalently, $\sigma \neq 1$, the solute will ultimately penetrate, and become equilibrated across, the membrane. In the long term, then, there can be no permanent concentration difference for a permeant solute across the membrane (i.e., with time, $\Delta C_{solute} \to 0$). Because Equation [4] indicates that the net osmotic pressure exerted by a solute is dependent on ΔC_{solute}, the concentration difference of the solute across the membrane, and, ultimately, $\Delta C_{solute} \to 0$ for a permeant solute, we understand that permeant solutes can give rise to temporary, but not permanent, changes in osmotic pressure. Moreover, because osmotic pressure drives the movement of water and consequent **changes in volume** (i.e., volume flow, Equation [5]), we can also say that permeant solutes can give rise only to temporary, not permanent, changes in volume.

Suppose a permeant solute is added to the extracellular fluid (ECF) bathing a cell. If the cell membrane is equally permeable to the added solute and to water, the reflection coefficient for the solute is $\sigma = 0$ and the solute should have no osmotic effect. If the cell membrane is less permeable to the added solute than to water, that is, $0 < \sigma < 1$, the solute will increase the osmotic pressure of the ECF relative to the intracellular fluid (ICF). In response, water will move out of the cell, with consequent cell shrinkage, which leads to a corresponding increase in the concentration of the impermeant solutes already trapped in the cell. Because the added extracellular solute is permeant, however, even as water is leaving the cell, the solute penetrates the cell to increase the solute concentration of the ICF. As a result, water will begin to follow the permeant solute back into the cell. The process continues until the cell has expanded back to its original volume, at which point the intracellular and extracellular concentrations of permeant, *as well as* impermeant, solutes are equalized. The time course of the entire process is shown qualitatively in Figure 3-4, which also shows recovery of the cell volume to its original value when normal ECF composition is restored. That permeant solutes can have no permanent osmotic effect and cannot cause permanent volume changes is demonstrated quantitatively in Box 3-6.

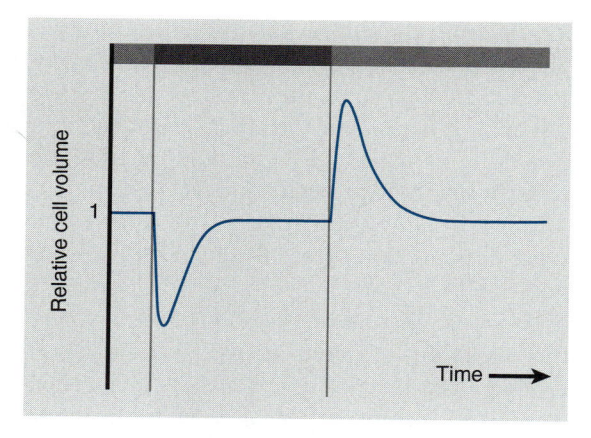

Figure 3-4 ■ Schematic representation of the time course of cell volume changes in response to changes in the concentration of permeant solute in the extracellular fluid (ECF). Solution composition is indicated by the long bar: light gray is normal ECF; dark gray is ECF with increased permeant solute concentration. The graph shows the response to a step increase in solute concentration and subsequent restoration of normal ECF.

Osmotic Pressure and Water Movement

BOX 3-6

Determining Volume Changes in Response to Osmotic Changes: Effect of Permeant Solutes

For a cell initially in osmotic equilibrium with a bath containing impermeant solute, what happens when the bath osmolarity is increased by adding a *permeant* solute, P? Qualitatively, we know that permeant solutes eventually equilibrate across the cell membrane until the inside and outside concentrations are equal. Thus the addition of permeant solutes to the bath should initially cause some water to leave the cell. Ultimately, however, the permeant solute concentration inside and outside should become equal. This means that, in the end, the permeant solute should have no permanent effect on the cell volume. We will demonstrate this quantitatively.

The cell is initially equilibrated with a bath containing impermeant (NP) solute. The total volume is

$$V_{Total} = V_{Cell,initial} + V_{Bath,initial} \quad [B1]$$

Because the osmotic pressures (and hence osmolarities) must be equal at equilibrium, we can say that

$$C_{NP,Cell,initial} = C_{NP,Bath,initial}$$

which also means that

$$\frac{n_{NP,Cell}}{V_{Cell,initial}} = \frac{n_{NP,Bath}}{V_{Bath,initial}} \quad [B2]$$

where n_{NP} is the number of moles of NP solute. Note that because NP solute cannot move from one compartment into another, the total number of moles in each compartment must remain the same. Thus, $n_{NP,Cell}$ and $n_{NP,Bath}$ remain unchanged regardless of osmotic conditions. If a permeant solute, P, is added to the outside and a new osmotic equilibrium is established, the intracellular and bath concentrations of P should be equal (and could be symbolized as C_P). The new osmotic balance between inside and outside can be written as

$$C_{NP,Cell,final} + C_P = C_{NP,Bath,final} + C_P$$

which, after canceling the C_P terms, is the same as

$$C_{NP,Cell,final} = C_{NP,Bath,final} \quad [B3]$$

If we assume that some permanent volume change ΔV had taken place as a result of equilibration, then, since any volume increase or decrease in either the cell or the bath is accompanied by the opposite change in the other compartment, Equation [B3] becomes

$$\frac{n_{NP,Cell}}{V_{Cell,initial} + \Delta V} = \frac{n_{NP,Bath}}{V_{Bath,initial} - \Delta V} \quad [B4]$$

Combining Equations [B2] and [B4] yields

$$(V_{Cell,initial} + V_{Bath,initial}) \cdot \Delta V = 0 \quad [B5]$$

The term in parentheses is the total volume, V_{Total}, which is constant and nonzero; therefore ΔV must be 0—no volume change could have taken place. We are thus forced to conclude that permeant solutes have no permanent osmotic effect and cannot cause permanent volume changes.

Persistent Changes in Cell Volume Occur in Response to Changes in the Extracellular Concentration of *Impermeant* Solutes

When the concentration of impermeant solutes in the ECF is increased, the extracellular osmotic pressure increases. Typically the volume of the ECF bathing a cell is much larger than the volume of the cell (this is known as the **infinite bath** condition). Because the cell membrane is essentially impermeable to most solutes present inside or outside the cell (see Chapter 2), only water will move out of the cell in response to the increase in ECF osmotic pressure, with a consequent drop in cell volume. This is illustrated in Figure 3-5, *A*, which also shows recovery of the cell volume to its original value when normal ECF composition is restored.

Conversely, if the impermeant solute concentration in the ECF is decreased, water would enter the cell and cause a lasting increase in cell volume, which would recover when normal ECF composition is restored. The corresponding time course is shown in Figure 3-5, *B*. That changes in impermeant solute concentration can cause persistent volume changes is demonstrated quantitatively in Box 3-7.

The Amount of *Impermeant* Solute Inside the Cell Determines the Cell Volume

Because impermeant solutes remain trapped inside the cell, when a cell is challenged by changing external osmotic conditions, the only changes that it can undergo rapidly are volume changes brought about by gain or loss of water. In other words, the cell gains or loses water to dilute or concentrate its impermeant solutes appropriately to match the osmolarity outside. For this reason it is the amount of impermeant intracellular solutes that ultimately determines cell volume.

■ SUMMARY

1. If a membrane is permeable to water but not to solute, and the solute concentration differs on the two sides of the membrane, water will move across the membrane from the side where the solute concentration is lower to the side where it is higher. This movement of water across a semipermeable membrane is called osmosis.
2. Osmotic movement of water leads to changes in fluid volume—the volume increases on the side of the membrane with higher solute concentration, and the volume decreases on the side with lower solute concentration.
3. Osmotic movement of water can be thought of as being driven by a difference in osmotic pressure on the two sides of a membrane. Osmotic pressure is proportional to solute concentration. Water moves from the side

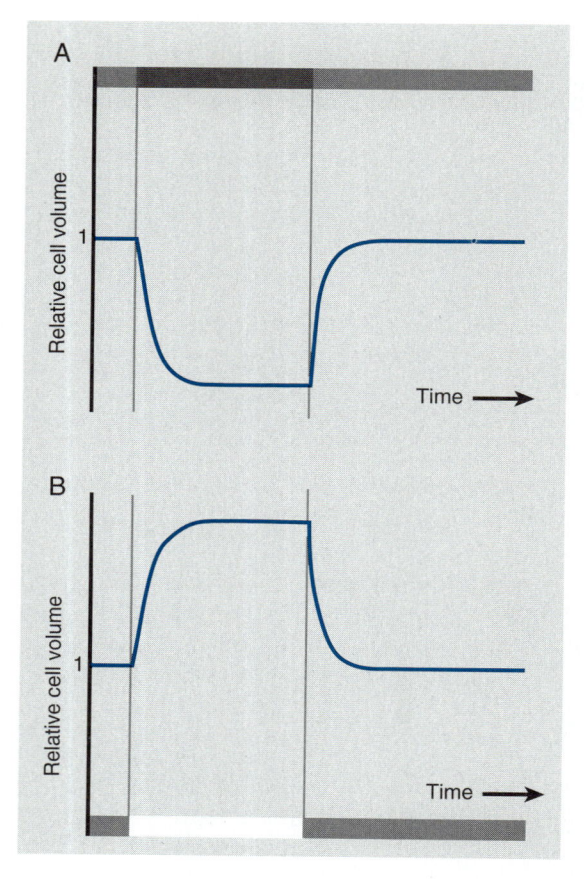

Figure 3-5 ■ Schematic representation of the time course of cell volume changes in response to changes in the concentration of impermeant solute in the extracellular fluid (ECF). Solution composition at any given time is indicated by the long bar: light gray is normal ECF; dark gray is ECF with increased impermeant solute concentration; white is ECF with decreased impermeant solute concentration. **A**, Response to a step increase in solute concentration and subsequent restoration of normal ECF. **B**, Response to a step decrease in solute concentration and subsequent restoration of normal ECF.

Osmotic Pressure and Water Movement

BOX 3-7

Determining Volume Changes in Response to Osmotic Changes: Effect of Impermeant Solutes

"Infinite Bath" Condition

A cell containing 200 mM impermeant (NP) solute is initially in osmotic equilibrium with a bath also containing 200 mM of NP solute. The bath volume is so large compared with the volume inside the cell that the bath can be considered "infinite." The osmolarity of the bath is then raised to 400 mM NP. What volume change will the cell undergo? We can deduce what should happen qualitatively. Because the solute is impermeant, it cannot move into or out of the cell. The difference in NP concentration inside and outside of the cell means that an osmotic driving force should move water out of the cell until a new osmotic equilibrium is established. That is, the cell should shrink. To determine the magnitude of the volume change, we have to do some calculation.

When osmotic equilibrium is established, no *net* movement of water should occur into or out of the cell, that is, the osmotic pressures (and osmolarities) outside and inside are equal. Therefore the initial condition of equilibrium (before the bath osmolarity was raised) and the final condition of equilibrium (after the cell had equilibrated with the new solution) are

$$C_{NP,Cell,initial} = C_{NP,Bath,initial} \quad \text{[B1]}$$
$$\text{and} \quad C_{NP,Cell,final} = C_{NP,Bath,final}$$

We also know that (1) $C_{NP,Bath,initial} = 200$, and (2) because the bath is "infinite" ($V_{Bath} \gg V_{Cell}$), the bath volume and concentration would essentially remain unchanged when a small amount of water moves out of the cell into the bath, that is, $C_{NP,Bath,final} = 400$. Substituting these two pieces of information into Equation [B1] gives

$$C_{NP,Cell,initial} = 200 \quad \text{and} \quad C_{NP,Cell,final} = 400 \quad \text{[B2]}$$

But the osmolarity, C, is just the number of millimoles (mmol), symbolized by n, divided by the volume, V. Moreover, because impermeant solute cannot enter or leave the cell, $n_{NP,Cell}$ remains unchanged throughout. Therefore Equation [B2] can be written as

$$\frac{n_{NP,Cell}}{V_{Cell,initial}} = 200 \quad \text{and} \quad \frac{n_{NP,Cell}}{V_{Cell,final}} = 400 \quad \text{[B3]}$$

Dividing the first equation in Equation [B3] by the second gives

$$\frac{V_{Cell,final}}{V_{Cell,initial}} = \frac{1}{2} \quad \text{[B4]}$$

When the osmolarity of an infinite bath is doubled by the addition of impermeant solute, the cell shrinks to one half of its initial volume.

Finite (Noninfinite) Bath Condition

Assume the solution conditions are the same as in the infinite bath case, except that the bath is no longer infinite. Now any water movement into or out of the cell will cause a corresponding volume change in the bath as well as the cell. If the bath osmolarity is suddenly doubled from 200 to 400 mM, we expect water movement out of the cell so that the bath osmolarity will drop as the cell osmolarity increases, until the osmolarity inside and outside is equalized.

The equilibrium conditions are always the same:

$$C_{NP,Cell,initial} = C_{NP,Bath,final} \quad \text{[B5]}$$
$$\text{and} \quad C_{NP,Cell,final} = C_{NP,Bath,final}$$

Since the bath is of finite size, any water flow into or out of the cell will change the bath volume. This means that after the new osmotic equilibrium is attained, the bath osmolarity will have changed from 400 mM. The way to take this change into consideration is as follows. If the cell undergoes volume change ΔV, the bath must undergo a corresponding volume change of $-\Delta V$. Thus the final cell volume will be $(V_{Cell,initial} + \Delta V)$. Correspondingly, the final bath volume is $(V_{Bath,initial} - \Delta V)$.

Continued

> **BOX 3-7**
>
> ### Determining Volume Changes in Response to Osmotic Changes: Effect of Impermeant Solutes—Cont'd
>
> Because of this volume change, the final bath osmolarity will be modified by the ratio $V_{Bath,initial}/(V_{Bath,initial} - \Delta V)$:
>
> $$C_{NP,Bath,final} = 400 \frac{V_{Bath,initial}}{V_{Bath,initial} - \Delta V} \quad [B6]$$
>
> Moreover, because $V_{Cell,final} = V_{Cell,initial} + \Delta V$ and $n_{NP,Cell}$ remains unchanged, the conditions of equilibrium (Equation [B5]) become
>
> $$\frac{n_{NP,Cell}}{V_{Cell,initial}} = 200 \quad \text{and} \quad [B7]$$
>
> $$\frac{n_{NP,Cell}}{V_{Cell,initial} - \Delta V} = 400 \frac{V_{Bath,initial}}{V_{Bath,initial} - \Delta V}$$
>
> Solving the two equations in Equation [B7] for ΔV gives the result
>
> $$\Delta V = \frac{-V_{Cell,initial} V_{Bath,initial}}{2V_{Bath,initial} + V_{Cell,initial}} \quad [B8]$$
>
> For example, assume that initially the bath and cell volumes are equal: $V_{Cell,initial} = V_{Bath,initial} = V$. Substitution into Equation [B8] gives $\Delta V = -V/3$. This means that the cell will shrink by $V/3$ and, correspondingly, the bath will expand by $V/3$. The bath osmolarity will be diluted from 400 by a factor of $V/(V + V/3) = 3/4$, to 300 mM. The cell osmolarity will be concentrated from 200 by a factor of $V/(V - V/3) = 3/2$, to 300 mM.
>
> In arriving at Equation [B8], we did not actually specify how large the bath was in relation to the cell volume. Equation [B8] should therefore apply to any volume. As a check, we apply Equation [B8] to the infinite bath case. Infinite bath means that $V_{Bath,initial} \gg V_{Cell,initial}$, which allows the denominator in Equation [B8] to be simplified: $(2V_{Bath,initial} + V_{Cell,initial}) \approx 2V_{Bath,initial}$. This leads to the result $\Delta V \approx -(V_{Cell,initial})/2$. That is, doubling the osmolarity of an infinite bath causes the cell to shrink by one half of its initial volume—exactly what we determined earlier.
>
> #### General Expression for Impermeant Solutes
>
> When the concentration of impermeant solutes in the bathing solution is changed from $C_{NP,initial}$ to $C_{NP,new}$, the volume change that occurs in a cell is given by
>
> $$\Delta V = \frac{(C_{NP,initial} - C_{NP,new})V_{Cell,initial}V_{Bath,initial}}{C_{NP,initial}V_{Cell,initial} + C_{NP,new}V_{Bath,initial}} \quad [B9]$$
>
> Equation [B9] is general; it applies to arbitrary bath and cell volumes and applies regardless of whether the bath osmolarity is increased or decreased. When the appropriate values are used in this general expression, we can easily verify that we get the same results as were obtained for the two specific examples discussed earlier in this box.

with low osmotic pressure (i.e., the side with higher water concentration) to the side with high osmotic pressure.

4. A difference in hydrostatic pressure on the two sides of a membrane can also drive water movement across the membrane barrier. Water moves from the side with high hydrostatic pressure to the side with low hydrostatic pressure.

5. The direction of net fluid flow across a capillary wall is controlled by the balance of hydrostatic and osmotic pressures, as described by the Starling equation.

6. A permeant solute can cross a membrane barrier and eventually abolish its own concentration gradient. Therefore a change in the extracellular concentration of a permeant solute can cause only a transient change in cell volume.

7. An impermeant solute cannot cross a membrane barrier to abolish its own concentration gradient. Therefore a change in the

concentration of an impermeant solute can cause a persistent change in cell volume.

■ KEY WORDS AND CONCEPTS

- Osmosis
- Osmotic pressure
- Osmolarity
- Tonicity
- van't Hoff's Law
- Reflection coefficient
- Hydrostatic pressure
- Volume flow
- Starling equation
- Colloid osmotic pressure (oncotic pressure)
- Hydraulic conductivity (filtration constant)
- Edema
- Permeant solute
- Impermeant solute
- Infinite bath
- Cell volume change

STUDY PROBLEMS

1. A cell is initially equilibrated with a very large volume of plasma that contains 300 mM *permeant* solute and 10 mM *impermeant* solute. The initial volume of the cell is V_0. Knowing that membrane permeability to water is higher than to solute, consider the three separate situations described below.
    a. The concentration of *impermeant* solute in the plasma is increased to 20 mM. Will water move into or out of the cell? When osmotic equilibrium is reestablished, what will be the final volume of the cell?
    b. The concentration of *permeant* solute in the plasma is increased to 400 mM. Describe the movement of water that is expected to take place. When equilibrium is reestablished, what will be the final volume of the cell?
    c. The concentration of *impermeant* solute in the plasma is increased to 20 mM *and* the concentration of *permeant* solute is decreased to 200 mM. Describe how the cell volume will change with time.

■ BIBLIOGRAPHY

Atkins PW: *Physical chemistry*, ed 5, New York, 1994, WH Freeman.
Gennis RB: *Biomembranes: molecular structure and function*, New York, 1989, Springer-Verlag.
Weiss TF: *Cellular biophysics*, Cambridge, Mass, 1996, MIT Press.

CHAPTER 4

Electrical Consequences of Ionic Gradients

Objectives:

1. Understand how the movement of ions can generate an electrical potential difference across a membrane.
2. Learn the concept of the equilibrium potential and how to use the Nernst equation to calculate it.
3. Understand how the resting membrane potential is generated in a cell and how to use the Goldman-Hodgkin-Katz (GHK) equation to calculate membrane potential.
4. Understand the relationship between the GHK equation and the Nernst equation.
5. Know how changes in membrane permeability to permeant ions can change the membrane potential.
6. Understand the Donnan effect and its consequences for living cells.

■ IONS ARE TYPICALLY PRESENT AT DIFFERENT CONCENTRATIONS ON OPPOSITE SIDES OF A BIOMEMBRANE

For any membrane in a living cell, biologically important ions are distributed asymmetrically on opposite sides of the membrane. In this chapter we focus on the plasma membrane of a cell, which separates the intracellular and extracellular environments. Across the plasma membrane, concentrations of the three common monovalent ions, Na^+, K^+, and Cl^-, are different. Ionic distributions for a "typical" mammalian cell are shown in Table 4-1. It is clear that the asymmetrical distributions of Na^+, K^+, and Cl^- ions give rise to concentration gradients of these ions across the plasma membrane. Such **ion concentration gradients** can drive the diffusional movement of the ions across the plasma membrane, which is selectively permeable to these ions. However, because ions carry electrical charge, their diffusional movement across the plasma membrane gives rise to electrical effects, which we now examine.

■ SELECTIVE IONIC PERMEABILITY THROUGH MEMBRANES HAS ELECTRICAL CONSEQUENCES: THE NERNST EQUATION

Consider a cell with the ion distributions shown in Table 4-1. Because the K^+ concentration is

TABLE 4-1

Intracellular and extracellular concentrations of the common monovalent ions for a typical mammalian cell

Ion	Intracellular (mM)	Extracellular (mM)
K^+	140	5
Na^+	10	145
Cl^-	6	106

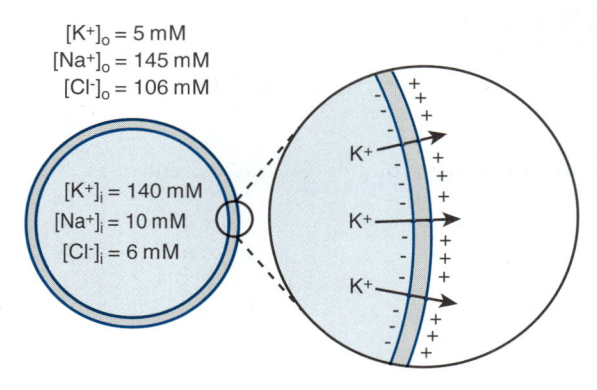

$[K^+]_o = 5$ mM
$[Na^+]_o = 145$ mM
$[Cl^-]_o = 106$ mM

$[K^+]_i = 140$ mM
$[Na^+]_i = 10$ mM
$[Cl^-]_i = 6$ mM

Plasma membrane permeable to K^+

Figure 4-1 ■ When the plasma membrane is selectively permeable only to K^+ ions, the K^+ concentration gradient (high concentration inside and low concentration outside) drives net movement of K^+ ions out of the cell.

higher inside the cell than outside, if the plasma membrane is selectively permeable *only* to K^+, we expect that K^+ ions will move down their concentration gradient, out of the cell (Figure 4-1).

When the positive K^+ ions leave the cell, however, they introduce positive charges to the exterior of the plasma membrane while leaving behind an equal number of negative charges on the intracellular side. This means that an electrical potential difference develops as a result of the diffusional movement of K^+ ions out of the cell. As K^+ ions exit the cell, the interior of the cell becomes progressively more negative while the exterior becomes correspondingly more positive. The effect of the developing electric field is to *oppose* further movement of K^+ ions (i.e., the negative interior tends to attract positive K^+ while the positive exterior tends to repel K^+). This analysis suggests that the "leakage" of K^+ ions cannot continue indefinitely because eventually a strong enough electric field will build up to exactly balance the tendency of K^+ to move out of the cell, down its concentration gradient. When the electrical forces exactly balance the driving force of the concentration gradient, we say that **electrochemical equilibrium** is reached. At electrochemical equilibrium, there can be no further *net* movement of K^+ ions into or out of the cell. The preceding discussion tells us that when K^+ ions are in electrochemical equilibrium across the plasma membrane, there is an electrical potential difference across the plasma membrane, with the inside being more negative than the outside. This electrical potential difference at which no net movement of K^+ occurs is the **equilibrium potential** for K^+ and is given the symbol E_K. For any ion whose extracellular and intracellular concentrations are C_{out} and C_{in}, respectively, the equilibrium potential can be calculated using the **Nernst equation*** (Box 4-1):

$$E_{eq} = \frac{RT}{zF} \ln\left(\frac{C_{out}}{C_{in}}\right) \quad [1]$$

where R is the universal gas constant, T is the absolute temperature in Kelvins (Celsius temperature plus 273.15), z is the electrical charge on the ion (+1 for K^+, −1 for Cl^-), and F is Faraday's

---

*Named after the German chemist Hermann Walther Nernst, who first derived the equation in 1889. Nernst received the Nobel Prize in Chemistry in 1920. Because the equilibrium potential for an ion is defined by the Nernst equation, the equilibrium potential is also known as the **Nernst potential**.

Electrical Consequences of Ionic Gradients

> **BOX 4-1**
>
> ### *Movement of Ions Driven by an Electrical Potential Gradient and the Origin of the Nernst Equation*
>
> In Chapter 2, diffusion, or the movement of molecules resulting from the presence of concentration gradients, was discussed. Here we examine, in an analogous way, the movement of ions (molecules carrying an electrical charge). Because an ion is charged, it will experience a force if it is placed in an electric field. This implies that an ion in an electric field in solution should move. It is reasonable to expect that the speed at which an ion in solution can move should depend on (1) the strength of the electric field: the stronger the electric field, the faster the ion will move; and (2) the charge on the ion: the higher the electrical charge on an ion, the faster it will move in an electric field. Within an electric field, a change in electrical potential, E, occurs with distance, x, that is, $\Delta E/\Delta x$. Analogous to the case of diffusion, where $\Delta C/\Delta x$ was a concentration gradient, the change in electrical potential with distance, $\Delta E/\Delta x$, is an *electrical potential gradient*. If the speed of ion movement is given the symbol s, the relationship between ion speed, the electrical potential gradient, and the charge on the ion can be represented as:
>
> $$s = uz \frac{\Delta E}{\Delta x} \quad \text{[B1]}$$
>
> where z is the number of charges on the ion (e.g., +1 for Na^+, +2 for Ca^{2+}, −2 for SO_4^{2-}) and u is a proportionality constant known as the "ionic mobility." Since $\Delta E/\Delta x$ has dimensions of volts per centimeter (V/cm) and s must have dimensions of centimeters per second (cm/s) and z is just the number of charges on an ion and therefore is dimensionless, u must have dimensions of (cm^2/s)/V for all the units to work out in Equation [B1].
>
> Knowing the speed of ion movement, we can easily figure out the flux of ions that are moving under the influence of an electric field. Imagine a cylindrical volume of solution containing the ions of interest (Figure B-1).
>
> **Figure B-1** ■ Flux of positive ions (cations) being driven by an electric field, $\Delta E/\Delta x$. The speed of movement of the ions is symbolized as s.
>
> In the figure the electrical potential gradient runs from right to left (i.e., left end more positive); positive ions (cations) would naturally move toward the right, that is, toward the negative end. Remembering that flux is the quantity of ions passing through unit area per unit time, to derive an expression for the flux, J, we need only to find out the quantity of ions flowing through area, A, in a given period of time, Δt. Because the ions are drifting with speed s toward the right, within the period Δt, any ion within a distance of $s \times \Delta t$ to the left of the area A would pass through A. The volume containing these ions that would pass through A is just $s \times \Delta t \times A$. The number of moles of ions in this volume is $C \times s \times \Delta t \times A$, where C is the concentration of the ion of interest. Taking the number of moles of ions that would pass through A and dividing by the area A and by the time interval, Δt, gives the flux of ions drifting in response to the electric field:
>
> *Continued*

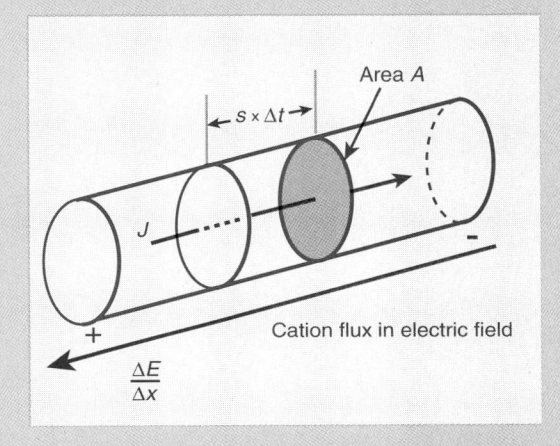

BOX 4-1

Movement of Ions Driven by an Electrical Potential Gradient and the Origin of the Nernst Equation—Cont'd

$J_{electr} = -[(C \times s \times \Delta t \times A)/A]/\Delta t = -C \times s$ [B2]

Substituting for s (use Equation [B1] in this box) the flux becomes

$$J_{electr} = -zuC \frac{\Delta E}{\Delta x} \quad [B3]$$

The minus sign takes into account the fact that for cations (z being a positive number), ion drift is toward the negative direction of the electric field, whereas for anions (z being a negative number), ion drift is toward the positive direction of the electric field.

If the electric field is not linear, $\Delta E/\Delta x$ can be replaced with dE/dx (a derivative):

$$J_{electr} = -zuC \frac{dE}{dx} \quad [B4]$$

Equation [B4] bears a strong resemblance to Equation [3] from Chapter 2 describing diffusion flux. Whereas a concentration gradient drives the diffusive flux of molecules or ions, an electrical potential gradient (an electric field) can drive the electrical flux of ions.

In view of the above, the total (net) flux of an ion is the sum of the flux caused by diffusion and the flux resulting from a driving electric field:

$$J_{total} = J_{diffusion} + J_{electr} = -D \frac{dC}{dx} - zuC \frac{dE}{dx} \quad [B5]$$

This equation quantifying the ionic flux driven by a concentration gradient as well as an electrical potential gradient is known as the Nernst-Planck equation.

At electrochemical equilibrium the flux driven by the concentration gradient is exactly balanced by the flux driven in the opposite direction by the electrical potential gradient, so the net flux must be zero. Therefore

$$J_{total} = J_{diffusion} + J_{electr} = -D \frac{dC}{dx} - zuC \frac{dE}{dx} = 0 \quad [B6]$$

which means that

$$zuC \frac{dE}{dx} = -D \frac{dC}{dx} \quad [B7]$$

Making use of a relationship, derived by Einstein, that relates the diffusion coefficient (D) and the mobility (u) of an ion,

$$D = \frac{uRT}{F} \quad [B8]$$

where R is the universal gas constant, T is the absolute temperature in Kelvins (Celsius temperature plus 273.15), and F is Faraday's constant (96,485 coulombs/mole), allows Equation [B7] to be rewritten in a form that is algebraically easier to manipulate:

$$zuC \frac{dE}{dx} = -\frac{uRT}{F} \frac{dC}{dx} \quad [B9]$$

Rearranging Equation [B9] gives

$$\frac{dE}{dx} = \frac{-RT}{zF} \frac{1}{C} \frac{dC}{dx} \quad [B10]$$

Such an equation can be integrated:

$$\int_{x_1}^{x_2} \frac{dE}{dx} dx = \frac{-RT}{zF} \int_{x_1}^{x_2} \frac{1}{C} \frac{dC}{dx} dx \quad [B11]$$

The result of integration is

$$E_2 - E_1 = \frac{-RT}{F} (\ln C_2 - \ln C_1) \quad [B12]$$

$$= \frac{-RT}{zF} \ln\left(\frac{C_2}{C_1}\right) = \frac{RT}{zF} \ln\left(\frac{C_1}{C_2}\right)$$

In other words, if a membrane is selectively permeable to a particular ion, and the ion is in electrochemical equilibrium across the membrane, we can calculate the membrane potential, ($E_2 - E_1$), that would be established just by knowing the concentration of the ion on the two sides of the membrane (C_1 and C_2).

The membrane potential of a cell is defined to be the potential of the inside relative to the outside

BOX 4-1

Movement of Ions Driven by an Electrical Potential Gradient and the Origin of the Nernst Equation—Cont'd

(i.e., $E_{in} - E_{out}$; subscripts 2 and 1 taken to be *in* and *out*, respectively). The membrane potential that is established when an ion is in electrochemical equilibrium across the membrane is referred to as the equilibrium potential for that ion and is given the symbol E_i, where the subscript *i* designates the particular ion under discussion (e.g., E_K is the equilibrium potential for K^+, E_{Cl} is the equilibrium potential for the Cl^- ion, and E_{Na} is the equilibrium potential for the Na^+ ion). By adopting these conventions, we can rewrite Equation [B12] in a form that is one of the most important equations in cellular physiology—the *Nernst equation*:

$$E_{eq} = \frac{RT}{zF} \ln\left(\frac{C_{out}}{C_{in}}\right) \quad [B13]$$

BOX 4-2

Alternative Forms of the Nernst Equation That May Be More Convenient for Calculations

If desired, the natural logarithm, ln, in the Nernst equation can be converted to base-10 logarithm: $\ln(C_{out}/C_{in}) = 2.303 \cdot \log(C_{out}/C_{in})$, to give the equivalent expression:

$$E_{eq} = \frac{2.303 RT}{zF} \log\left(\frac{C_{out}}{C_{in}}\right) \quad [B1]$$

At 37° C, the group of constants $RT/F = 26.7$ mV. For computation at 37° C, either of the following two forms of the Nernst equation could be used:

$$E_{eq} = \frac{26.7}{z} \ln\left(\frac{C_{out}}{C_{in}}\right) \quad \text{or} \quad [B2]$$

$$E_{eq} = \frac{61.5}{z} \log\left(\frac{C_{out}}{C_{in}}\right)$$

E is in units of mV.

---

constant (96,485 coulombs/mole). Some alternative forms of the Nernst equation that might be more convenient for use in computation are shown in Box 4-2. It is important to note here that a **membrane potential** for a cell is defined as the electrical potential *inside* the cell measured relative to the electrical potential *outside*. Because the extracellular electrical potential is a reference level against which the intracellular potential is measured, we can define the extracellular electrical potential to be zero (0).

Using the concentrations given in Table 4-1, we calculate the equilibrium potential for K^+ to be

$$E_K = \frac{61.5}{+1} \log\left(\frac{5}{140}\right) = 61.5\,(-1.45) = -89.1 \text{ mV}$$

This is the potential inside the cell relative to the outside, and it is negative, as we deduced earlier.

The Nernst equation can be used to calculate the equilibrium potential for any permeant ion, as long as the inside and outside concentrations for that ion are known. For example, for the ionic distributions shown in Table 4-1, if the plasma membrane were permeable only to Na$^+$ ions, the sodium equilibrium potential, E_{Na}, for our cell would be

$$E_{Na} = \frac{61.5}{+1} \log\left(\frac{145}{10}\right) = 61.5 \, (1.16) = +71.5 \text{ mV}$$

at 37° C. The sign for E_{Na} is positive because as positively charged Na$^+$ ions leak into the cell, down their concentration gradient, they make the inside of the cell more positive, while leaving behind a corresponding excess of negative charges on the outside. That is, the inside of the cell becomes more positive relative to the outside, hence the positive equilibrium potential for Na$^+$. It is equally straightforward to verify that for chloride ions, $E_{Cl} = -76.8$ mV at 37° C for our cell.

Some ion movement is required to establish physiological membrane potentials. Therefore we are justified in asking whether such movements significantly alter the ion concentrations inside the cell. After all, if ions enter or leave the cell, the intracellular ion concentration *must* change. In turn, we may ask whether the concentrations used in the Nernst equation should be corrected for the effect of such ion movements. The calculation in Box 4-3 shows that the number of ions that move into or out of the cell in order to establish a membrane potential is so small that the cellular ion concentrations are essentially undisturbed.

At first sight the magnitudes of the electrical potentials calculated above seem somewhat small. However, it must be remembered that these potentials exist across the plasma membrane, which is only ~50 angstroms thick (1 angstrom = 1×10^{-10} meter). Box 4-4 gives some observations about the membrane potential and the strength of electrostatic forces acting on oppositely charged ions separated by the plasma membrane.

The most important observation from the preceding discussion is that selective permeability of the plasma membrane to ions can have profound electrical consequences. For a typical cell (with ionic concentrations similar to those in Table 4-1), if the plasma membrane is selectively permeable to K$^+$, the resulting K$^+$ efflux will tend to drive the cell's membrane potential negative. Alternatively, if the plasma membrane is selectively permeable to Na$^+$, the resulting Na$^+$ influx will tend to drive the cell's membrane potential positive. The linkage between the membrane potential and the selective ionic permeabilities of a cell underlies the mechanism by which living cells regulate their electrical properties. This linkage is more fully explored in Chapter 7.

■ THE STABLE RESTING MEMBRANE POTENTIAL IN A LIVING CELL IS ESTABLISHED BY BALANCING MULTIPLE IONIC FLUXES

Cell Membranes Are Permeable to Multiple Ions

The concept of the equilibrium, or Nernst, potential for a particular ion (e.g., Na$^+$, K$^+$, or Cl$^-$) was developed by examining the fluxes of that ion in an idealized cell whose membrane is permeable *only* to that ion. The plasma membrane of a real cell is not permeable to only one ion; rather, it shows moderate to significant permeability to all of the three common monovalent ions. During the earlier discussion on the Nernst potential, we noted that it is the selective permeability of the plasma membrane to various ions that allows the cell to regulate its membrane potential. Just how does this regulation take place? How do the permeabilities of K$^+$, Na$^+$, and Cl$^-$ contribute to the cell's **resting membrane potential**?

If the cell is permeable to all three ionic species, fluxes of all three ions will occur across the plasma membrane. As we have seen, **ion fluxes** into and out of the cell have electrical consequences; namely, they change the membrane potential (V_m) of the cell. For example,

BOX 4-3

The Ion Movement Needed to Establish a Physiological Membrane Potential Does Not Significantly Change Ion Concentration Inside the Cell

Realizing that selective ion movements across the plasma membrane are necessary for establishing a membrane potential, we might ask whether such ion movements (e.g., leakage of K^+) will significantly disturb the intracellular concentration of the ion in question. To answer this question, we need to know one important property of biological membranes: the membrane capacitance, C. The capacitance is a measure of the amount of charge, q, that is separated by the membrane at a given membrane potential, V_m:

$$C = \frac{q}{V_m} \quad \text{[B1]}$$

The amount of charge is then just $q = C \cdot V_m$. The relevant units are the coulomb for electrical charge, the volt for electrical potential, and the farad (symbol F) for capacitance; 1 farad is equal to 1 coulomb per volt. The capacitance of biological membranes is typically 1 µF per cm² of membrane area (1×10^{-6} F/cm²). A spherical cell with a radius of 10 µm has a membrane surface area of

$$A_{cell} = 4\pi r^2 = 1257 \text{ µm}^2 = 1.257 \times 10^{-5} \text{ cm}^2$$

The capacitance for such a cell is

$$C = 1 \times 10^{-6} \text{ F/cm}^2 \times (1.257 \times 10^{-5} \text{ cm}^2)$$
$$= 1.257 \times 10^{-11} \text{ F}$$

If the membrane potential of this cell, V_m, is taken to be equal to the value of $E_K = -89.1$ mV (i.e., -0.0891 V) calculated for the example in the main text, the amount of charge separated by the cell membrane is

$$q = C \cdot E_K = (1.257 \times 10^{-11} \text{ F}) \times (0.0891 \text{ V})$$
$$= 1.120 \times 10^{-12} \text{ coulomb}$$

To convert the amount of electrical charge into the quantity of K^+ ions that had to move to establish E_K, we make use of Faraday's constant ($F = 96,485$ coulombs/mole; note the distinction between Faraday's constant, F, and the farad, F, the unit of capacitance):

Amount of K^+ moved $= q/F = (1.120 \times 10^{-12} \text{ coul})/$
$(96,485 \text{ coul/mol}) = 1.161 \times 10^{-17}$ **mol**

To assess whether the leakage of 1.161×10^{-17} mol of K^+ ions out of the cell significantly lowers the K^+ content of the cell, we need to calculate the moles of K^+ originally present in the cell. The number of moles of K^+ present inside the cell is just $[K^+]_{in} \times Vol_{cell}$. The volume of our cell is

$$Vol_{cell} = 4\pi r^3/3 = 4189 \text{ µm}^3 = 4.189 \times 10^{-12} \text{ L}$$

(1 Liter = 10^{15} µm³). The total amount of K^+ initially present in the cell must have been

K^+ content $= (0.140 \text{ mole/L}) \times (4.189 \times 10^{-12} \text{ L})$
$= 5.864 \times 10^{-13}$ **mol**

The fraction of the K^+ content that had to move out of the cell in order to establish the K^+ equilibrium potential is simply

$$\frac{\text{Amount of } K^+ \text{ moved}}{K^+ \text{ content in cell}} = \frac{1.160 \times 10^{-17} \text{ mol}}{5.864 \times 10^{-13} \text{ mol}}$$
$$= 1.979 \times 10^{-5} \approx \frac{20}{1,000,000} = 0.002\%$$

This calculation tells us that for every 1 million K^+ ions in the cell, roughly 20 must leak out of the cell in order to establish $E_K = -89.1$ mV. This amount of outward K^+ movement will diminish the intracellular K^+ content by only ~0.002%, an insignificantly small fraction. Therefore it is clear that the ion movement needed to establish a membrane potential, although electrically significant, does not change ion concentrations much.

> **BOX 4-4**
>
> ### The Electrical Forces Between Ions Separated by the Plasma Membrane Are Very Strong
>
> Typical physiological membrane potentials are on the order of many tens of millivolts across a membrane that is approximately 50 angstroms in thickness (1 Å = 10^{-8} cm = 10^{-10} m). Because the *electric field*, $\mathcal{E}$, is defined as the electrical potential per unit distance, the electric field across the plasma membrane when the membrane potential is 80 mV is
>
> $$\mathcal{E} = \frac{80 \times 10^{-3} \text{ V}}{50 \times 10^{-10} \text{ cm}} = 16{,}000{,}000 \; \frac{\text{V}}{\text{m}}$$
>
> This is about a thousand times stronger than typical field strengths used in electrophoresis.
>
> One can appreciate the strength of the electrostatic (or "Coulombic") interaction by calculating the attractive force between oppositely charged ions separated on the two sides of the plasma membrane. The magnitude of the electrostatic force, $F_{electrostatic}$, depends on q, the amount of charge separated by the membrane, and $\mathcal{E}$, the electric field across the membrane:
>
> $$F_{electrostatic} = \frac{q \times \mathcal{E}}{2} \quad\quad [B1]$$
>
> In Box 4-3, it was shown that to establish a potassium equilibrium potential, E_K, of -89.1 mV (or -0.0891 V) across the plasma membrane of a 20-μm spherical cell, 1.12×10^{-12} C of charges are separated on the two sides of the membrane. By using Equation B1, we can estimate the magnitude of the attractive force exerted by the separated charges on each other across the 50 Å thickness of the plasma membrane:
>
> $$F_{electrostatic} = \frac{1}{2} \cdot (1.12 \times 10^{-12} \text{ C}) \times \frac{0.0891 \text{ V}}{50 \times 10^{-10} \text{ m}}$$
> $$= 9.98 \times 10^{-6} \text{ N}$$
>
> We recall from Box 4-3 that the membrane area of the 20-μm spherical cell is 1.257×10^{-9} m². Therefore, the force per unit area of membrane is 7,940 N·m⁻². Since each newton (N) is equal to 0.225 pounds of force, this means that for a square meter of membrane area, the attractive force between the charges would be about 1,800 pounds, or nine tenths of a ton! Incidentally, this remarkable strength of the electrical forces underlies the *principle of electroneutrality*, which states that, in a solution, the number of positive ions are balanced by an equal number of negative ions, so that overall, the solution carries no net electrical charge.

efflux of K^+ tends to drive V_m toward more negative values, whereas influx of Na^+ tends to drive the V_m toward more positive values. Similarly, influx of Cl^- brings negative charges into the cell and would drive V_m toward more negative values. With all these fluxes occurring simultaneously (and "fighting" with each other), eventually a steady state will be established—a steady state in which the cell will have a stable, nonvarying membrane potential. What is the implication of a stable, nonvarying V_m? We know that whenever *net* movement of electrically charged ions into or out of the cell occurs, V_m will change. We can therefore conclude that a stable, nonvarying V_m implies that no *net* charge movement occurs into or out of the cell in the steady state. In other words, all fluxes tending to make the cell more negative are exactly balanced by fluxes that tend to make the cell more positive.

The Resting Membrane Potential Can Be Quantitatively Estimated by Use of the Goldman-Hodgkin-Katz Equation

The stable, resting membrane potential of a cell that is permeable to all three of the common monovalent ions is given quantitatively by the **Goldman-Hodgkin-Katz (GHK) equation**[*]:

$$V_m = \frac{RT}{F} \ln \frac{P_K[K^+]_o + P_{Na}[Na^+]_o + P_{Cl}[Cl^-]_i}{P_K[K^+]_i + P_{Na}[Na^+]_i + P_{Cl}[Cl^-]_o} \quad [2]$$

where P_K, P_{Na}, and P_{Cl} are the cell membrane **ionic permeabilities** for K^+, Na^+, and Cl^-, respectively.

We can examine the GHK equation to understand its meaning in terms of a physical picture. Recall that the product of a membrane permeability coefficient and a concentration is a unidirectional flux (see Chapter 2); for example,

$$K^+ \text{ efflux} = J_K^{in \to out} = P_K[K^+]_i \quad \text{and}$$
$$K^+ \text{ influx} = J_K^{out \to in} = P_K[K^+]_o$$

Keeping this point in mind, we see that the three terms summed in the numerator of the GHK equation correspond to K^+ influx, Na^+ influx, and Cl^- *efflux*. All three fluxes represent ion movements that tend to drive the membrane potential more *positive* (positively charged K^+ and Na^+ entering and negatively charged Cl^- leaving the cell). The three terms summed in the denominator, however, correspond to K^+ efflux, Na^+ efflux, and Cl^- *influx*, all of which represent ion movements that tend to drive the membrane potential more *negative* (positive K^+ and Na^+ leaving and negative Cl^- entering). The GHK equation, therefore, describes the behavior of the membrane potential, V_m, when all the ion fluxes that tend to drive V_m in the positive direction are balanced against all the ion fluxes that tend to drive V_m in the negative direction. These observations can also be stated in electrical terms. Because a flux of ions is equivalent to a flow of electrical charges, an ionic flux is also an ionic current. Therefore we can say that the GHK equation gives the value of the membrane potential when no *net* current is flowing through the membrane. The precise **relationship between ionic flux and ionic current** is defined in Box 4-5.

If we know the intracellular and extracellular concentrations, as well as the permeabilities, of the permeant ions, it is straightforward to use the GHK equation to calculate the resting membrane potential of the cell. It is customary and convenient to take the permeability coefficient for K^+ as a reference and normalize the other ionic permeabilities relative to that of K^+. The membrane of a resting cell has relatively high permeability to K^+ and Cl^- ions and relatively low permeability to Na^+ ions. Thus, typical relative permeabilities for a resting cell might have the following values: $P_K = 1$, $P_{Na} = 0.02$, and $P_{Cl} = 0.5$. Knowing these permeability coefficients and the fact that $RT/F = 26.7$ mV at 37° C, we can use the GHK equation and the concentrations given in Table 4-1 to calculate V_m for our typical cell:

$$V_m = 26.7 \times \ln \frac{1(5) + 0.02(145) + 0.5(6)}{1(140) + 0.02(10) + 0.5(106)}$$
$$= -76.8 \text{ mV}$$

The value of the resting membrane potential calculated from the GHK equation can be compared with the equilibrium potential for K^+ calculated previously by use of the Nernst equation: $E_K = -89.1$ mV. The resting membrane potential is about 12 mV more positive than the equilibrium potential for K^+. This situation is typical; most cells have a resting membrane potential that is 5 to 20 mV more *positive* than the K^+ equilibrium potential.

---

[*]The GHK equation was first derived by the American biophysicist David E. Goldman for his PhD dissertation research. Later, it was rederived and cast into its present, more physiologically useful form by the British physiologists Alan L. Hodgkin and Bernard Katz, recipients of the Nobel Prize in Physiology or Medicine in 1963 and 1970, respectively.

BOX 4-5

The Relationship Between Ionic Fluxes and Ionic Currents

Up to this point, the movement of ions through the cell membrane has been discussed in terms of flux, J, which is the number of moles of ion moving through a unit area of membrane per unit time. In future discussions that deal with the electrical behavior of cells, it is more convenient to use the concept of electrical *current* flowing through the membrane (symbolized as I), rather than ion flux. The two concepts are equivalent and are related in a simple way. Electrical current is the movement of *charges* per unit time. Converting flux into current involves figuring out the relationship between moles of ions and the amount of charge they carry. Each mole of ions represents z moles of electrical charge if each ion has charge z. Moreover, to convert molar units to electrical units, we need to use the Faraday constant, $F = 96,480$ coulombs per mole of charge. The relationship between ionic flux and current through the membrane is then

$$I = zF \times J \times A_{mem} \quad \text{[B1]}$$

where A_{mem} is the membrane area across which the flux/current is occurring. The two quantities, flux and current, are seen to be directly related through conversion factors and can be thought of as the same quantity in different units.

Different sign conventions are used in describing fluxes and currents in cellular physiology. Whereas in flux theory, flow of any kind of "particle" (i.e, positive ions, negative ions, or molecules) *into* the cell is defined to be a positive flux, flow of *positive* charges *out of* the cell is defined to be positive current in electrical theory. The four physically possible scenarios are summarized in Table B-1.

TABLE B-1

Sign conventions for fluxes and currents

Flow of positive or negative ions relative to cell	Direction and sign of flux, J	Direction and sign of current, I
Positive ion, outward	Outward, negative ($J < 0$)	Outward, positive ($I > 0$)
Positive ion, inward	Inward, positive ($J > 0$)	Inward, negative ($I < 0$)
Negative ion, inward	Inward, positive ($J > 0$)	Outward, positive ($I > 0$)
Negative ion, outward	Outward, negative ($J < 0$)	Inward, negative ($I < 0$)

A Permeant Ion Already in Electrochemical Equilibrium Does Not Need to Be Included in the GHK Equation

Earlier in the chapter the equilibrium potential for Cl⁻ was calculated for a cell with the ionic distributions shown in Table 4-1, and the result was E_{Cl} = −76.8 mV. Comparing E_{Cl}, calculated with the Nernst equation, with V_m calculated with the GHK equation above, we see that the equilibrium potential for Cl⁻ happens to be the same as the resting membrane potential—both are equal to −76.8 mV. Thus, at the resting membrane potential, V_m, Cl⁻ ions are in electrochemical equilibrium in this cell. This situation is characteristic of many cells in which Cl⁻ is not actively transported and yet its membrane permeability is high: Cl⁻ simply distributes *passively* in accordance with the resting membrane potential until it is in electrochemical equilibrium.

We can use the fact that Cl⁻ ions are in electrochemical equilibrium in our cell to illustrate another aspect of the GHK equation. Recall that a stable resting membrane potential is achieved by balancing the fluxes of various permeant ions. When an ion is already in electrochemical equilibrium, however, no net flux occurs for that ion. Because the GHK equation incorporates the balance of permeant ion fluxes to arrive at a resting membrane potential, any ion whose net flux is already zero does not really have to be included in the calculation. In our cell, since Cl⁻ is already in electrochemical equilibrium, the Cl⁻ terms need not be included in the GHK equation for calculating the resting membrane potential. This is easy to verify:

$$V_m = \frac{RT}{F} \ln \frac{P_K[K^+]_o + P_{Na}[Na^+]_o}{P_K[K^+]_i + P_{Na}[Na^+]_i}$$

$$= 26.7 \ln \frac{1(5) + 0.02(145)}{1(140) + 0.02(10)} = -76.8 \text{ mV}$$

Indeed, in this particular case the GHK equation gives the same resting membrane potential even when the Cl⁻ terms are left out of the numerator and denominator.

We can conclude that if a permeant ion is already in electrochemical equilibrium, that ion need not be included in the GHK equation for calculating the membrane potential. Said in another way, if V_m is equal to the equilibrium potential for a particular permeant ion, terms involving that ion can be dropped from the GHK equation without any effect.

The Nernst Equation May Be Viewed as a Special Case of the GHK Equation

The GHK equation predicts the membrane potential when the cell membrane is permeable to all three common monovalent ions. The Nernst equation, on the other hand, predicts the membrane potential when the membrane is permeable to only *one* ion. Therefore the Nernst equation should be a limiting case of the GHK equation. In other words, if the permeability coefficients of all but one ion are made zero in the GHK equation (corresponding to the membrane being permeable only to a single type of ion), the GHK equation should give the equilibrium potential for that permeant ion. This expectation is easy to verify. For example, if P_{Na} = P_{Cl} = 0 (so the membrane is permeable only to K⁺), the GHK equation can be simplified:

$$V_m = \frac{RT}{F} \ln \frac{P_K[K^+]_o + 0 \times [Na^+]_o + 0 \times [Cl^-]_i}{P_K[K^+]_i + 0 \times [Na^+]_i + 0 \times [Cl^-]_o}$$

$$V_m = \frac{RT}{F} \ln \frac{P_K[K^+]_o}{P_K[K^+]_i} = \frac{RT}{F} \ln \frac{[K^+]_o}{[K^+]_i} = E_K$$

Indeed, when the membrane is permeable only to K⁺, the GHK equation simplifies to the Nernst equation for K⁺. Similarly, if P_K = P_{Cl} = 0 (membrane permeable only to Na⁺), the GHK equation simplifies to the Nernst equation for Na⁺.

THE CELL CAN CHANGE ITS MEMBRANE POTENTIAL BY SELECTIVELY CHANGING MEMBRANE PERMEABILITY TO CERTAIN IONS

The relationship between the GHK and Nernst equations immediately suggests that if Na^+ permeability predominates, the membrane potential should approach the equilibrium potential of Na^+. If K^+ permeability predominates, the membrane potential should approach the equilibrium potential for K^+. The above inference holds true for any permeant ion. As a demonstration, assume that the relative permeability coefficients are $P_K = 1, P_{Na} = 20$, and $P_{Cl} = 0.5$, so that now the membrane permeability to Na^+ is 20 times that of K^+, whereas in the earlier case the Na^+ permeability was only 1/20 that of K^+. Using the same ionic distributions as before, the GHK equation now yields

$$V_m = 26.7 \times \ln\frac{1(5) + 20(145) + 0.5(6)}{1(140) + 20(10) + 0.5(106)}$$
$$= +53.5 \text{ mV}$$

Recalling that the equilibrium potential for Na^+ in this cell is $E_{Na} = +71.5$ mV, we see that with the vastly increased Na^+ permeability, the membrane potential is now quite positive and rather close to E_{Na}, as anticipated.

The preceding observations suggest that the cell can change its membrane potential just by manipulating the relative permeabilities of the common permeant ions through the cell membrane—an important mechanism that underlies the ability of nerve cells to transmit electrical signals.

THE DONNAN EFFECT IS AN OSMOTIC THREAT TO LIVING CELLS

If a cell were merely a bag of simple ions, such as K^+, Na^+, and Cl^-, immersed in an extracellular solution containing similar ions, nothing complex or interesting could ever happen; real biology requires something else. To carry out any real

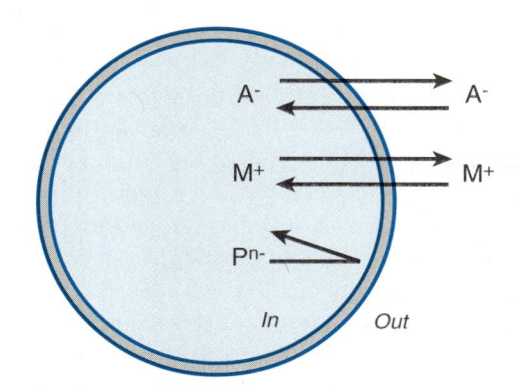

Figure 4-2 ■ A cell containing permeant cations and anions (M^+ and A^-) and impermeant polyanions (P^{n-}) bathed in extracellular solution containing only permeant cations and anions.

biological process, a cell must have in it, in addition to simple ions, more complex machinery. Biological machinery takes the form of proteins and nucleic acids, all of which are macromolecules that (1) carry multiple electrical charges and (2) are membrane impermeant and therefore trapped inside the cell. It is important to know the ionic consequences of the presence of impermeant, multiply charged macromolecules for the cell.

The situation to be considered is schematically represented in Figure 4-2, where M^+ represents a singly charged cation (e.g., Na^+, K^+), A^- represents a singly charged anion (e.g., Cl^-), and P^{n-} represents a macromolecule bearing n negative charges. The plasma membrane of a living cell always has finite permeability to the common small ions; therefore M^+ and A^- can permeate the plasma membrane, but the large polyanion P^{n-} cannot. Because P^{n-} cannot leave the cell and yet each negative charge on P^{n-} must be balanced with a positive charge, each molecule of P^{n-} will retain n M^+ ions inside the cell, just to maintain electroneutrality. The remaining "free" M^+ and A^- will equilibrate across the plasma membrane. Therefore a cell contains impermeant solute inside (all the P^{n-} macromolecules with their entourage of M^+ ions), while being bathed in a solution of permeant ions (M^+ and A^-). Recalling the discussion of osmosis from Chapter 3, we recognize that the imbalance of impermeant solute will tend to drive water into the cell continuously. Thus the presence of impermeant solutes inside the cell (but not outside) puts the cell in danger of uncontrolled swelling and rupture. This and other consequences of having multiply charged macromolecules trapped inside a compartment enclosed by a semipermeable membrane are collectively referred to as the **Donnan effect** (for a more quantitative treatment, see Box 4-6).

Because the Donnan effect gives rise to osmotic imbalance, water will enter the cell by osmosis and cause swelling and rupture. To forestall this kind of osmotic catastrophe, the cell can potentially adopt one of two survival strategies. The first is to pump water out as quickly as it enters, but no evidence has shown that this occurs in the cells of higher organisms. The second strategy is, in effect, to make an extracellular solute impermeant, so that the impermeant solute inside the cell is balanced by impermeant solute outside. How can the cell "transform" a permeant solute (e.g., Na^+ ions) into an impermeant solute? The cell can render a solute effectively impermeant by pumping the solute out as soon as it enters. In this way no net gain or loss of the solute occurs, which means that the solute behaves *as if* it is impermeant. Indeed, this is the major mechanism for regulating cell volume—all living cells pump out permeant cations as quickly as they enter the cell. For living cells at steady state, Na^+ ions, the major permeant cations outside the cell, are extruded from the cell by active transport as rapidly as they leak in. This is functionally equivalent to making the cell membrane impermeable to Na^+ ions. Thus the plasma membrane sodium pump (Na^+/K^+-ATPase; see Chapter 11), by constantly removing a small ionic solute from the interior of the cell with the expenditure of ATP energy, maintains cellular osmotic balance.

■ SUMMARY

1. Biologically important ions (e.g., Na^+, Ca^{2+}, Cl^-) typically are asymmetrically distributed across a biological membrane. That is, an ionic species is typically present at different concentrations on opposite sides of a biomembrane. This implies that a concentration gradient exists for each type of ion across the membrane.
2. Movement of ions (which carry electrical charge) across a membrane changes the electrical potential across the membrane.
3. If a cell membrane is selectively permeable to only a *single* type of ion, the concentration gradient of the ion will drive diffusion of that ion across the membrane. Within a very short time such ion movement will generate an electrical potential across the membrane that will be strong enough to oppose any further net movement of ions across the membrane. The membrane potential that is reached is known as the equilibrium potential of the ion. At the equilibrium potential of an ion, no *net* flux of that ion occurs across the membrane.
4. The equilibrium potential of an ion can be calculated by using the Nernst equation, as long as the concentrations of the ion on the two sides of the membrane are known. The equilibrium potential is also known as the Nernst potential.
5. In reality, a cell membrane is permeable to multiple types of ions, each of which will have a flux across the membrane. The steady-state *resting membrane potential* of a cell is achieved when all of the ionic fluxes balance each other (when no *net* movement of ionic charges across the membrane occurs).

BOX 4-6

A Calculation Illustrating the Donnan Effect

The Nernst equation and the concept of the equilibrium potential for a permeant ion can be used to examine the Donnan effect. With reference to Figure 4-2, we adopt the following symbols: $[M^+]_i$ and $[M^+]_o$ are the concentrations of M^+ inside and outside the cell, respectively, while $[A^-]_i$ and $[A^-]_o$ are the concentrations of A^- inside and outside the cell, respectively. $[P^{n-}]$ is the concentration of impermeant macromolecules inside the cell. We have already shown that if a permeant ion is allowed to move and redistribute across a cell membrane, eventually a membrane potential will be established that *just* balances any movement of the ion that is driven by concentration differences between the inside and the outside of the cell. At this balance point there is no longer a net flux of the permeant ion across the membrane. The membrane potential at the balance point is the Nernst, or equilibrium, potential for that ion. In the present situation both M^+ and A^- permeate the cell membrane. This implies that eventually the equilibrium potential will be established for each ion:

$$E_M = \frac{RT}{(+1)F} \ln\left(\frac{[M^+]_o}{[M^+]_i}\right) \quad \text{and} \quad \text{[B1]}$$

$$E_A = \frac{RT}{(-1)F} \ln\left(\frac{[A^-]_o}{[A^-]_i}\right)$$

Because both ionic species (M^+ and A^-) are simultaneously in equilibrium across the *same* cell membrane, the equilibrium potentials achieved must be *identical*. That is, $E_M = E_A$. This means that

$$\frac{RT}{(+1)F} \ln\left(\frac{[M^+]_o}{[M^+]_i}\right) = \frac{RT}{(-1)F} \ln\left(\frac{[A^-]_o}{[A^-]_i}\right) \quad \text{[B2]}$$

Algebraic simplification gives

$$\frac{[M^+]_i}{[M^+]_o} = \frac{[A^-]_o}{[A^-]_i} \quad \text{[B3a]}$$

or, the equivalent expression

$$[M^+]_i \times [A^-]_i = [M^+]_o \times [A^-]_o \quad \text{[B3b]}$$

Equation [B3] is known as the Donnan condition. In other words, at equilibrium the presence of the multiply charged macromolecules gives rise to an asymmetrical distribution of the permeant small cations and anions across the membrane. It can be seen from the Donnan condition (Equation [B3]) that the distribution (and gradient) of permeant cations across the membrane is the *inverse* of the distribution (and gradient) of permeant anions across the same membrane. Thus the presence of impermeant macromolecules that carry multiple negative charges results in a higher concentration of permeant cations inside the cell relative to the outside, while the concentration of permeant anions is correspondingly higher outside relative to the inside of the cell. Any system in which the permeant cations and anions obey the Donnan condition is said to be in Donnan equilibrium.

The situation can now be analyzed with respect to the principle of electroneutrality: In any solution the total number of positive and negative charges must be equal, so that the solution remains electrically neutral overall. Electroneutrality thus dictates that all the positive charges inside the cell must be balanced by all the negative charges inside the cell. Referring to Figure 4-2, we see that

$$[M^+]_i = [A^-]_i + n[P^{n-}] \quad \text{[B4]}$$

because each A^- needs only one M^+ to balance it, whereas each P^{n-} must have n M^+ for charge balance. Charge balance must also hold for the extracellular fluid; therefore

$$[M^+]_o = [A^-]_o \quad \text{[B5]}$$

If the ratio in Equation [B3a], commonly referred to as the Donnan ratio, is given the symbol R_D (i.e., $R_D = [M^+]_i/[M^+]_o = [A^-]_o/[A^-]_i$), Equation [B4] can be rewritten as

$$R_D [M^+]_o = \frac{[M^+]_o}{R_D} + n[P^{n-}] \quad \text{[B6]}$$

Multiplying through by R_D and moving all the terms to the same side of the equal sign gives the quadratic equation

BOX 4-6

A Calculation Illustrating the Donnan Effect—Cont'd

$$[M^+]_o R_D^2 - n[P^{n-}]R_D + [M^+]_o = 0 \quad [B7]$$

which has the solution

$$R_D = \frac{n[P^{n-}]}{2[M^+]_o} + \sqrt{1 + \left(\frac{n[P^{n-}]}{2[M^+]_o}\right)^2} \quad [B8]$$

As reasonable estimates, we can take $[M^+]_o = [A^-]_o = 150$ mM. In addition, we assume that $n = 50$ and $[P^{n-}] = 5$ mM. That is, we assume that the cell contains approximately 5 mM of macromolecules bearing 50 negative charges each, on average. For these estimates,

$$R_D = \frac{50(5)}{300} + \sqrt{1 + \left(\frac{50(5)}{300}\right)^2} = 2.14 \quad [B9]$$

This means that

$$R_D = \frac{[M^+]_i}{[M^+]_o} = \frac{[A^-]_o}{[A^-]_i} = 2.14 \quad [B10]$$

This calculation verifies that the presence of the negatively charged macromolecules inside the cell causes excess accumulation of permeant cations in the cell relative to the extracellular fluid, while there is a corresponding deficit of permeant anions in the cell relative to the extracellular fluid. This reciprocal asymmetrical distribution of the permeant cations and anions resulting from the presence of impermeant charged macromolecules is one aspect of the *Donnan effect*.

The second, more important, consequence of the presence of impermeant charged macromolecules in the cell can be seen by examining the total concentration of solutes inside and outside the cell. For the extracellular fluid, the estimates

$$[M^+]_o = [A^-]_o = 150 \text{ mM}$$

were used; therefore (with use of the Donnan ratio, R_D, just calculated):

$$[M^+]_i = 2.14[M^+]_o = 2.14(150) = 321 \text{ mM}$$

$$[A^+]_i = [A^-]_o/2.14 = 150/2.14 = 70 \text{ mM}$$

In addition,

$$[P^{n-}] = 5 \text{ mM}$$

The total concentration of solutes outside the cell is

$$[\text{Solute}]_o = [M^+]_o + [A^-]_o = 150 + 150 = 300 \text{ mM}$$

while the total concentration of solutes inside the cell is

$$[\text{Solute}]_i = [M^+]_i + [A^-]_i + [P^{n-}]_i = 321 + 70 + 5 = 396 \text{ mM}$$

We see that the total intracellular solute concentration is significantly higher than the total extracellular solute concentration. The conclusion is that the presence of multiply charged macromolecules inside the cell will always cause the intracellular osmolarity to *exceed* the extracellular osmolarity. This osmotic imbalance will always drive water movement into the cell, which leads to increased cell volume and eventual rupture. Therefore, to survive, a living cell must have evolved mechanisms to correct or counteract this osmotic imbalance.

---

6. The resting membrane potential of a cell can be quantitatively estimated by using the *Goldman-Hodgkin-Katz equation*, as long as the concentrations of the relevant ions, as well as the relative membrane permeabilities for the ions, are known.
7. A cell can change its membrane potential by controlling the relative permeabilities of the cell membrane to certain ions (principally Na^+, K^+, and Cl^-).
8. The presence of impermeant, multiply charged macromolecules (e.g., nucleic acids, proteins) inside the cell gives rise to the Donnan effect, one aspect of which is that intracellular osmolarity will tend to be higher relative to the extracellular environment. This would

cause water to move into the cell, which would swell and rupture. The sodium pump (Na^+,K^+-ATPase; see Chapter 11), by continually pumping out Na^+ ions, reduces the intracellular osmolarity to match the extracellular osmolarity and thus counteracts the osmotic consequences of the Donnan effect.

■ KEY WORDS AND CONCEPTS

- Ion concentration gradient
- Electrochemical equilibrium
- Equilibrium (Nernst) potential
- Nernst equation
- Membrane potential
- Ionic permeability
- Resting membrane potential
- Ion flux
- Goldman-Hodgkin-Katz (GHK) equation
- Donnan effect
- Relationship between ionic flux and ionic current

STUDY PROBLEMS

1. In a particular cell, the equilibrium potential of Na^+ was found to be $E_{Na} = +20$ mV. If the intracellular concentration of Na^+ was found to be $[Na^+]_i = 5$ mM, what was the extracellular Na^+ concentration?

2. For a particular cell, the intracellular and extracellular concentrations of the common monovalent ions are shown in the table below.

Ion	Intracellular (mM)	Extracellular (mM)
K^+	140	3
Na^+	15	145
Cl^-	5	105

    a. If the relative permeabilities of the cell membrane to the three ions are $0.8 : 1.0 : 0.5$ ($P_K : P_{Na} : P_{Cl}$), what is the membrane potential of this cell?
    b. What is the equilibrium potential for Cl^-?
    c. What is the expected direction of the net *flux* of Cl^-?
    d. What is the direction and sign of the Cl^- *current*?

3. If Na^+ extrusion by the Na^+ pump in the plasma membrane of a cell is inhibited, how is the volume of the cell expected to change? Explain.

■ BIBLIOGRAPHY

Atkins PW: *Physical chemistry*, ed 5, New York, 1994, WH Freeman.

Byrne JH, Schultz SG: *An introduction to membrane transport and bioelectricity*, ed 2, New York, 1994, Raven Press.

Ferreira HG, Marshall MW: *The biophysical basis of excitability*, Cambridge, Eng, 1985, Cambridge University Press.

Gennis RB: *Biomembranes: molecular structure and function*, New York, 1989, Springer-Verlag.

Weiss TF: *Cellular biophysics*, Cambridge, Mass, 1996, MIT Press.

CHAPTER 5

SECTION II Ion Channels and Excitable Membranes

Ion Channels

Objectives:

1. Understand that ion channels are gated, water-filled pores that increase the permeability of the membrane to selective ions.
2. Describe the function of the selectivity filter in an ion channel.
3. Understand that ion channels can be grouped into gene families on the basis of structural homology.
4. Describe the structural features of the voltage-gated channel superfamily.

■ ION CHANNELS ARE CRITICAL DETERMINANTS OF THE ELECTRICAL BEHAVIOR OF MEMBRANES

This chapter and the following three chapters focus on the properties of the cell membrane that determine the overall electrical behavior of the cell. To put this material in its proper context, consider a typical neuron, such as the α motor neuron illustrated in Figure 5-1. The cell body (soma) contains the nucleus, mitochondria, and the endoplasmic reticulum, which is the site of protein synthesis. Two types of processes usually extend from the cell body. *Dendrites* are relatively short, small-diameter processes that branch extensively and receive signals from other neurons. The *axon* is a long cylindrical process that can be more than 3 m in length and is responsible for transmitting signals to other neurons. The axon begins at a region of the soma called the *axon hillock* and terminates in several small branches that make contact with as many as 1000 other neurons. Specialized junctions *(synapses)* are formed at the points of contact between neurons and are sites of communication between the cells (see Chapter 8). The main electrical functions of this type of cell are (1) to sum, or integrate, electrical inputs from a large number of other neurons; (2) to generate an *action potential,* which is a rapid, transient membrane depolarization, if the inputs reach a critical level; and then (3) to propagate this signal to the nerve terminals. All of these processes depend on the activity of several types of **ion channels**. The channels are integral membrane proteins that form water-filled (aqueous) pores, which permit ions to permeate.

The primary role of the neuronal cell body and dendrite membranes (Figure 5-1) is to integrate, over both space and time, the activity of all synaptic inputs impinging on the cell. The characteristics of this integrative process are determined largely by the passive electrical properties of the membrane, which are described in Chapter 6. When the membrane potential at the axon hillock (Figure 5-1) reaches threshold, an action potential is generated. Threshold behavior and the generation of the action potential are caused primarily by two types of ion channels in nerves, voltage-gated Na^+ and K^+ channels. The properties of these channels and their roles in the generation of the action potential are presented in Chapter 7. Once the action potential has been generated, it is conducted, or *propagated,* at full amplitude (i.e., it is "*all-or none*"; see Chapter 7) along the axon to the nerve terminals. Action potential propagation is a process that involves both the passive properties of the membrane and the dynamic activity of the voltage-gated Na^+ and K^+ channels.

■ DISTINCT TYPES OF ION CHANNELS HAVE SEVERAL COMMON PROPERTIES

Ion Channels Increase the Permeability of the Membrane to Ions

The permeability of a pure phospholipid bilayer membrane to ions (e.g., Na^+, K^+, Cl^-, and Ca^{2+}) is extremely small: the permeability coefficients for these ions are in the range of 10^{-11} to 10^{-13} cm/sec (see Chapter 2). Because of this low intrinsic permeability, ions must cross membranes by one of two types of mechanism: by reversibly binding to a carrier, or transporter, molecule (see Chapters 10 and 11) or by diffusion through

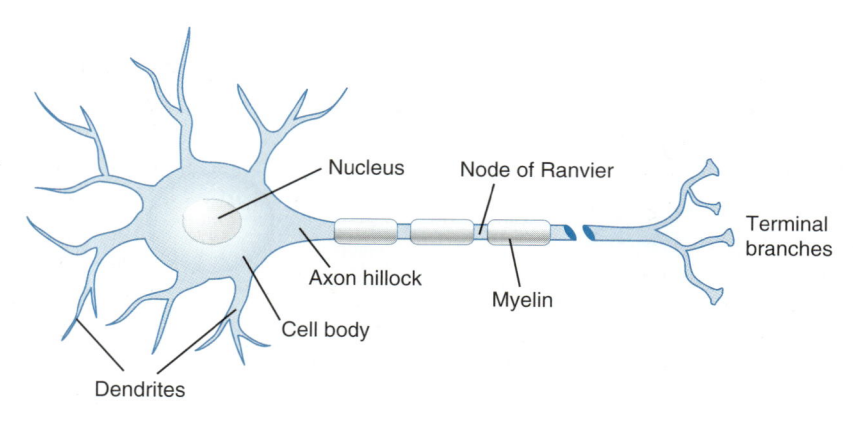

Figure 5-1 ■ Structure of a myelinated neuron. The cell body gives rise to two types of neuronal processes: dendrites and axons. The dendrites and the cell body (or soma) form the receptive surfaces of the neuron. They receive inputs from other neurons. The axon begins at the axon hillock and can be more than 3 m in length. The axon represents the output element of the neuron. Many axons, like the one shown in this figure, are myelinated: they are surrounded by a fatty sheath of myelin that insulates the axon from the surrounding solution. The myelin is interrupted by the nodes of Ranvier. The terminal branches of the axon make synaptic contacts with other neurons, or in the case of the α motor neuron, with skeletal muscle cells.

Ion Channels and Excitable Membranes

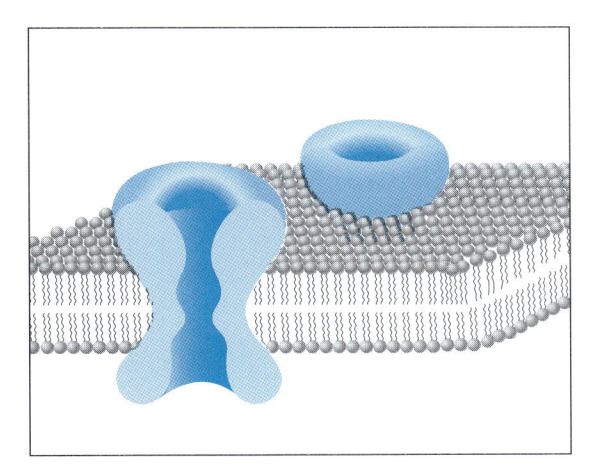

Figure 5-2 ■ An open ion channel embedded in a lipid bilayer membrane. The ion channel is a protein macromolecule that extends across the membrane and is in contact with the aqueous environment on both sides of the membrane. The channel provides an aqueous pathway for selective ions to move through the membrane. (Redrawn from Hille B: *Ionic channels of excitable membranes,* ed 3, Sunderland, Mass, 2001, Sinauer.)

an aqueous pore (Figure 5-2). The maximum transport rate for carriers is on the order of 5000 ions per second. This is much too slow to generate the rapid changes in membrane potential that are required for neuronal signaling. Nerve and muscle excitation (i.e., the generation and propagation of the action potential; see Chapter 7) and neuronal signaling require much faster ion movements. The rate of ion movement by diffusion through a small-diameter pore is usually several orders of magnitude faster than the transport rate supported by carriers (Box 5-1).

Ion Channels Are Integral Membrane Proteins That Form Gated Pores

Ion channels are large macromolecular proteins that often consist of several peptide subunits.

These channel proteins extend across the lipid bilayer and are in contact with the aqueous environment on both sides of the membrane. The channel peptide forms a water-filled pore that allows ions to cross the membrane by diffusion. A single channel can conduct ions at the rate of 1 to 100 million ions per second, which is several orders of magnitude faster than carrier transport.

The pore in an ion channel is not open all the time. Channels open and close spontaneously and in response to various stimuli. The channel functions as if it had a gate that could close and prevent ions from moving through the pore or could open to allow ion movement. **Voltage-gated** ion channels have an *open probability* (the fraction of time the channel is open) that depends on the membrane potential (see Chapter 7). **Ligand-gated** channels are activated after the binding of a neurotransmitter to a receptor located on the channel (see Chapter 8). In the latter case, open probability is related to ligand binding, which in turn is related to ligand concentration.

Ion Channels Exhibit Ionic Selectivity

One of the more remarkable properties of ion channels is their ability to conduct ions *selectively* at very high rates. For example, K^+-selective ion channels that conduct about 10 million K^+ ions per second are 100 times more permeable to K^+ than to Na^+. This, at first, seems remarkable, in view of the fact that the crystal radius of Na^+ (0.095 nm) is actually less than that of K^+ (0.133 nm). If the channel is simply an aqueous pathway for ion movement, how does it accomplish ion selectivity?

A proposed explanation of selectivity is that the channel has a narrow region within the pore that acts as a **selectivity filter**. The selectivity filter has a certain size and shape and acts as a molecular sieve to prevent larger ions from passing through. However, selectivity also re-

> **BOX 5-1**
>
> ### Calculation of the Rate of Ion Movement Through an Aqueous Pore
>
> The diffusion equation described in Chapter 2 can be used to calculate the rate of ion movement across a membrane through an aqueous pore. The equation is
>
> $$J = -D \frac{\Delta C}{\Delta x}$$
>
> where J is the flux per unit area (in moles/cm^2/sec), D is the diffusion coefficient, ΔC is the concentration difference across the membrane, and Δx is the pore length. We will assume that the pore is a cylinder with radius r_p and length Δx. To calculate a flux in units of moles/sec, we multiply both sides of the flux equation by the cross-sectional area of the pore ($\pi \times r_p^2$):
>
> $$J \text{ (moles/sec)} = -\pi \times r_p^2 \times D \frac{\Delta C}{\Delta x} \quad \text{[B1]}$$
>
> Let us assume that the diffusion coefficient for the ion in the pore is the same as in bulk solution (2×10^{-5} cm^2/sec). We will further assume that the pore radius is 3×10^{-8} cm, the concentration difference is 100 mM, and the pore length is 5×10^{-7} cm. Plugging these values into Equation [B1] gives
>
> $$J = \pi \times (3 \times 10^{-8} \text{ cm})^2 \times 2 \times 10^{-5} \frac{\text{cm}^2}{\text{sec}} \times \frac{0.1 \frac{\text{mole}}{10^3 \text{ cm}^3}}{5 \times 10^{-7} \text{ cm}} \approx 1 \times 10^{-17} \frac{\text{moles}}{\text{sec}}$$
>
> Multiplying by Avogadro's number (6.023×10^{23} ions/mole) gives the flux as 6 million ions/sec, which is 1000 times faster than the maximum rate of carrier-mediated transport (see Chapter 11).

quires *specific interaction* between the ion and the selectivity filter. Ions bind water molecules tightly (i.e., they are *hydrated*), and they must shed some waters of hydration to move through the narrow selectivity filter. A specific ion type will move through the channel only if the ion's binding interaction with the selectivity filter compensates for the loss of waters of hydration (Box 5-2).

ION CHANNELS SHARE STRUCTURAL SIMILARITIES AND CAN BE GROUPED INTO GENE FAMILIES

Channel Structure Is Studied with Biochemical and Molecular Biological Techniques

To understand fully how an ion channel works, we must know the **ion channel structure** in detail. In the early 1970s, channels were identified as peptides. Over the next three decades, various protein biochemical and molecular biological techniques were developed to isolate and characterize the structure of channel peptides. Channel proteins were purified on affinity columns, making use of their ability to bind specific ligands with high affinity. Channels isolated in this way were found to be large, glycosylated proteins often composed of more than one protein subunit. For example, the voltage-gated Na$^+$ channel (see Chapter 7) was first purified on the basis of its ability to bind tetrodotoxin* (TTX) with high affinity. The principal subunit of the Na$^+$ channel (the α-subunit) has a molecular weight of about 250 kDa and consists of a linear sequence of about 1800 amino acids. The α-subunit contains all the functional characteristics of Na$^+$ channels, including the pore-forming region and the TTX-binding site. The Na$^+$ channel also contains two smaller, auxiliary

---

*Tetrodotoxin is a puffer fish toxin that selectively blocks voltage-gated Na$^+$ channels with high affinity.

Ion Channels and Excitable Membranes

> **BOX 5-2**
>
> ### Selectivity Involves Interaction of an Ion with the Selectivity Filter
>
> Water is a dipolar molecule because charge is separated within the molecule. The oxygen atom has a slight negative charge, and the hydrogen atoms have a slight positive charge. As a result, an ion in aqueous solution is hydrated; that is, the ion floats around with a cloud of water molecules that are electrostatically attracted to the ion. This is a stable configuration: the hydration energy is of the same magnitude as a covalent bond. Thus energy must be expended to remove waters of hydration from an ion. The selectivity filter in an ion channel is a narrow region containing carboxyl or carbonyl groups that can substitute for some of the ion's water molecules. An ion will move through the narrow region only if the energy of interaction with the selectivity filter compensates for the loss of waters of hydration. For example, a K^+ ion in a rigid 0.3-nm diameter pore lined with carbonyl oxygen atoms might have the same energy as a K^+ ion in water. However, the smaller diameter Na^+ ion would have a higher energy in the pore than in water, so it would not shed its water molecules. Therefore it could not enter the pore.

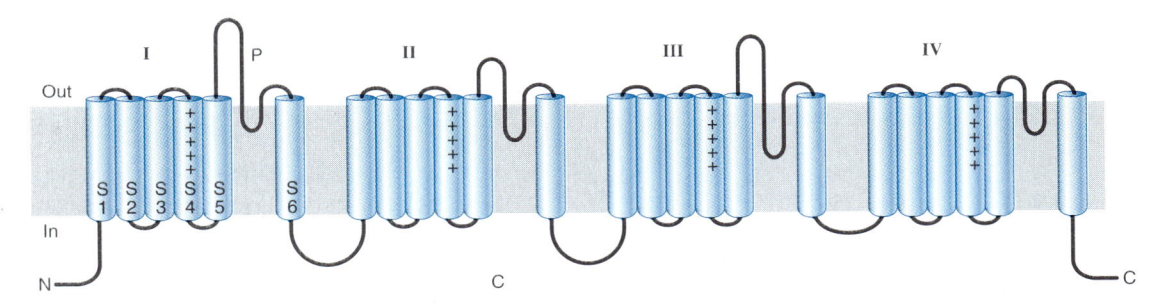

Figure 5-3 ■ The voltage-gated Na^+ channel. The Na^+ channel α-subunit is a single polypeptide chain that contains four homologous domains (I, II, III, and IV). Each domain contains six α-helical segments (S1 to S6) that span the membrane (shown as cylinders). Segment S4 contains a positive amino acid at every third position. Each domain also contains a P region between S5 and S6 on the extracellular side, which dips partway into the membrane and forms part of the pore.

peptide subunits. The function of the auxiliary subunits is not completely clear.

In 1984, the α-subunit of the voltage-gated Na^+ channel was cloned, revealing its primary amino acid sequence. On the basis of this sequence a model of the secondary structure (i.e., the protein folding pattern) of the channel was developed, which was later confirmed by various biochemical and functional studies. The current model of the Na^+ channel α-subunit (Figure 5-3) shows that it contains four homologous domains (designated I, II, III, and IV), each with six α-helical membrane-spanning segments (S1 to S6). Segment S4 has a positively charged amino acid at every third residue and is the voltage sensor (see Chapter 7). A sequence of residues from S5 to S6 on the extracellular side of the channel, called the P region or P loop, dips partway into the membrane and lines the pore of the channel.

Voltage-gated Ca^{2+} and K^+ channels are structurally similar to Na^+ channels: they are composed of four repeats of the basic motif containing S1 to S6 and the P loop. Voltage-gated Ca^{2+} channels, like Na^+ channels, have the four repeats on a single α-subunit. In contrast, **voltage-gated K^+ channels** are composed of four peptide subunits, each containing a single repeat of the basic motif (Figure 5-4, *A*). The remarkably similar amino acid sequences of the voltage-gated ion channels indicate that they are members of a **gene superfamily** and probably evolved from a common ancestral gene.

The voltage-gated K^+ channels are also related to two other families of K^+-selective ion channels (Figure 5-4). The inward-rectifier K^+ channel* subunit has only two α-helical transmembrane segments, which are connected by a pore-forming P loop. The channel is formed by four of these subunits. The twin-pore K^+ channel subunit has four transmembrane segments and two P loops, and the channel is composed of two of these subunits.

Structural Details of a K^+ Channel Are Revealed by X-Ray Crystallography

The most direct method for determining protein structure is analysis of the x-ray diffraction pattern obtained from a protein crystal. Ion channel proteins have been difficult to crystallize, in part because of the large amount of

---

*In electronics, a rectifier is a device that allows current to flow in one direction, but not in the opposite direction. Inward-rectifier K^+ channels allow K^+ ions to flow freely into, but not out of, the cell.

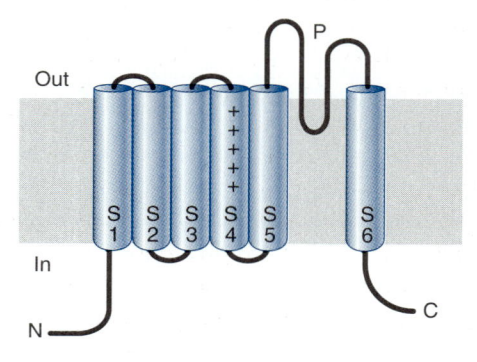

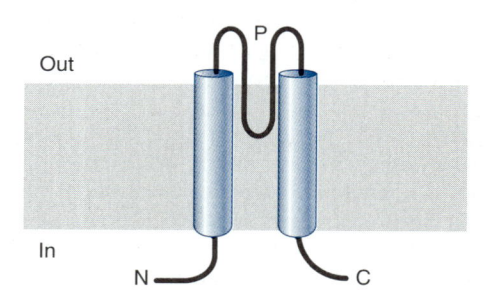

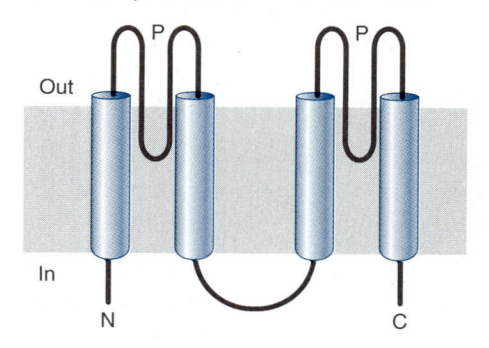

Figure 5-4 ■ Potassium channels are formed by separate subunits. **A,** A voltage-gated K^+ channel subunit is homologous to one of the domains of the voltage-gated Na^+ channel. It contains six membrane-spanning segments and a P region between S5 and S6. A voltage-gated K^+ channel is formed by four of these subunits. **B,** An inward rectifier K^+ channel subunit has only two membrane-spanning segments with a P region between them. The channel is formed by four of these subunits. **C,** A two-pore domain K^+ channel subunit has four transmembrane segments and two P regions. A K^+ channel is formed by two of these subunits.

protein required. MacKinnon and his colleagues recently succeeded in crystallizing a member of the inward-rectifier K^+ channel family, KcsA, from the bacterium *Streptomyces lividans*.* This channel protein has substantial sequence homology to mammalian K^+ channels, which indicates that the bacterial and mammalian channels were derived from a common ancestor. The KcsA channel protein was relatively easy to crystallize because it is not glycosylated, has a small size, and could be produced in large quantities by overexpression in *Escherichia coli*.

The crystal structure of KcsA provides a detailed picture of the channel structure and critical clues to the mechanism of K^+-selective permeation. The KcsA channel is a tetramer, composed of four identical subunits that form a central aqueous pore (Figure 5-5, *A*). Each subunit has two transmembrane segments: an inner helix that lines the pore near the intracellular surface of the membrane and an outer helix that faces the lipid bilayer (Figure 5-5, *B*). The P (pore) region connects the two helices on the extracellular side and consists of three components: (1) the turret region is a chain of residues that surrounds the extracellular mouth of the channel; (2) the pore helix, which is inserted into the membrane between inner helices, provides contacts that hold the four subunits together; and (3) a loop of amino acids that forms the selectivity filter of the channel (Figure 5-5, *B* and *C*). The selectivity filter is formed by three main-chain carbonyl oxygen atoms of three amino acids: glycine (G), tyrosine (Y), and glycine (G). The side chains of these amino acids point away from the pore and interact with other residues to stabilize the pore at the optimum diameter for K^+ permeation.

---

*The American physiologist Roderick MacKinnon shared the 2003 Nobel Prize in Chemistry for this work.

■ SUMMARY

1. An ion channel is a large macromolecular protein that extends across the lipid bilayer and forms a water-filled pore, which allows ions to cross the membrane by diffusion. By controlling the membrane permeability to ions, channels play a primary role in the electrical behavior of the cell.

2. Many distinct types of ion channels exist, but they all share some common properties. The primary function of all ion channels is to increase, selectively, the permeability of the membrane to ions. A specific type of ion channel transports ions *selectively* at very high rates. For example, a K^+-selective ion channel conducts about 10 million K^+ ions per second and is 100 times more permeable to K^+ than to Na^+.

3. All ion channels function as if they have a gate that can close and prevent ions from moving through the channel or can open to allow ion movement. Voltage-gated channels are opened by changes in the membrane potential. Ligand-gated channels are opened after the binding of a neurotransmitter to a receptor on the channel.

4. Molecular cloning of voltage-gated Na^+, K^+, and Ca^{2+} channels reveals that they have remarkably similar amino acid sequences, indicating that they are members of a gene superfamily. The three-dimensional structure of these channels contains four homologous domains (or four subunits in the case of K^+ channels), each with six α-helical membrane-spanning segments (S1 to S6). Segment S4 is the voltage sensor. A sequence of residues from S5 to S6 forms the P loop that lines the pore of the channel.

5. A bacterial K^+ channel (KcsA) has been crystallized, allowing its detailed structure to be determined by x-ray crystallography. The KcsA channel is a tetramer, composed of four

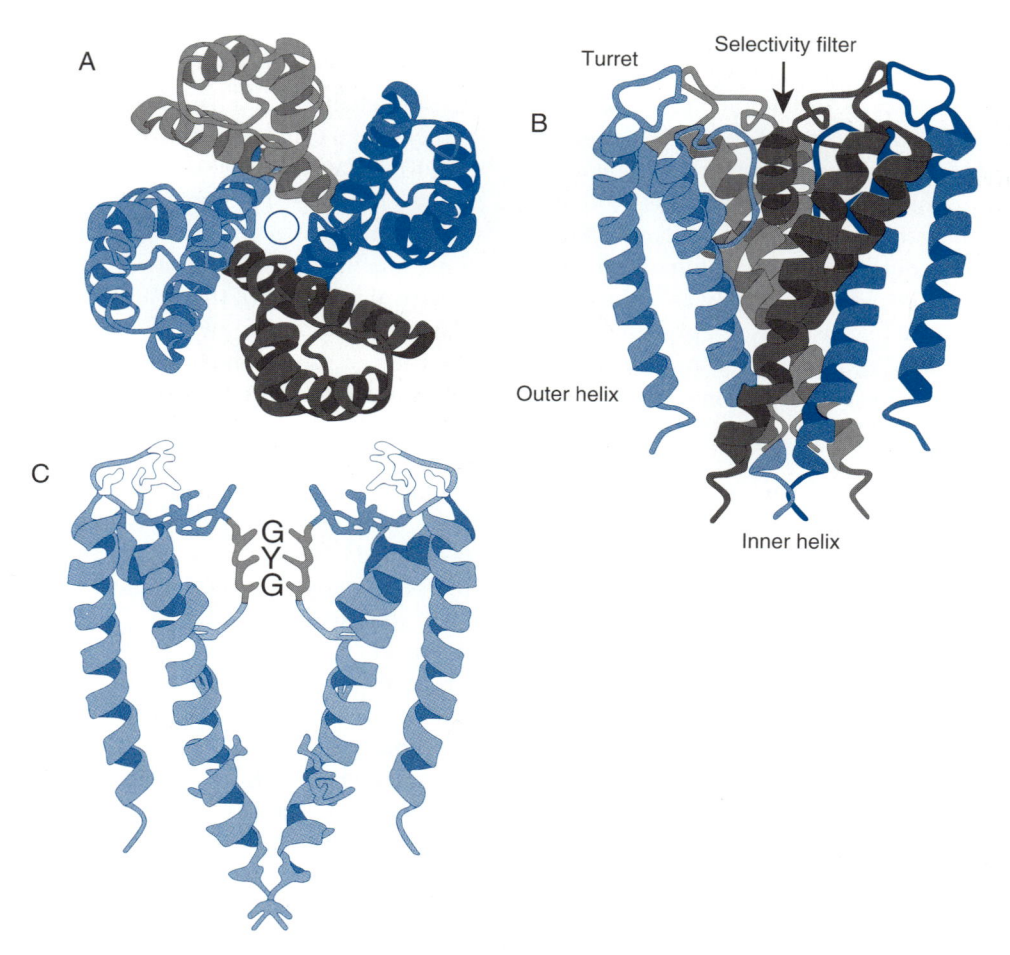

Figure 5-5 ■ **Structure of an inward-rectifying K⁺ channel. A,** This view of the channel is looking down at the pore from outside of the membrane. Each of the four subunits is shown in a different shade of blue or gray, and each contributes a P region to the lining of the pore. A K⁺ ion is shown in the middle of the pore. **B,** A view of the channel parallel to the plane of the membrane. An inner helix from each subunit forms the inner part of the pore, and they are arranged as an inverted teepee. **C,** This is the same view as in B with two of the subunits removed. The gray region is the selectivity filter that is formed by three main chain carbonyl oxygen atoms from the amino acids glycine (G), tyrosine (Y), and glycine (G). (Modified from Doyle DA, Cabral JM, Pfuetzner RA, et al: *Science* 280:69, 1998.)

identical subunits that form a central aqueous pore. The P region of each KcsA subunit contains a loop of amino acids that contains the main chain carbonyl oxygen atoms of three consecutive amino acids: glycine (G), tyrosine (Y), and glycine (G). The GYG carbonyl oxygen atoms from the four KcsA subunits form a pore with an optimum diameter for K⁺ permeation; this region is called the "selectivity filter."

Ion Channels and Excitable Membranes

■ KEY WORDS AND CONCEPTS

- Ion channel
- Voltage-gated channel
- Ligand-gated channel
- Selectivity filter
- Ion channel structure
- Voltage-gated K^+ channel
- Gene superfamily

STUDY PROBLEMS

1. The resting K^+ permeability of the pancreatic β-cell membrane is determined mainly by a specific population of K^+ channels. Describe at least three ways that the β-cell could change the properties of these K^+ channels and thereby change the K^+ permeability of the membrane.

2. A point mutation in the gene coding for a voltage-gated Na^+ channel results in a single amino acid substitution in the channel protein and causes the channel to change from an Na^+-selective channel to a Ca^{2+}-selective channel. What is the most likely location of the substituted amino acid in the channel structure? Describe a possible mechanism that could explain the change in selectivity resulting from a single amino acid substitution.

■ BIBLIOGRAPHY

Catterall WA: Structure and function of voltage-gated ion channels, *Annu Rev Biochem* 64:493, 1995.

Doyle DA, Cabral JM, Pfuetzner RA, et al: The structure of the potassium channel: molecular basis of K^+ conduction and selectivity, *Science* 280:69, 1998.

Hille B: *Ionic channels of excitable membranes,* ed 3, Sunderland, Mass, 2001, Sinauer.

CHAPTER 6

Passive Electrical Properties of Membranes

Objectives:

1. Understand that passive membrane electrical properties refer to properties that are constant near the resting potential of the cell.
2. Understand that membranes behave, electrically, like a resistor in parallel with a capacitor.
3. Understand that open ion channels are electrically equivalent to conductors (or resistors).
4. Describe Ohm's Law as it relates to current flow through ion channels.
5. Understand that membranes have capacitive properties because the lipid bilayer is an insulator that allows ions to accumulate at the surface of the membrane.
6. Define membrane time constant and length constant, and describe the passive properties that influence them.

■ THE TIME COURSE AND SPREAD OF MEMBRANE POTENTIAL CHANGES ARE PREDICTED BY THE PASSIVE ELECTRICAL PROPERTIES OF THE MEMBRANE

The steady-state membrane potential of a membrane permeable to more than one ion can be estimated by use of the Goldman-Hodgkin-Katz (GHK) equation (see Chapter 4). One of the main limitations of this approach, however, is that it cannot be used to predict how the membrane potential *changes* as a function of time or distance. In neurons, skeletal muscle cells, and other electrically excitable cells, certain changes in membrane potential have well-defined time courses. For example, the nerve action potential, which is described in detail in Chapter 7, is a "spike" of depolarization that lasts 1 to 2 msec. In addition, postsynaptic potentials (membrane potential changes that result from neurotransmitter release at chemical synapses; see Chapter 8) have relatively fast rising phases and exponential decays. The membrane properties that help to determine the time course of these signals are described in this chapter. The passive spread of a change in membrane potential with distance along a membrane surface is also discussed.

Passive electrical properties refer to properties that are fixed, or constant, near the resting potential of the cell. Three such properties play important roles in determining the time course and spread of electrical activity: the membrane resistance, the membrane capacitance, and the internal or "axial" resistance of long thin processes or cells such as nerve axons and dendrites and skeletal muscle cells. By examining the membrane as an electrical circuit, we can deduce how these parameters can be used to describe changes in the membrane potential. Equivalent circuit models of membranes are used to analyze potentials that vary with time and distance in a manner that depends only on the passive membrane properties. These potentials are called **electrotonic potentials**.

■ THE EQUIVALENT CIRCUIT OF AN EXCITABLE MEMBRANE HAS A RESISTOR IN PARALLEL WITH A CAPACITOR

Membrane Conductance Is Established by Open Ion Channels

Many ion channels behave, in electrical terms, like conductors (or resistors, since **conductance** = 1/resistance). Each channel (Figure 6-1, *A*) can be modeled as a resistor, or conductor, with a *single-channel* conductance, γ, when the channel is open (Figure 6-1, *B*). Naturally, when the channel is closed, the conductance is zero.

Most permeant ions are distributed asymmetrically across the plasma membrane (see Chapter 4). This results in a chemical driving force that tends to push the ion through the open channel. This chemical force functions as a battery (with voltage equal to the equilibrium potential of the ion, E_K in this case). The battery is in series with the resistor (γ_K) representing the open channel, as shown for K$^+$ in Figure 6-1, *B*. The current flow through the open channel obeys **Ohm's Law** (see Appendix C), which for current flow through a resistor of R ohms (or g = 1/R siemens) is

$$V = I \times R \quad \text{or} \quad I = \frac{V}{R} = g \times V \quad [1]$$

where I is the current in amperes for a potential difference of V volts. For ion channels, Ohm's

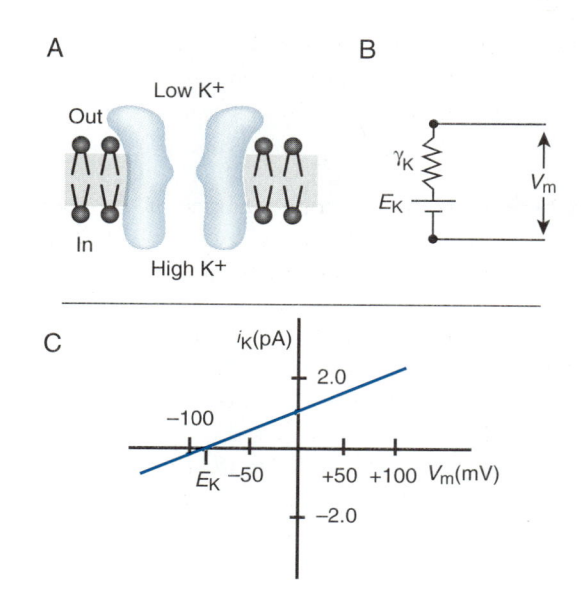

Figure 6-1 ■ Ion channels behave like electrical conductors. **A**, Schematic of a single, open K$^+$ channel, with a conductance of γ_K, embedded in a lipid bilayer that has an outwardly directed K$^+$ gradient. **B**, The equivalent electrical circuit of the channel is a resistor, or conductor, in series with a battery (E_K) that represents the concentration gradient for K$^+$ ions. **C**, Current through the channel (i_K) varies linearly with membrane potential (V_m).

Law must be modified because the net ionic flux (and therefore the current) will be zero when the membrane potential is equal to the equilibrium potential of the ion. Because the equilibrium potential is almost never zero mV, Ohm's Law for a single K$^+$ channel is

$$i_K = \gamma_K (V_m - E_K) \quad [2]$$

where i_K is the current through a single channel and $V_m - E_K$ is called the **driving force**. Ohm's Law predicts that the potassium current is directly proportional to the driving force (Figure 6-1, *C*).

Membranes usually contain several different types of ion channels that are each present in large numbers. In electrical terms, single channels

Passive Electrical Properties of Membranes

in the membrane represent conductors arranged in parallel; in this case the individual conductances are additive. In other words,

$$g_{Na} = N_o \times \gamma_{Na} \quad [3]$$

where g_{Na} is the total conductance of the open **sodium** (Na^+) **channels** present in a unit area of membrane, γ_{Na} is the conductance of a single Na^+ channel, and N_o is the number of open Na^+ channels per unit area. In the equivalent circuit, we can then model a group of Na^+ channels as a resistor with conductance equal to g_{Na}, in series with a battery of voltage E_{Na} (Figure 6-2). A similar resistor-battery pair can be used to model a population of **potassium** (K^+) **channels,** or any other ion channels, in the membrane (Figure 6-2).

Capacitance Reflects the Ability of the Membrane to Separate Charge

To complete the equivalent circuit, we need to account for the ability of the lipid bilayer to act as an electrical insulator that allows charges (ions such as K^+, Na^+, and Cl^-) to accumulate at the surface of the membrane. In electrical circuits a **capacitor** is an element that stores, or separates, charges across an insulator. Thus the equivalent circuit of the membrane has a capacitor (C_m) connected in parallel with the elements representing the ion channels (Figure 6-2).

The amount of charge (q in coulombs) that can be separated across the membrane is directly proportional to the membrane potential:

$$q = C_m \times V_m \quad [4]$$

where V_m is the potential difference in volts and C_m is the capacitance in farads. A 1-farad capacitor can store 1 coulomb of charge per volt of potential difference. A farad (F) is a very large quantity; all biological membranes have capacitances of about 1×10^{-6} F (1 µF) per cm^2 of membrane surface area (Box 6-1).

■ PASSIVE MEMBRANE PROPERTIES PRODUCE LINEAR CURRENT-VOLTAGE RELATIONSHIPS

The passive properties of cell membranes can be studied by the injection of current into the cell through a microelectrode (Box 6-2 and Figure 6-3, *A*). When an inward pulse of current is passed across the membrane (Figure 6-3, *B*), the membrane potential approaches a more negative, or *hyperpolarized*, value following an exponential time course (Figure 6-3, *C*) and eventually reaches a constant, steady-state level. The larger the applied current, the greater the hyperpolarization. A graph of the current versus the steady-state membrane potential is a straight line (Figure 6-3, *D*). Therefore, in the steady state, the resting membrane behaves electrically like a resistor. The slope of the **linear current-voltage relationship** (i.e., $\Delta I/\Delta V_m$) is a measure of the resting conductance of the membrane.

■ MEMBRANE CAPACITANCE AFFECTS THE TIME COURSE OF VOLTAGE CHANGES

Ionic and Capacitive Currents Flow When a Channel Opens

When current starts to flow across the membrane, the membrane potential does not instantaneously reach a new steady-state level. Instead,

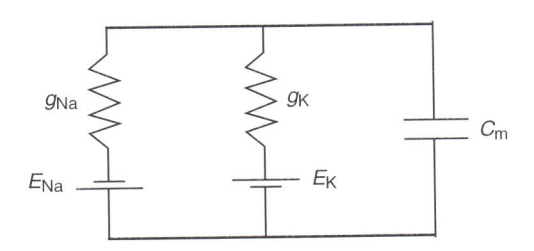

Figure 6-2 ■ Equivalent circuit of a membrane containing many open Na^+ and K^+ channels. The resistors labeled g_{Na} and g_K are the conductances of the membrane to Na^+ and K^+, respectively; E_{Na} is the sodium equilibrium potential; E_K is the potassium equilibrium potential; and C_m is the membrane capacitance.

BOX 6-1

Cell Size and Total Cell Capacitance

The capacitance of a pure phospholipid bilayer is roughly the same as that of all biological membranes: the *specific membrane capacitance* (C_m, capacitance per unit surface area) is commonly given as 1 µF/cm². It is important to note, however, that with respect to total cell capacitance, even 1 µF is a large quantity. A calculation of the total cell capacitance of a 10-µm diameter spherical cell (slightly larger than a red blood cell) illustrates the point. The surface area of a sphere is equal to πd^2, where d is the diameter of the sphere. For the 10-µm diameter cell:

Surface area $= \pi d^2$; $d = 10 \times 10^{-6}\,m = 10 \times 10^{-4}\,cm = 10^{-3}\,cm$

Surface area $= \pi \times 10^{-3} \times 10^{-3}\,cm^2 = 3.1 \times 10^{-6}\,cm^2$

and

Total cell capacitance $= C_m \times$ Surface area

$$= 10^{-6}\,\frac{F}{cm^2} \times 3.1 \times 10^{-6}\,cm^2$$

$$= 3.1 \times 10^{-12}\,F = 3.1\,pF$$

Because cell surface area is on the order of hundreds of µm², it may be more relevant to use units of F/µm² for C_m, that is,

$$C_m = 1.0\,\frac{\mu F}{cm^2} = 0.01\,\frac{pF}{\mu m^2}$$

BOX 6-2

Measuring and Manipulating the Membrane Potential

The most common technique for recording the membrane potential involves the use of microelectrodes. The microelectrode is a glass capillary tube tapered to a fine, sharp tip with a diameter <1 µm. The electrode is filled with a concentrated salt solution, and a wire is placed in the back of the electrode to allow connection to electronic devices. The sharp tip of the microelectrode allows it to be pushed through the cell membrane without damaging the cell, thereby allowing the measurement of the intracellular potential. A pair of these electrodes (one intracellular and one extracellular) is connected to an amplifier to record the cell membrane potential, as shown in Figure 6-3, *A*.

A second pair of electrodes can be used to inject current into the cell. Figure 6-3, *A*, shows an inward current being passed into the cell: positive charges flow out of the extracellular electrode and are deposited on the outside surface of the cell, while positive charges move away from the inside surface of the membrane and enter the intracellular electrode. Thus this inward current makes the membrane potential become more negative.

the presence of **membrane capacitance** causes the membrane potential to approach the steady-state level gradually (Figure 6-3, *C*). To understand the effect of the membrane capacitance, we will first examine the currents that flow across the membrane when a channel opens. Consider a cell that contains only a single closed K⁺ channel (Figure 6-4, *A*). If the initial membrane potential is 0 mV when the K⁺ channel opens, and the K⁺ equilibrium potential

Passive Electrical Properties of Membranes

is −90 mV, K$^+$ ions will flow out of the cell down their electrochemical gradient. The removal of positive charge from the cell makes the membrane potential move in the negative direction. Because the cell is permeable only to K$^+$, the membrane potential will eventually reach E_K and stop changing. In terms of current flow in the equivalent circuit (Figure 6-4, B), we say that an *outward* **ionic current**, I_i (K$^+$ ions moving out of the cell), produces an *inward* **capacitive current**, I_c. This capacitive current consists of positive charges moving away from the inside surface of the membrane and an equal number of positive charges moving up to the outside surface of the membrane. Because it takes time for ions to move through the channel and accumulate at the membrane surface, V_m can change only gradually.

The Exponential Time Course of the Membrane Potential Can Be Understood in Terms of the Passive Properties of the Membrane

The resting (passive) membrane can be represented by an equivalent circuit. This circuit (Figure 6-5, A) can help to explain the role of the membrane capacitance in the exponential time course of the membrane potential change (Figure 6-3, C). All open ion channels have been combined into a single conducting pathway, R_m, in series with battery E_{RP}, which represents the resting potential of the cell. The membrane is connected to a constant current generator and to a device to monitor membrane potential. With no current flowing from the external source, the membrane potential will be at E_{RP} with an excess of negative charges at the inside surface of the capacitor. A constant inward current (I_m) is then passed into this circuit. At the instant the current is turned on, all of the current flows to the capacitor (Figure 6-5, B). Perhaps the simplest way to understand this is to recognize that at the instant the current is turned on, there

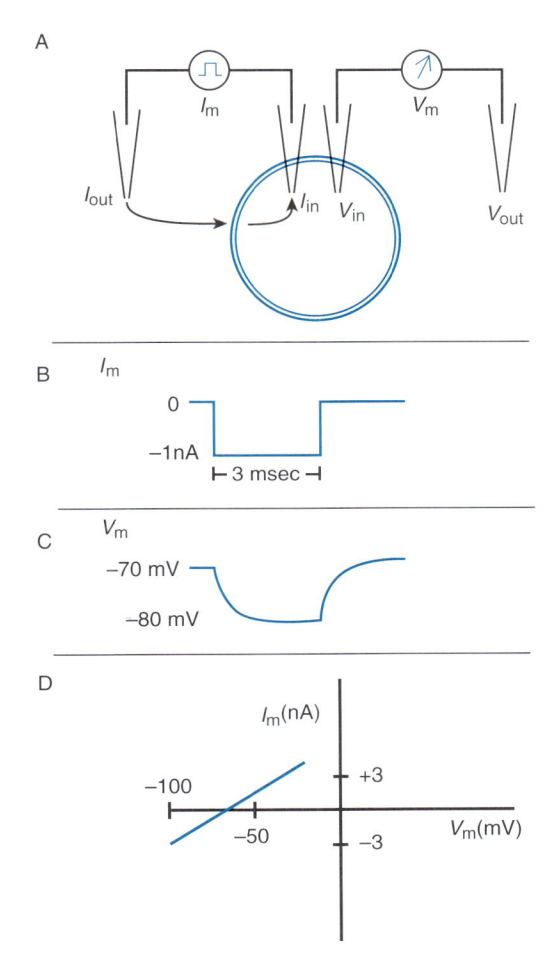

Figure 6-3 ■ Experimental arrangement used to study the passive properties of membranes. **A**, One intracellular microelectrode (I_{in}) is used to pass current across the membrane from a constant current source, I_m. The arrows illustrate an inward current flowing from the extracellular current electrode (I_{out}) through the membrane to I_{in}. A second intracellular electrode (V_{in}) is used to monitor the membrane potential, V_m. When a constant inward current is passed across the membrane (**B**), V_m approaches a new steady-state level along an exponential time course (**C**). **D**, The steady-state current voltage relationship for a resting cell is a straight line.

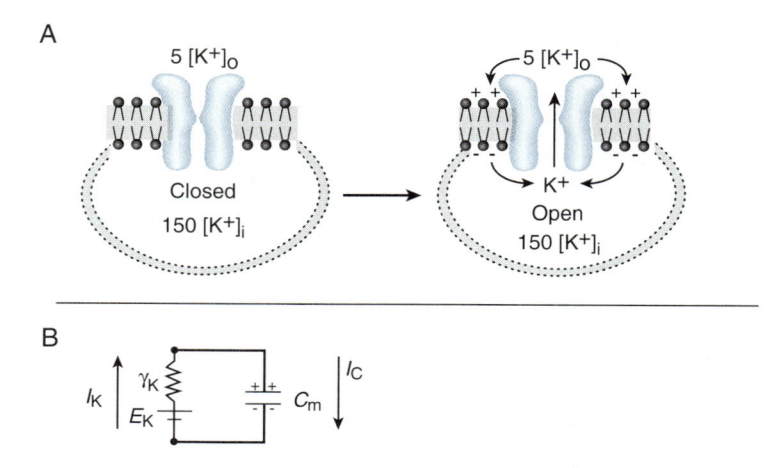

Figure 6-4 ■ Current flow through a single K⁺ channel alters the charge distribution across the membrane. A, When the K⁺ channel opens (*right*), K⁺ ions flow out of the cell, making the outside more positive and leaving the inside of the cell more negative. B, In terms of the equivalent circuit, the outward K⁺ current (I_K) produces an inward capacitive current (I_c).

is no driving force for current flow through the resistor (i.e., $V_m - E_{RP} = 0$). The inward capacitive current further increases the charge separation across the capacitor because positive charges build up at the external surface and move away from the internal surface. As a result, the membrane potential moves in the negative direction, which in turn produces a driving force for current flow through the resistor. Because the total current being controlled by the constant current generator must remain constant, the capacitive current decreases in magnitude as the resistive (ionic) current increases (Figure 6-5, *C*). Finally, a new steady-state membrane potential is reached, and all of the applied current flows through the resistor. Analysis of this circuit (see Appendix C) produces the following relationship between membrane potential and time:

$$\Delta V_m(t) = \Delta V_{m,\infty}\left[1 - \exp\left(\frac{-t}{\tau_m}\right)\right] \quad [5]$$

$\Delta V_m(t)$ is the change in V_m at time t, $\Delta V_{m,\infty}$ is the change in V_m in the steady state ($t = \infty$), and $\tau_m = R_m \times C_m$ is called the **membrane time constant**. The units for τ are seconds if R_m and C_m are ohms and farads, respectively. Note that $\Delta V_{m,\infty} = I_m \times R_m$. This is a formal statement of the fact that in the steady state all of the current flows through the resistor and none through the capacitor. In addition to the membrane potential, both the capacitive and ionic currents follow an exponential time course (Figure 6-6; see Appendix C).

When the external current pulse is turned off, the ionic and capacitive currents are equal in magnitude but opposite in direction (Figure 6-6). Before the external current is turned off, all of the applied current flows through channels (i.e., $I_i = I_m$; Figure 6-5, *D*). At this time the return pathway for current flow is through the external current generator. When the external current is turned off, the return pathway for the current is through the membrane capacitor; thus $I_i = -I_c$. The resulting outward I_c causes the membrane potential to become less negative, and this decreases I_i because of a reduction in the driving

Passive Electrical Properties of Membranes

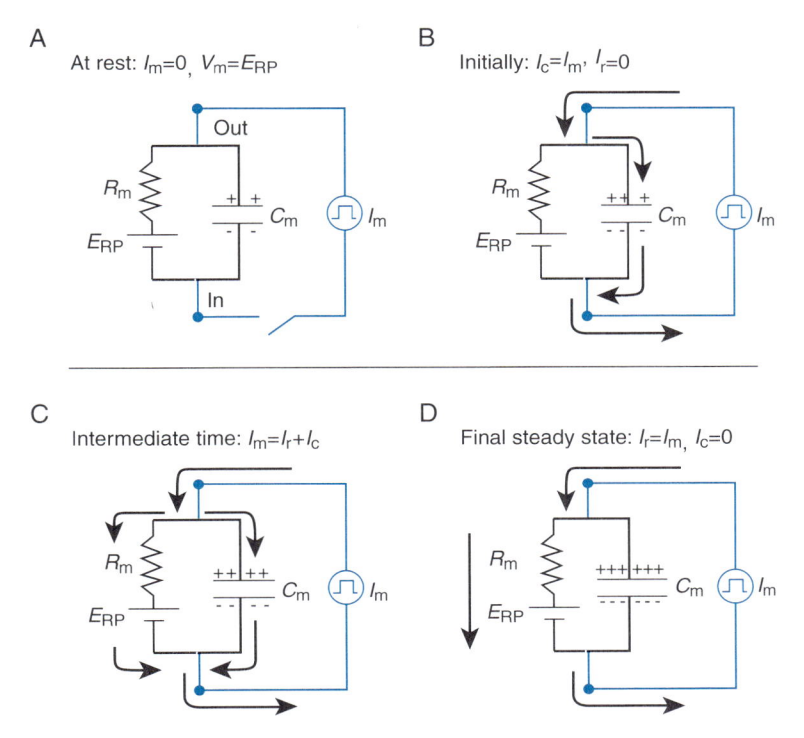

A At rest: $I_m=0$, $V_m=E_{RP}$

B Initially: $I_c=I_m$, $I_r=0$

C Intermediate time: $I_m=I_r+I_c$

D Final steady state: $I_r=I_m$, $I_c=0$

Figure 6-5 ■ An equivalent circuit of passive, resting membrane used to analyze current flow across the membrane. A, The membrane is modeled as a single resistor, R_m, which represents all open channels, in series with a battery that has a voltage equal to the resting potential of the cell (E_{RP}). B, At the instant a constant inward current, I_m, is turned on, all of the current goes through the capacitor, and the membrane potential begins to hyperpolarize. C, As soon as V_m begins to change, some of the current starts to flow through open channels. D, Eventually, V_m reaches a new steady-state level and all current flows through open ion channels.

---

force. When $V_m = E_{RP}$, there is no driving force for current flow; thus I_i and I_c will both be zero and the membrane potential will stop changing.

The membrane time constant is a measure of the time scale over which changes in membrane potential occur. Consider the value of ΔV_m at a time equal to τ_m. If $t = \tau_m$,

$$\Delta V_m = \Delta V_{m,\infty}[1 - \exp(-1)] = \Delta V_{m,\infty}(1 - 0.37) \quad [6]$$
$$= 0.63 \Delta V_{m,\infty}$$

In other words, the time constant is the length of time required for 63% of the total change in V_m to occur.

■ MEMBRANE AND AXOPLASMIC RESISTANCES AFFECT THE PASSIVE SPREAD OF SUBTHRESHOLD ELECTRICAL SIGNALS

As small-amplitude membrane potentials spread along the surface of a cell, they decrease in amplitude. This effect can be conveniently studied in an elongated structure, such as an axon, with the experimental arrangement shown in Figure

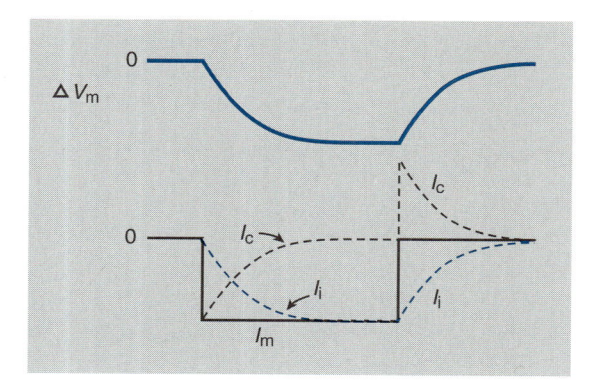

Figure 6-6 ■ In response to a pulse of constant current (I_m), the membrane potential (ΔV_m) follows an exponential time course to a new level. Initially, the capacitive current (I_c) is equal to I_m. I_c decays along an exponential time course as the ionic current (I_i) increases from zero to a steady-state level equal to I_m. When the current pulse is turned off ($I_m = 0$), the ionic and capacitive currents are equal in magnitude, but opposite in direction. Both I_c and I_i then decline to zero as the membrane potential returns to its initial level.

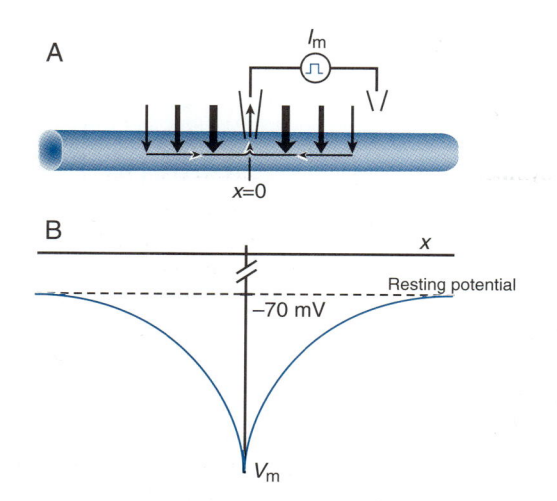

Figure 6-7 ■ A subthreshold change in membrane potential decreases in amplitude as an exponential function of distance along an axon. A, An external current source (I_m) passes a constant inward current pulse across the membrane. The current follows the path of least resistance: the largest membrane current density is closest to the current passing electrode. B, As a result, the change in V_m is largest at the site of current injection ($x = 0$), and it decreases as an exponential function of distance (x) away from this site.

6-7. One microelectrode is inserted into the axon to pass a constant subthreshold current across the membrane. The term "subthreshold" refers to the fact that the membrane potential stays below the level required to initiate an action potential. A second electrode is used to measure the change in membrane potential at various distances away from the current passing electrode. If an inward (hyperpolarizing) current pulse of long duration is used, the membrane potential will reach a new, hyperpolarized steady-state level. A plot of the *steady-state* membrane potential as a function of *distance* reveals that the hyperpolarization is maximal at the site of current injection. The membrane potential becomes progressively less hyperpolarized as we move along the axon away from this point (Figure 6-7). Far away from the site of current injection the membrane is at the resting potential and is unaffected by the current. Such passive spread of small-amplitude signals along the surface of the cell is called **electrotonic conduction**.

The Decay of Subthreshold Potentials with Distance Can Be Understood in Terms of the Passive Properties of the Membrane

Because the axon can be idealized as a cylindrical structure, it is convenient to normalize the units for resistance and capacitance to a 1-cm *length* of axon (we use lower case *r* and *c* to represent these parameters). The relevant parameters, and their units, are shown in Table 6-1. Box 6-3 describes the origin of the resistance units used here.

Passive Electrical Properties of Membranes

TABLE 6-1
Parameters used in the equivalent circuit of an axon

Symbol	Circuit component	Units
r_o	Extracellular resistance	Ohms/cm
r_i	Intracellular resistance	Ohms/cm
r_m	Membrane resistance	Ohms × cm
c_m	Membrane capacitance	Farads/cm

BOX 6-3

Origin of Resistance Units Used in the Cable Equation

Physiological resistances can be given in various units. The resistance of a conductor, such as a length of wire or a length of axoplasm, depends on the geometry of the conductor and on a parameter called the resistivity of the material (ρ). The resistivity depends on the physical properties of the material that determine its ability to conduct current. The resistance of the wire increases with the length of the wire and decreases with the diameter, or cross-sectional area. The following equation shows this relationship:

$$R = \rho \frac{L}{A_c} \quad \text{[B1]}$$

In this equation R is the resistance of the conductor in ohms, ρ is the resistivity in ohms × cm, L is the length of the conductor in cm, and A_c is the cross-sectional area of the conductor in cm².

To study the passive properties of an axon, we can conveniently consider the axon in similar terms and express resistances for a 1-cm length of axon. For the internal, or axial, resistance of the axoplasm (which is equivalent to the resistance of a wire), we combine R and L (from Equation [B1]) into a single parameter r_i:

$$r_i = \frac{R}{L} = \frac{\rho}{A_c} \quad \text{units:} \frac{\text{ohms} \times \text{cm}}{\text{cm}^2} = \frac{\text{ohms}}{\text{cm}}$$

Thus r_i has units of ohms/cm. Identical units would apply to the longitudinal resistance of the extracellular solution (r_o). To convert the normalized resistance r_i or r_o into ohms, we must multiply r_i or r_o by the length of the axon. In other words, the longitudinal internal (or external) resistance, in units of ohms, increases with the length of the axon.

The resistance equation (Equation [B1]) cannot be applied as easily to *membrane* resistance because the length of the conductor is now the membrane thickness, which is usually not known precisely. Therefore a new parameter is defined, $R_m = \rho \times L$, which combines the resistivity and length into a single parameter with units of ohms × cm². Thus, for membrane resistance, Equation [B1] can be rewritten:

$$R = \frac{\rho \times L}{A_c} = \frac{R_m}{A_s} = \frac{R_m}{\text{Circumference} \times L}$$

where R_m has units of ohms × cm² and the cross-sectional area of the "resistor" (the membrane) is the membrane surface area in cm² (A_s). For a cylindrical axon the surface area is circumference × length (both parameters in cm). Finally, we can combine R and L into a single parameter (r_m) that represents the membrane resistance per cm length of axon:

$$r_m = R \times L = \frac{R_m}{\text{Circumference}}$$

$$\text{units:} \frac{\text{ohms} \times \text{cm}^2}{\text{cm}} = \text{ohms} \times \text{cm}$$

and clearly r_m has units of ohms × cm.

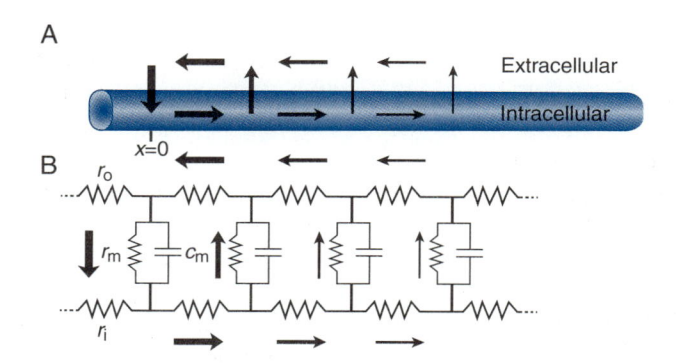

Figure 6-8 ■ The equivalent electrical circuit of an axon. **A,** The arrows indicate the steady-state current flowing in different regions of the axon during the injection of a constant current at the point $x = 0$. The relative thickness of the arrow represents the relative magnitude of the current. **B,** The equivalent circuit of the axon consists of patches of membrane, represented by parallel r_m-c_m circuits, connected together by resistors r_o and r_i. All parameters are normalized to a 1-cm length of axon: r_o is the resistance of extracellular fluid, r_i is the resistance of axoplasm, r_m is the membrane resistance, and c_m is the membrane capacitance.

The axon can be modeled, in electrical terms, by the circuit depicted in Figure 6-8, *B*. This circuit consists of several parallel r_m-c_m circuits connected together. Each r_m-c_m "patch" of membrane is connected through an internal resistance, r_i, and an external resistance, r_o, to the adjacent patch.

An intuitive explanation for the decay of amplitude with distance is provided by consideration of the circuit in Figure 6-8. As the applied current moves along the axon through r_i, some of the current "leaks" out through r_m, leaving less current available to affect more distant patches of membrane. Analysis of this circuit in the *steady state* predicts that the change in membrane potential, ΔV_m, should decrease exponentially with distance away from the current injection site, according to the relation,

$$\Delta V_m(x) = \Delta V_0 \exp(-x/\lambda) \quad [7]$$

$$\text{where} \quad \lambda = \sqrt{\frac{r_m}{r_i + r_o}} \approx \sqrt{\frac{r_m}{r_i}}$$

ΔV_0 is the change in membrane potential at the site of current injection (i.e., at $x = 0$). Nerve fibers are usually bathed in a very large volume of conducting (low-resistance) extracellular fluid. Thus the total resistance to current flow in the external part of the loop (r_o) is negligible compared to the resistance along the corresponding stretch of axoplasm (r_i) inside the axon. Consequently $r_o \ll r_i$; thus r_o may be dropped out of the expression for λ. Equation [7] is often called a **cable equation** because a similar equation was derived to explain the decrease in the amplitude of signals transmitted through underwater transatlantic cables. We note that the membrane capacitance, c_m, has no effect on λ. This is because we are considering steady-state membrane potentials, and in the steady state no current flows through the capacitor.

The parameter λ is the **length constant** with units of cm. We can think of λ in physically descriptive terms. If the membrane resistance, r_m, is raised, the current has more difficulty escaping through the membrane. Hence a larger fraction of the total current flows farther from the stimulus site before escaping through the membrane; in quantitative terms, λ is increased. Similarly, if r_i is lowered, the current flows more easily along the axoplasmic path and λ is also increased.

The Length Constant Is a Measure of How Far Away from a Stimulus Site a Membrane Potential Change Will Be Detectable

At a distance λ cm from the point of current injection, ΔV_m would be reduced by 63% to about 37% of its value at the stimulus site:

$$\Delta V(\lambda) = \Delta V_0 \exp(-\lambda/\lambda) = \Delta V_0 \exp(-1) = 0.37 \Delta V_0 \quad [8]$$

Thus, when λ is increased, the change in V_m requires a longer distance to decay by a given amount. In other words, a larger length constant means that the change in membrane potential will be detectable farther away from the stimulation site. In the next chapter we show that changes in λ affect the conduction velocity of the action potential.

■ SUMMARY

1. Passive electrical properties refer to membrane properties that are constant near the resting potential of the cell. Three such properties, the membrane resistance, the membrane capacitance, and the internal resistance of long thin processes or cells, help to determine the time course and spread of electrical activity.
2. The cell membrane is electrically equivalent to a capacitor connected in parallel with a resistor and a battery connected in series.
3. Ion channels behave, in electrical terms, like conductors (or resistors). The current flow through an open channel obeys Ohm's Law.
4. The membrane is like a capacitor because the lipid bilayer acts as an electrical insulator, allowing charges to accumulate at the surface of the membrane. Capacitance is a measure of the amount of charge that can be separated across the membrane per unit of membrane potential. All biological membranes have a capacitance of about 1×10^{-6} F (1 µF) per cm^2 of membrane surface area.
5. When ionic current flows through channels, the membrane capacitance causes the membrane potential to come to a new steady-state level gradually. In response to a pulse of constant current, the membrane potential follows an exponential time course to a new level. The time constant of this exponential curve is called the membrane time constant, τ_m, and is equal to the membrane capacitance times the membrane resistance.
6. The passive spread of small-amplitude, subthreshold signals along the surface of an axon is affected by membrane and axoplasmic resistances. The amplitude of these signals decreases as an exponential function of distance along the axon. The length constant, λ, provides a measure of how far subthreshold signals propagate. An increase in membrane resistance increases λ, and an increase in axoplasmic resistance decreases λ.

■ KEY WORDS AND CONCEPTS

- Passive electrical properties
- Electrotonic potentials
- Conductance
- Ohm's Law
- Driving force
- Sodium channels and potassium channels
- Capacitor
- Linear (ohmic) current-voltage relationship
- Membrane capacitance
- Ionic and capacitive currents
- Membrane time constant (τ_m)
- Cable equation
- Membrane length constant (λ)
- Electrotonic conduction

STUDY PROBLEMS

1. A small spherical cell has a total membrane surface area of 10 μm² (1 μm = 10^{-4} cm) and a capacitance of 1 × 10^{-6} F/cm². Initially the cell has a membrane potential of zero mV, and there are no open channels in the membrane. Assume that $[Cl^-]_i$ = 10 mM, $[Cl^-]_o$ = 140 mM, RT/F = 26.7 mV, and γ_{Cl} = 10^{-11} S.
   a. What happens to the membrane potential when a single Cl^- channel opens?
   b. Draw a graph of the membrane potential as a function of time following the opening of the channel. Indicate the values of the initial and final membrane potential. What is the value of the membrane time constant in the presence of the open Cl^- channel?

2. A 100-μm diameter nonmyelinated nerve axon has the following properties: r_m = 2.5 × 10^4 ohms × cm, r_i = 1 × 10^5 ohms/cm, r_o = 0, and c_m = 3 × 10^{-8} farads/cm. For this axon the permeability to Cl^- (P_{Cl}) is very high and Cl^- ions are at equilibrium at the resting potential of −70 mV. A steady inward current is injected into the axon, which results in a V_m of −100 mV at the site of current injection.
   a. What would V_m be at a distance of 4 mm from the site of current injection?
   b. If P_{Cl} now became zero (by blocking all of the open Cl^- channels), what would happen to the membrane potential at 4 mm from the site of current injection? (Assume that V_m remains at −100 mV at the site of current injection.)

3. Two different-diameter cylindrical dendrites on a cerebellar Purkinje neuron have the following passive membrane properties (r_m is membrane resistance per unit length, r_i is internal resistance per unit length, and c_m is membrane capacitance per unit length). Assume that the external resistance is zero and that the dendrites are cylindrical structures with homogeneous membrane properties along their entire length.

	r_m, ohms/cm	r_i, ohms/cm	c_m, F/cm
Dendrite 1	2 × 10^6	1 × 10^{10}	2 × 10^{-10}
Dendrite 2	2 × 10^4	1 × 10^6	2 × 10^{-8}

   a. An excitatory synaptic input impinges on each of these dendrites at a distance of 2 cm from the cell body. Activation of these synapses causes a depolarization of the postsynaptic cell, which is called an excitatory postsynaptic potential (EPSP). When a subthreshold EPSP occurs at this synapse, the amplitude of the EPSP decays along an exponential time course back to the resting potential. Would the decay rate in dendrite 1 be faster, slower, or the same as in dendrite 2? Explain your answer.
   b. The amplitude of the EPSP decreases as a function of distance away from the synapse. In which dendrite would the amplitude decrease more with distance away from the synapse? Explain your answer. Would a subthreshold EPSP in either dendrite produce a detectable depolarization of the cell body? Why?

■ BIBLIOGRAPHY

Aidley DJ: *The physiology of excitable cells*, ed 2, Cambridge, Eng, 1978, Cambridge University Press.

Hodgkin AL, Rushton WAH: The electrical constants of a crustacean nerve fibre, *Proc R Soc Lond Ser B* 133:444, 1946.

Jack JJB, Noble D, Tsien RW: *Electric current flow in excitable cells*, Oxford, Eng, 1975, Clarendon.

Katz B: *Nerve, muscle and synapse*, New York, 1966, McGraw-Hill.

Rall W: Core conductor theory and cable properties of neurons. In Kandel ER, editor: *Handbook of physiology: a critical, comprehensive presentation of physiological knowledge and concepts.* Sect 1. *The nervous system.* Vol 1. *Cellular biology of neurons,* Part 1, pp 39-97, Bethesda, Md, 1977, American Physiological Society.

CHAPTER 7

Generation and Propagation of the Action Potential

Objectives:

1. Describe the properties of the voltage clamp, and explain why it is useful for the study of ion channels.
2. Describe the properties of voltage-gated Na^+ and K^+ channels.
3. Understand the terms "conductance," "ionic current," and "driving force," and use Ohm's Law to calculate these quantities.
4. Define inactivation and describe some functional properties of neurons that result from Na^+ channel inactivation.
5. Explain how the activity of voltage-gated Na^+ and K^+ channels generates the action potential.
6. Explain how local circuit currents produce action potential propagation in nonmyelinated axons.
7. Describe how propagation in myelinated axons differs from that in nonmyelinated axons, and explain why the conduction velocity is much faster as a result of myelination.

■ THE ACTION POTENTIAL IS A RAPID AND TRANSIENT DEPOLARIZATION OF THE MEMBRANE POTENTIAL IN ELECTRICALLY EXCITABLE CELLS

Action potentials are observed in "excitable cells" (neurons, muscle cells, some endocrine cells). An action potential is caused by a sudden selective alteration in the permeability of the membrane to small ions. In neurons or skeletal muscle cells the membrane rapidly increases its permeability to Na^+ ions, thereby allowing Na^+ to flow into the cell down its electrochemical gradient, making the inside potential more positive. The Na^+ permeability then decreases and the K^+ permeability rises. This allows K^+ to flow out of the cell and return the membrane potential toward its resting level. The membrane permeability to Na^+ and K^+ ions is controlled, at the molecular level, by voltage-gated Na^+ and K^+ channels, respectively.

The Properties of the Action Potential Can Be Studied with Intracellular Microelectrodes

Many properties of the action potential in a nerve axon can be illustrated by use of the experimental arrangement shown in Figure 7-1, *A*. One intracellular electrode is used to pass a

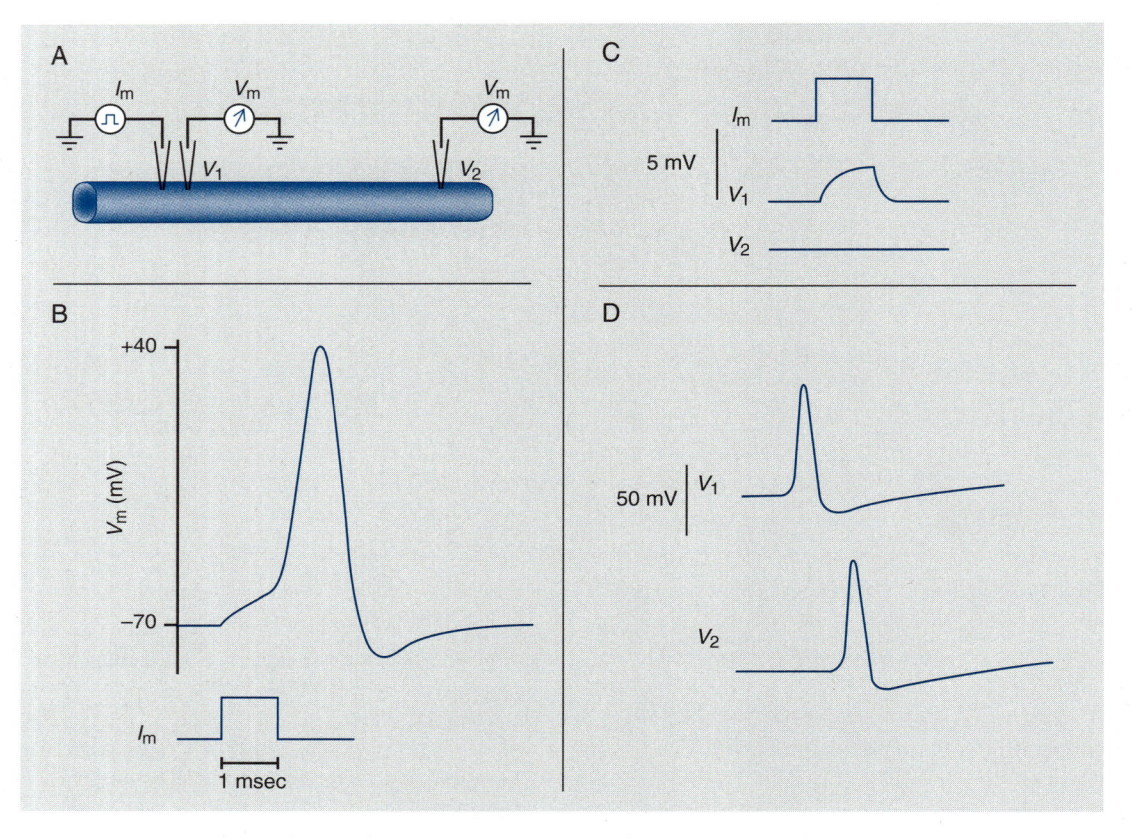

Figure 7-1 ■ Properties of the action potential in axons. A, One voltage-recording electrode (V_1) is placed close to the current passing electrode (I_m), and a second voltage electrode (V_2) is placed at a distance that is at least three to four times the length constant. B, The time course of the action potential in a squid giant axon. C, A subthreshold voltage change recorded at V_1 is not seen at V_2. D, An action potential initiated at V_1 is transmitted at full amplitude to V_2.

current pulse across the membrane. A second electrode (the "recording electrode") is used to monitor the resulting changes in membrane potential. When a hyperpolarizing, or small depolarizing, current step is passed across the membrane, the membrane potential exponentially approaches a new steady-state level (see Chapter 6). If a depolarizing stimulus exceeds a critical level (termed **threshold**), the membrane potential responds with an action potential (Figure 7-1, B). During an axonal action potential the membrane potential depolarizes to a value near E_{Na} in about 1 msec (1/1000 of a second). The membrane potential then returns to the resting value in the next 1 to 2 msec. Further increases in stimulus intensity beyond the threshold level have no additional effect on the action potential. If an action potential is generated, its time course and amplitude are independent of the stimulus intensity; therefore the response is said to be **"all-or-none."** Because of the sharp, pointy appearance of an action potential, it is often referred to as a "spike."

To examine the characteristics of action potential propagation along the nerve axon, we can place a second recording electrode in the axon at a position that is 3 to 4 length constants away from the stimulating electrode (Figure 7-1, *A*). Under these circumstances subthreshold membrane potential changes are not observed at the second recording electrode (Figure 7-1, *C*) because of the electrotonic decay of such subthreshold signals caused by the passive properties of the axon (see Chapter 6). However, the action potential is transmitted *at full amplitude* to the second recording electrode (Figure 7-1, *D*). Thus the action potential is propagated along the axon without decrement in size despite the passive properties of the axon.

If a pair of just-threshold stimuli is given with a long enough interval between them, both produce action potentials (Figure 7-2, *A*). If the interval between stimuli is short enough, however, the second stimulus fails to evoke an action potential. The nerve is said to be *refractory*. The interval of time following an action potential during which a second stimulus, regardless of its amplitude, is unable to evoke a response is called the **absolute refractory period** (Figure 7-2, *B*). The **relative refractory period** is the interval of time following an action potential during which the second stimulus must be increased in intensity to evoke a second action potential (Figure 7-2, *B*).

■ ION CHANNEL FUNCTION IS STUDIED WITH A VOLTAGE CLAMP

Ionic Currents Are Measured at a Constant Membrane Potential with a Voltage Clamp

In the late 1940s, Hodgkin and Huxley pioneered the study of ion channels using a technique called the **voltage clamp** to study the ionic basis of the action potential in squid giant axons.* With this technique they could measure the **ionic currents** that flow across a membrane at a constant membrane potential. To appreciate the advantages of a voltage clamp, consider the following parameters that have complex interdependencies during a propagated action potential in an axon: current, voltage, distance, and time. As illustrated in Figure 7-1, the membrane potential changes as a function of distance during propagation. The ionic and capacitive currents that flow during the action potential must also change as a function of distance. Furthermore, both the currents and the membrane potential change as a function of time. By eliminating some of these variables while controlling others (see Box 7-1 for details of the method), the voltage clamp simplifies the situation in the following ways: (1) Distance is eliminated as a variable when the voltage clamp ensures that the membrane potential is the same over the entire membrane surface under study; this condition is called "space-clamp." (2) The voltage clamp apparatus allows the membrane potential to be held, or clamped, at a constant level. Except for a very brief time immediately after a step change in membrane potential, the membrane potential is constant,

$$\frac{dV_m}{dt} = 0 \qquad [1]$$

so the capacitive current

$$I_c = C\frac{dV_m}{dt} \qquad [2]$$

is zero. (3) As a result, the ionic current is measured as a function of time at a constant membrane potential. Because the ionic current flows through open ion channels, we can investigate the functional properties of the channels by analyzing the current.

---

*The British physiologists Alan Hodgkin and Andrew Huxley were awarded the Nobel Prize in Physiology or Medicine in 1963 for this work.

BOX 7-1

The Voltage Clamp Is Used to Maintain a Constant Membrane Potential

The voltage clamp, which uses an electronic device that allows control, or "clamping," of the membrane potential at a desired level, is an example of a negative feedback control system. In this type of system, like the thermostat controlling the temperature in your home, a variable (temperature) is measured and compared with a "command level," or set point (the temperature setting of the thermostat). The difference between the measured variable and the set point creates an "error signal." The error signal activates an effector system (heater or air conditioner) that decreases the magnitude of the error (i.e., brings the temperature closer to the set point).

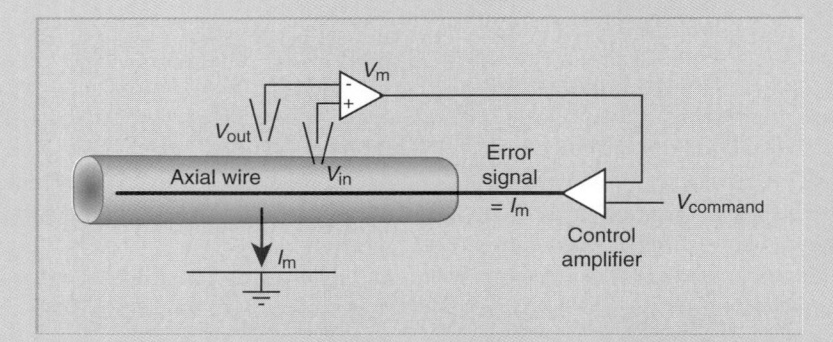

Figure B-1 ■ Schematic diagram of an axial wire voltage clamp. A wire is inserted longitudinally down the axon ("axial wire"). The membrane potential (V_m) is measured as the difference between the intracellular (V_{in}) and the extracellular (V_{out}) potential. The control amplifier compares V_m to a command potential ($V_{command}$). The output of the control amplifier passes the current (I_m) that is required to hold V_m at $V_{command}$.

A schematic of the squid giant axon axial wire voltage clamp is shown in Figure B-1. An amplifier measures the potential difference between an intracellular electrode (V_{in}) and an extracellular electrode (V_{out}). The output of this amplifier (V_m) is the controlled variable and is compared with the command potential ($V_{command}$), or set point, by an amplifier called the control amplifier. If V_m is not equal to $V_{command}$, an error signal causes a current to flow through an axial wire that is connected to the output of the control amplifier and inserted longitudinally through the axon. The current then flows out through the membrane to a grounded electrode to complete the circuit. The current passing through the axial wire rapidly and continuously causes V_m to remain equal to $V_{command}$. One way to measure the membrane current (I_m) in the voltage clamp is simply to measure the current flowing out of the control amplifier.

An important benefit of the low-resistance axial wire is that it greatly reduces the internal, axial resistance of the axoplasm. Thus the length constant

$$\lambda = \sqrt{\frac{r_m}{r_i}}$$

is greatly increased. The result is that V_m is constant over the membrane surface under study, or in other words, the membrane potential is "space clamped."

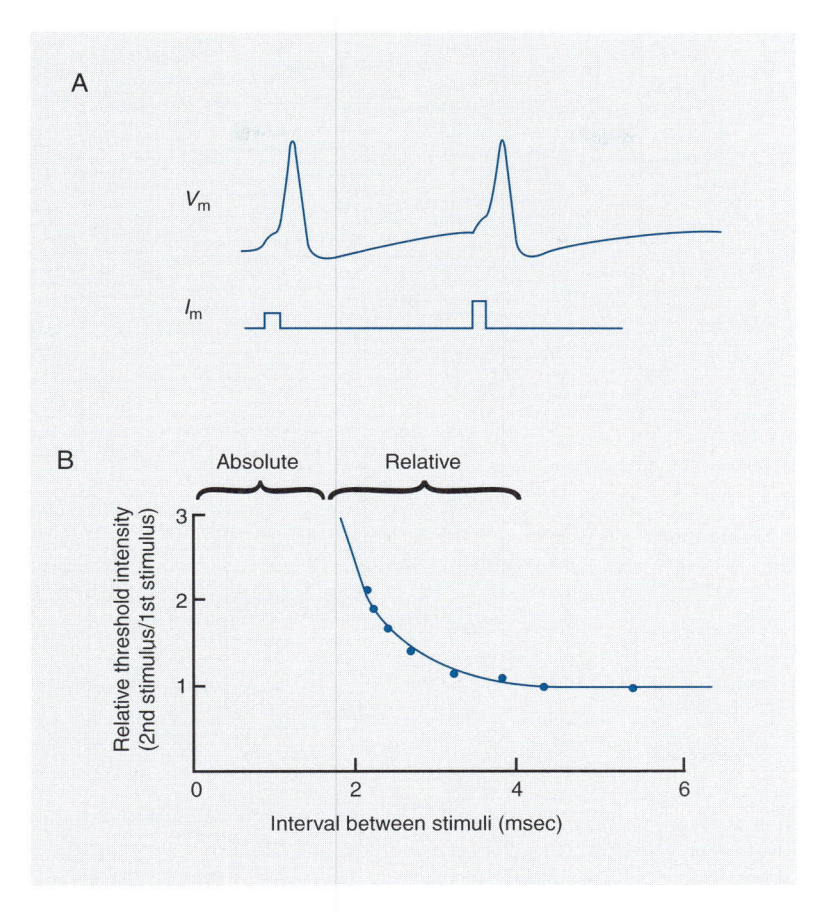

Generation and Propagation of the Action Potential

Figure 7-2 ■ Absolute and relative refractory periods. **A,** As the interval between two stimuli is decreased, the intensity of the second stimulus must be increased to generate an action potential. **B,** The relative threshold intensity (defined as the threshold intensity of the second stimulus divided by the threshold intensity of the first stimulus) graphed as a function of the interval between stimuli. During the relative refractory period the intensity of the second stimulus must be increased to generate an action potential. During the absolute refractory period an increase in stimulus intensity is ineffective: an action potential cannot be generated. (Redrawn from Tasaki I, Takeuchi T: *Pflügers Arch* 245:764, 1942.)

Ionic Currents Are Dependent on Voltage and Time

In a typical voltage clamp experiment the membrane potential is changed in stepwise fashion from a negative "holding" potential (−70 mV, for example), which is near the cell's resting potential, to some new level. When the membrane potential of the squid giant axon is stepped to a more negative potential (e.g., −100 mV), the current shown in Figure 7-3, *A*, is recorded. The current consists of an initial very brief "spike" of inward current followed by a

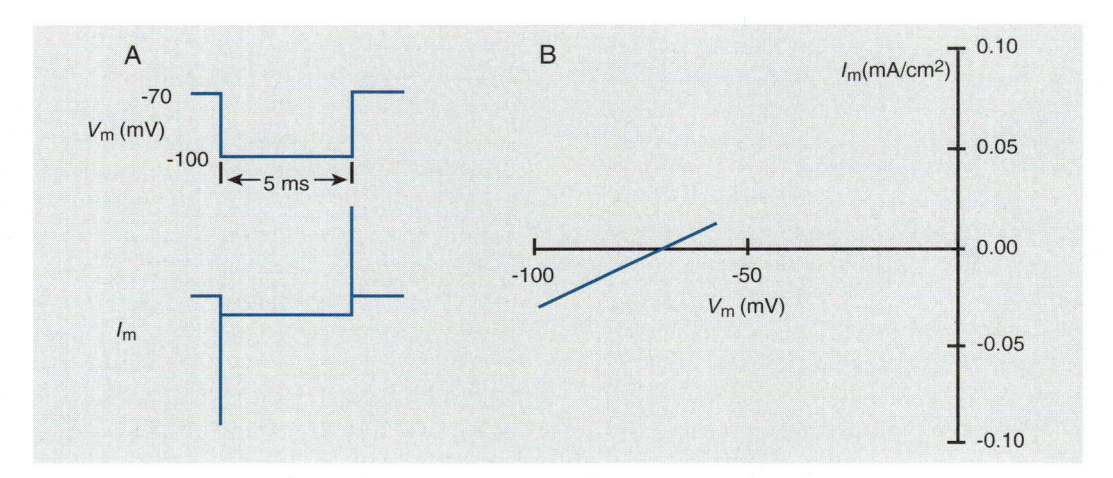

Figure 7-3 ■ **Hyperpolarizing and small depolarizing voltage clamp steps produce passive responses. A,** A voltage clamp step from −70 mV to −100 mV results in an inward current that consists of an initial spike of capacitive current, followed by a steady inward ionic current. When the clamp step ends and V_m rapidly returns to the original level, there is a spike of outward capacitive current. **B,** The magnitude of the ionic current varies as a linear function of the membrane potential, V_m.

steady (time-independent) inward current. The spike of current is capacitive current, which reflects the addition of negative charges at the inside membrane surface as the potential goes from −70 to −100 mV. The steady inward current is ionic current that flows through ion channels that are already open under resting conditions. After this steady ionic current is measured at different membrane potentials (e.g., over a negative voltage range from −100 to −70 mV), a plot of the current as a function of voltage reveals a linear, or ohmic (i.e., it obeys Ohm's Law), relationship (Figure 7-3, B). This is consistent with the result shown in Figure 6-3, which was obtained by injecting current and measuring the change in membrane potential.

For small depolarizations from −70 mV, the membrane continues to behave ohmically; that is, a spike of outward capacitive current is followed by a steady outward ionic current. For larger depolarizations, however, the current pattern is strikingly different, as illustrated by the current recorded during a voltage clamp step to 0 mV (Figure 7-4, A). Shortly after the spike of outward capacitive current, an inward current develops and reaches a maximum in about 1 msec. This inward current then declines in amplitude and is followed by an outward current that reaches a maximum and is maintained throughout the remainder of the voltage clamp step. This total membrane current recording contains three separable components of current (Box 7-2):

1. A linear component, similar to that shown in Figure 7-3, A, contains capacitive and ionic currents (Figure 7-4, B).
2. A time-dependent inward ionic current is carried by Na^+ ions flowing through **voltage-gated Na^+ channels** (Figure 7-4, C).
3. A time-dependent outward ionic current develops more slowly than the Na^+ current and is carried by K^+ ions flowing through **voltage-gated K^+ channels** (Figure 7-4, D).

The total current flowing through multiple channels is commonly referred to as a *macroscopic* current. The macroscopic Na^+ and K^+ currents shown in Figure 7-4 can be described in terms of the gating (channel opening and

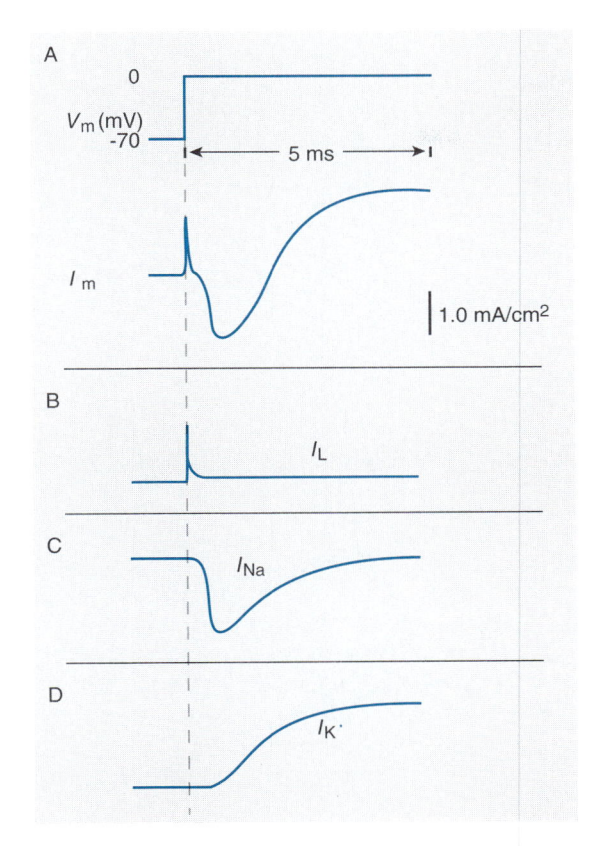

Generation and Propagation of the Action Potential

Figure 7-4 ■ **Current recorded during a voltage clamp step to 0 mV.** The total membrane current (I_m) recorded at 0 mV, A, contains three separable components (see Box 7-2): B, capacitive and ionic leakage currents (I_L), C, current flow through voltage-gated Na⁺ channels (I_{Na}), and, D, current flow through voltage-gated K⁺ channels (I_K).

closing) kinetics and current flow through individual channels. Because the size of the current flowing through a single open channel is constant at a constant membrane potential (see below), the size of the macroscopic current is proportional to the number of open channels. Thus the macroscopic Na⁺ current (Figure 7-4, C) indicates that, shortly after the depolarization, the Na⁺ channels rapidly open. This permits Na⁺ to flow into the cell down its electrochemical gradient (at 0 mV, the net driving force on Na⁺ is inward and therefore the Na⁺ current is inward in direction). The Na⁺ current reaches a maximum in about 1 msec and then becomes smaller as the Na⁺ channels close. This closure of the Na⁺ channels during maintained depolarization is called **inactivation**. The macroscopic K⁺ current (Figure 7-4, D) indicates that the gates on K⁺ channels open much more slowly than the Na⁺ channel gates. Moreover, the K⁺ channel gates stay open during the remainder of the depolarization. Thus the time-dependent characteristics of the macroscopic currents provide a measure of the kinetics of channel gating. The Na⁺ current reaches a maximum in about 1 msec, indicating that the Na⁺ channels open rapidly. The K⁺ current increases more slowly, reaching a maximum in about 3 to 4 msec because the K⁺ channels open more slowly.

Voltage-Gated Channels Exhibit Voltage-Dependent Conductances

Permeability and **conductance** both provide a measure of the ease with which ions cross cell membranes (see Chapter 4). Conductance is the more appropriate measure of ease of ion movement when electrical measurements are used, such as with the voltage clamp. By analogy to the permeability ($P = J/\Delta C$), according to Ohm's Law (Chapter 6, Equation [1]), conductance is the ratio between the rate of charge movement (current) and the potential difference across the membrane (i.e., $g = I/\Delta V$). The unit of conductance is the siemen: a 1-siemen conductor passes 1 ampere of current per volt of potential difference.

Ohm's Law can be used to calculate conductance from the Na⁺ and K⁺ ionic currents (I_{Na} and I_K) measured in a voltage clamp:

$$I_{Na} = g_{Na}(V_m - E_{Na}) \qquad [3]$$

$$I_K = g_K(V_m - E_K) \qquad [4]$$

The membrane potential, V_m, is known (it is

BOX 7-2

Current Components in Axons Are Separated and Identified with Ionic Substitutions

The most straightforward way to separate the ionic currents is to perform ionic substitution experiments, in which permeant ions are replaced by larger, impermeant ions. In the isolated squid giant axon the axoplasm can be removed and the axon interior perfused with a solution of known composition. Thus the ionic composition of both the internal and external solutions is under experimental control. If Na^+ is replaced with the larger, impermeant cation choline, the early inward current carried by Na^+ ions is eliminated (Figure B-1, B), and if the remaining current is subtracted from the total current (Figure B-1, A), the isolated Na^+ current is obtained (Figure B-1, C). If cesium ions (Cs^+) are then substituted for intracellular and extracellular K^+, the outward K^+ current is abolished and only linear capacitive and leakage currents remain (Figure B-1, D). By subtracting the linear current (Figure B-1, D) from the current shown in Figure B-1, B, the isolated K^+ current is obtained (Figure B-1, E).

Figure B-1 ■ Ionic substitutions can be used to separate current components. A, The current recorded during a voltage clamp step to 0 mV contains Na^+ (I_{Na}), K^+ (I_K), leak (I_L), and capacitive (I_c) currents. B, After all of the Na^+ is replaced with choline$^+$, the Na^+ current is abolished. C, The isolated I_{Na} is calculated by subtraction of the current shown in B from that in A. D, In the absence of Na^+, substitution of Cs^+ for K^+ abolishes I_K. E, The isolated I_K is calculated by subtraction of the current shown in D from that in B.

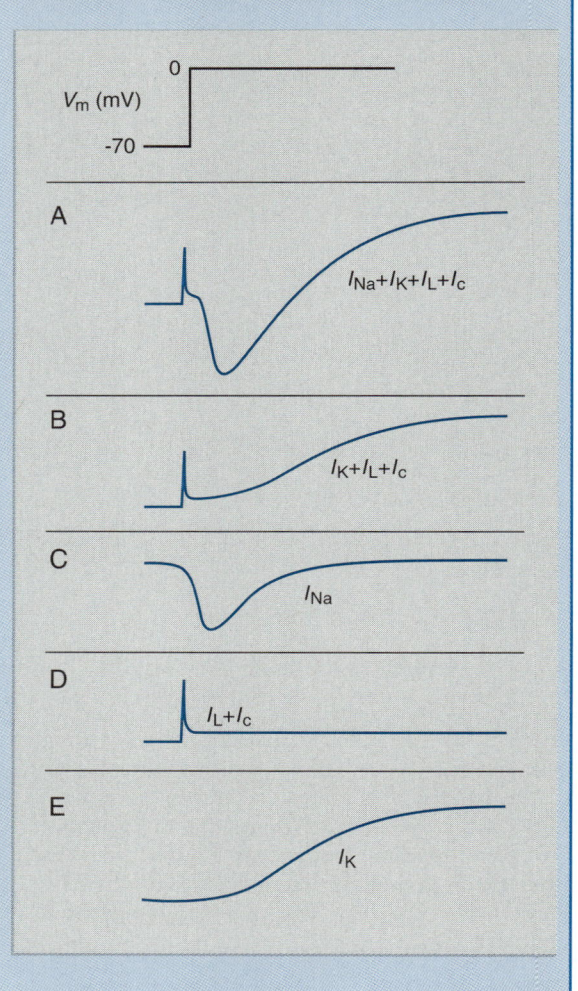

controlled by the voltage clamp). E_{Na} and E_K can be calculated from the Nernst equation. The time courses of g_{Na} and g_K at 0 mV, calculated from the currents at 0 mV, are shown in Figure 7-5. Note that the conductances are always positive. After a brief delay, g_{Na} rapidly rises to a peak and then declines back toward zero, even though the membrane is still depolarized.

The rising phase of the conductance is termed **activation**, and the declining phase is termed inactivation. The K^+ conductance, g_K, begins to increase (or activate) after a much longer delay and rises more slowly than g_{Na}. After reaching a plateau, g_K remains at that level during the remainder of the depolarization (i.e., it does not inactivate).

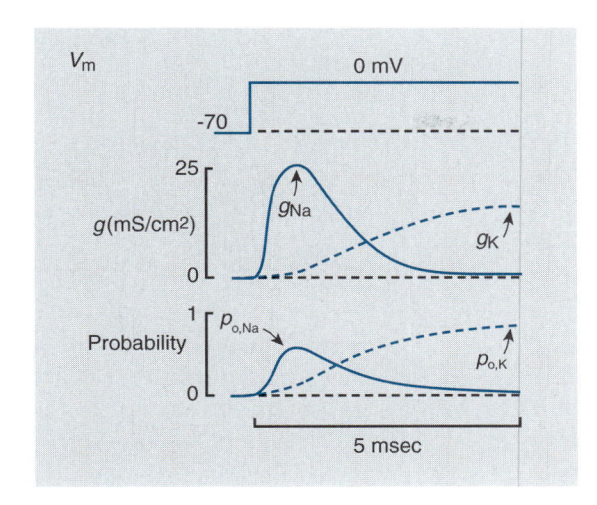

Generation and Propagation of the Action Potential

Figure 7-5 ■ The time course of g_{Na}, g_K, $p_{o,Na}$, and $p_{o,K}$ during a voltage clamp step to 0 mV. g_{Na} and g_K are the membrane conductances to Na$^+$ and K$^+$, respectively. $p_{o,Na}$ is the Na$^+$ channel open probability, and $p_{o,K}$ is the K$^+$ channel open probability.

At the molecular level, open ion channels are responsible for the conductance of the membrane, so the macroscopic conductance, g_{Na} or g_K, is proportional to the number of open channels:

$$g_{Na} = N_o\, \gamma_{Na} \qquad [5]$$

where N_o is the number of open Na$^+$ channels and γ_{Na} is the conductance of a single Na$^+$ channel. If all Na$^+$ channels have the same average **open probability** and they behave independent of one another, it follows that

$$g_{Na} = N_T\, p_o\, \gamma_{Na} \qquad [6]$$

where N_T is the total number of Na$^+$ channels and p_o is the probability that a channel is open. Since N_T and γ_{Na} are constants, it is clear that g_{Na} varies as a function of time (and voltage, as we will see later) because of variations in the probability that a Na$^+$ channel is open. The traces at the bottom of Figure 7-5 show how the probability of channel opening varies as a function of time during a voltage clamp step to 0 mV. The fact that Na$^+$ channels activate and then inactivate during maintained depolarization suggests that there are *two* gates controlling the open and closed states of the channel: an activation gate and an inactivation gate (see below). The closure of Na$^+$ channel activation gates upon repolarization from a depolarizing voltage clamp step is called **deactivation**.

For voltage-gated ion channels the probability that a gate is in the open configuration depends on the membrane potential (V_m). For Na$^+$ channels in the squid axon the fraction of open activation gates (i.e., p_o for the activation gate) in the steady state begins to increase at about –40 mV, then increases rapidly with small changes in voltage, and reaches a maximum at about 0 mV (Figure 7-6). This is one of the most important, fundamental properties of the *voltage-gated* Na$^+$ (and K$^+$) channels found in nerve axons and other excitable cells: the probability that a channel will open increases as the membrane potential is made more positive.

How does a voltage-gated channel work? The answer to this question is now being clarified. The S4 region in voltage-gated channels contains a series of positive amino acids (see Chapter 5) that acts as the voltage sensor. Movement of S4, caused by depolarization, induces a conformational change in the channel protein that causes it to go from the closed to the open conformation. Movement of the voltage sensor (S4) itself produces a current because the charged amino acid residues are moving in response to the electric field (the voltage gradient) across the membrane. This *gating current* has in fact been measured (Box 7-3).

■ INDIVIDUAL ION CHANNELS HAVE TWO CONDUCTANCE LEVELS

The current that flows through an individual ion channel is very small (about 1 to 5 pA) and

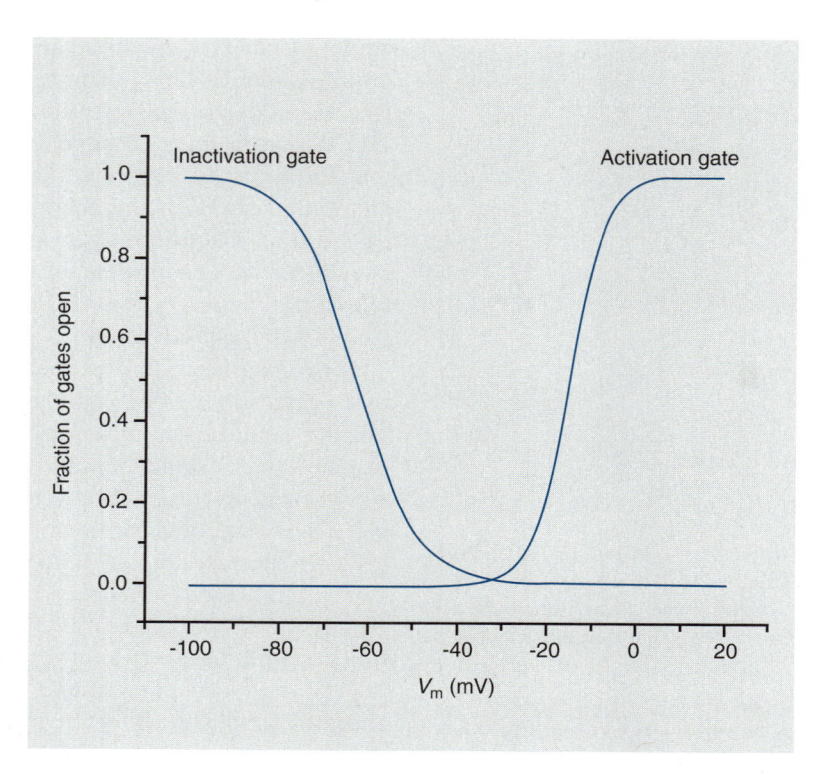

Figure 7-6 ■ **Graph of the fraction of Na⁺ channel activation and inactivation gates that are open *in the steady state,* as a function of V_m, in a squid axon. As the membrane depolarizes (i.e., membrane potential moves in the positive direction), the Na⁺ channel activation gates open and the inactivation gates close. The fraction of open gates changes along a sigmoidal curve as V_m moves in the positive direction.** (Modified from Hodgkin AL, Huxley AF: *J Physiol* 116:473, 1952.)

---

cannot be resolved with a classical voltage clamp. These small *single-channel currents* can be measured, however, by use of a **patch clamp** to electrically isolate a small patch of membrane (Figure 7-7, *A*).* Patch clamp recordings reveal that a single channel has two conductance levels: zero when the channel is closed and a constant conductance, γ, when the channel is open. Thus individual ion channels gate in an all-or-none manner and pass a "pulse" of current when they are open (Figure 7-7, *D*).

■ SODIUM CHANNELS INACTIVATE DURING MAINTAINED DEPOLARIZATION

The time course of the Na⁺ conductance change (Figure 7-5) shows that membrane voltage has a dual effect on Na⁺ channels. First, voltage causes the gates on some of the Na⁺ channels to open rapidly, giving rise to the activation phase of g_{Na}. Later on during the depolarization, g_{Na} declines

---

*The German biophysicists Erwin Neher and Bert Sakmann developed the patch clamp to measure ionic currents through single channels. They were awarded the Nobel Prize in Physiology or Medicine in 1991 for this achievement.

Generation and Propagation of the Action Potential

> **BOX 7-3**
>
> ### *Gating Currents Directly Reflect Movement of the Voltage Sensor*
>
> Hodgkin and Huxley correctly predicted the existence of a voltage sensor in voltage-gated channels. They reasoned that the voltage sensor would move passively in response to a change in membrane potential. This movement of the voltage sensor would change the conformation of the channel protein and would cause the channel gate to open or close. Movement of the gating charge generates a gating current. So that the relatively small-amplitude gating current can be measured, ionic Na^+ and K^+ currents must be blocked and the spike of capacitive current that charges the membrane must be subtracted. The gating current has been measured as a brief outward current that flows before the opening of the Na^+ channels (Figure B-1).
>
> **Figure B-1** ■ **Na^+ channel gating current is a direct measure of the movement of the voltage sensor. Following a depolarization, the gating current (I_g) is a brief outward current that flows before the opening of the Na^+ channels (note the time scale compared with Figure 7-4). The time course of Na^+ channel opening is illustrated by I_{Na}.** (From Armstrong CM, Bezanilla F: *J Gen Physiol* 63:533, 1974.)

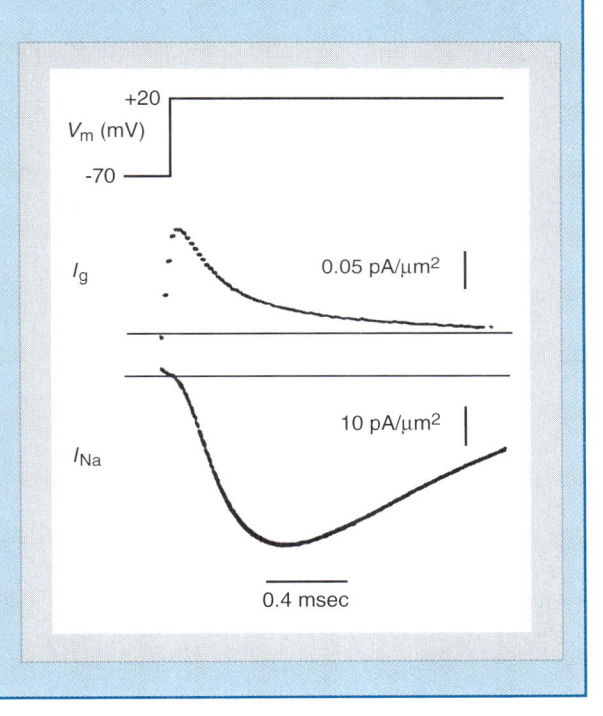

back toward zero as if the gates on the channels are closing. This dual behavior occurs because Na^+ channels have two gates. These gates, the activation gate and the inactivation gate, together control the open and closed states of the channel. The diagrams in Figure 7-8 illustrate the configuration of the gates in the closed, open, and inactivated states of the channel. At negative voltages the activation gate is closed and the inactivation gate is open. When the membrane is depolarized, the activation gate in most Na^+ channels opens before the inactivation gate closes, allowing the channel to open and conduct Na^+ ions. In time the inactivation gate will close, thereby closing the channel through inactivation.

Na^+ channel inactivation is physiologically important for at least three reasons:
1. The Na^+ conductance automatically begins to turn off at the peak of the action potential. This allows more rapid repolarization and potentially more rapid repetitive firing of action potentials.
2. A slowly depolarizing stimulus can be ineffective in evoking an action potential because the membrane can *accommodate* to

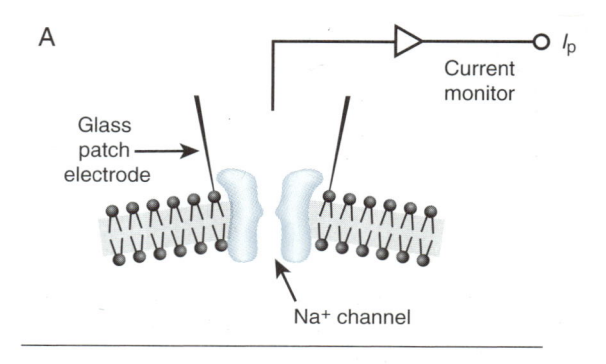

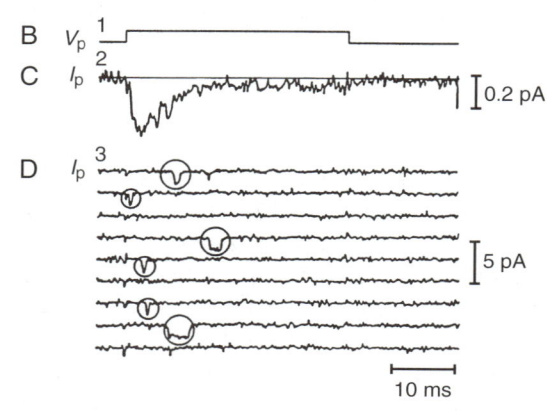

Figure 7-7 ■ Measurement of currents through single Na⁺ channels. A, A glass "patch electrode" is used to isolate, electrically, a small patch of membrane containing a single Na⁺ channel. The current flowing through the electrode, and thus through the channel, is recorded by a current monitor. B, Repetitive identical depolarizing voltage clamp steps (V_p) are applied to the membrane. C, The current summed from a large number of traces, such as those in D. D, Each trace is the current recorded from the patch of membrane during a single voltage clamp step. (B, C, and D from Sigworth FJ, Neher E: *Nature* 287:447, 1980.)

a slowly rising stimulus. Accommodation occurs when the rate of rise of the stimulus is sufficiently slow, so that many Na⁺ channels inactivate before enough of them open to produce an action potential.

3. The time course of inactivation is a determinant of the absolute and relative refractory periods.

A change in the inactivation gating of the skeletal muscle Na⁺ channel is responsible for the temporary weakness or paralysis experienced by patients with *hyperkalemic periodic paralysis* (Box 7-4).

■ THE ACTION POTENTIAL IS GENERATED BY VOLTAGE-GATED Na⁺ AND K⁺ CHANNELS

The Equivalent Circuit of a Patch of Membrane Can Be Used to Describe Action Potential Generation

To explain how the activity of Na⁺ and K⁺ channels can produce an action potential, we can use the equivalent electrical circuit for a patch of axonal membrane (Figure 7-9). The equivalent circuit includes a variable resistor representing voltage-gated Na⁺ channels (labeled g_{Na}), a variable resistor representing K⁺ channels (g_K), a resistor representing other, non-voltage-gated ("leak") channels (g_L), and a capacitor for the membrane capacitance (C_m). At the resting potential the capacitor is charged to −70 mV, and in this steady state the sum of all ionic currents is zero. To change the membrane potential, charge must flow onto, or off of, the capacitor.

To initiate an action potential, an external current source connected to the patch of membrane depolarizes the membrane just beyond threshold by adding positive charges to the inside surface of the membrane (Figure 7-9, *B*). This depolarization causes some Na⁺ channels to open quickly. Thus the membrane conductance to Na⁺ ions increases and Na⁺ flows into the cell down its electrochemical gradient. This gives rise to an inward Na⁺ current (I_{Na}). Current must flow in a loop, and the return pathway for the inward ionic current is through the membrane capacitor. The outward capacitive current is

Generation and Propagation of the Action Potential

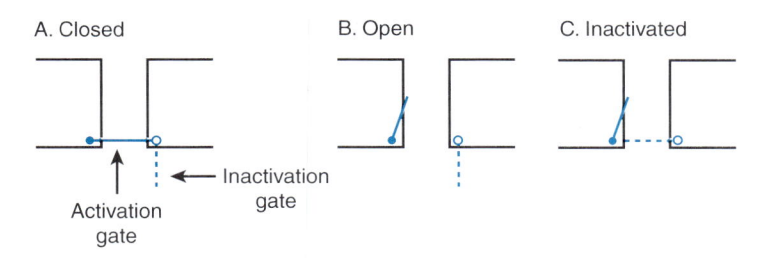

Figure 7-8 ■ Voltage-gated Na⁺ channels behave as if they have two gates: an activation gate and an inactivation gate. A, At negative membrane potentials the channel is closed, with the activation gate closed and the inactivation gate open. B, On depolarization the activation gate opens and the channel is open. C, Later during depolarization the inactivation gate closes and the channel is inactivated.

depolarizing, since positive charge flows onto the inside surface of the capacitor. Thus the entry of positively charged Na⁺ ions depolarizes the membrane further (Figure 7-9, C). This opens more Na⁺ channels and permits more Na⁺ to flow in. This phase of inward Na⁺ current accounts for the upstroke of the action potential. After about 1 msec the Na⁺ conductance begins to decrease (as Na⁺ channels inactivate) and K⁺ channels begin to open. Because the driving force on K⁺ ($V_m - E_K$) is outward, the increase in K⁺ conductance gives rise to an outward K⁺ current. This outward ionic current produces an inward capacitive current that repolarizes the membrane over the next 1 to 2 msec, thereby accounting for the falling phase of the action potential and the undershoot (Figure 7-9, D).

The Action Potential Is a Cyclical Process of Channel Opening and Closing

The cycle of events involved in the generation of an action potential is shown in Figure 7-10. The rapid rising phase of the spike is the result of positive feedback; that is, membrane depolarization opens Na⁺ channels (increases g_{Na}), which increases the Na⁺ current, and this further depolarizes the membrane, thus opening more Na⁺ channels, and so on. The result is an explosive response. The depolarization stops when the membrane potential approaches E_{Na} and the Na⁺ current decreases because (1) the driving force on Na⁺ becomes small ($V_m \approx E_{Na}$) and (2) Na⁺ channels start to inactivate. Repolarization occurs when the developing outward K⁺ current exceeds the declining inward Na⁺ current. If the stimulus is maintained, the cycle can be repeated so that action potentials can be generated repetitively.

Both Na⁺ Channel Inactivation and Open Voltage-Gated K⁺ Channels Contribute to the Refractory Period

During the later phases of the action potential, both Na⁺ channel inactivation and the activation of K⁺ channels contribute to the production of the refractory period. As a result of inactivation a fraction of the Na⁺ channels are unavailable for opening in response to a depolarizing stimulus. Moreover, open K⁺ channels tend to "pull" the membrane potential toward E_K, which is more negative than the normal resting potential (see discussion of the Goldman-Hodgkin-Katz equation in Chapter 4). Therefore the current

BOX 7-4

Hyperkalemic Periodic Paralysis Results from Genetically Defective Skeletal Muscle Sodium Channels

Hyperkalemic periodic paralysis (HPP) is a relatively rare genetic disease that is caused by a defect in the voltage-dependent Na^+ channel isoform that is expressed in skeletal muscle. Neuronal Na^+ channels are not affected. The disease has autosomal dominant inheritance and is characterized by episodes of skeletal muscle weakness or paralysis. These episodes are preceded by a normally occurring increase in the concentration of extracellular K^+ ions, thus the name HPP. Electrophysiological experiments have shown that the resting potential of skeletal muscle fibers from HPP patients is *abnormally* depolarized in the presence of elevated extracellular K^+ (Figure B-1). Maintained depolarization of skeletal muscle causes it to become inexcitable and unable to contract. The result is weakness or paralysis (see Chapter 14).

The molecular mechanisms underlying HPP are now understood. Patients with HPP have a single point mutation in the gene coding for the skeletal muscle Na^+ channel. The mutation leads to a single amino acid substitution in the Na^+ channel. An important change in function results: the defective Na^+ channels do not inactivate completely (Figure B-2). The noninactivating Na^+ channels give rise to the abnormal depolarization of HPP-affected skeletal muscle fibers.

The following chain of events occurs during a period of paralysis in patients with HPP: Some

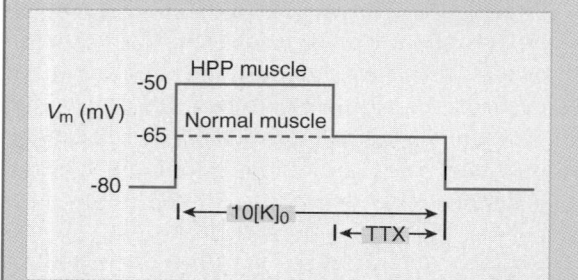

Figure B-1 ■ Diagram of resting membrane potential changes caused by an increase in $[K^+]_o$ in normal muscles and in muscle from a person with hyperkalemic periodic paralysis (HPP). When $[K^+]_o$ is increased from 5 mM to 10 mM, HPP-affected muscle depolarizes more than normal muscle. Tetrodotoxin (TTX) abolishes the additional depolarization observed in HPP-affected muscle. This demonstrates that the depolarization is due to I_{Na} through voltage-gated (TTX-sensitive) Na^+ channels.

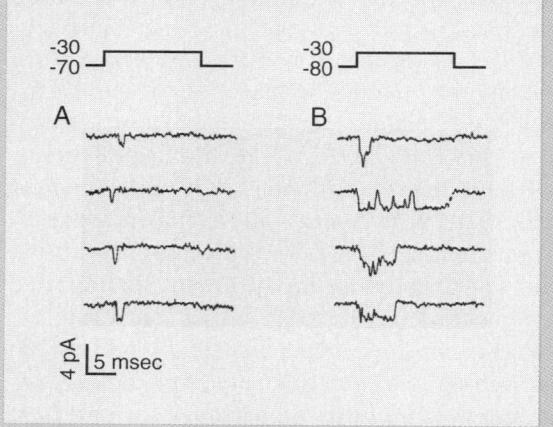

Figure B-2 ■ Currents through single Na^+ channels recorded from, A, normal muscle and, B, skeletal muscle affected by hyperkalemic periodic paralysis (HPP) during a depolarizing voltage clamp step (shown at the top). The Na^+ channels from normal muscle open briefly at the beginning of the depolarization and then inactivate. The Na^+ channels from HPP-affected muscle can continue to open and close throughout the depolarization; thus they do not inactivate normally. (From Cannon SC, Brown RH Jr, Corey DP: *Neuron* 6:619, 1991.)

> **BOX 7-4**
>
> ### Hyperkalemic Periodic Paralysis Results from Genetically Defective Skeletal Muscle Sodium Channels—Cont'd
>
> normal event, such as exercise, leads to an increase in extracellular K^+. This elevated extracellular K^+ level causes membrane depolarization, which activates some voltage-gated Na^+ channels. In normal individuals the Na^+ channels then rapidly inactivate, but in patients with HPP they do not. An inward current flowing through the non-inactivating Na^+ channels produces an additional depolarization. This inactivates the muscle contraction apparatus (see Chapter 14), and a temporary paralysis occurs.

required to reach threshold is larger than in a resting nerve.

Pharmacological Agents That Block Na^+ or K^+ Channels, or Interfere with Na^+ Channel Inactivation, Alter the Shape of the Action Potential

Thousands of chemical agents can alter current flow through ion channels either by changing the single channel conductance or by altering the gating of the channel. Agents that block voltage-gated Na^+ or K^+ channels or that impede Na^+ channel inactivation change the shape of the action potential in predictable ways. Blocking a fraction of the Na^+ channels with a low concentration of *tetrodotoxin* or *saxitoxin* decreases the magnitude of the Na^+ current (Box 7-5). This results in an action potential that has a higher threshold, a slower rate of rise, and a lower peak amplitude (Figure 7-11, *A*). A similar effect is produced by *local anesthetics* (Figure 7-11, *B*), which also block Na^+ channels. The rate of action potential repolarization is decreased by agents that intereferewith Na^+ channel inactivation, such as sea anemone toxin (Figure 7-11, *C*), or that block voltage-gated K^+ channels, such as tetraethylammonium ions (Figure 7-11, *D*).

■ ACTION POTENTIAL PROPAGATION OCCURS AS A RESULT OF LOCAL CIRCUIT CURRENTS

In Nonmyelinated Axons an Action Potential Propagates as a Continuous Wave of Excitation Away from the Initiation Site

Propagation occurs because an active patch of membrane that is undergoing the upstroke of the action potential can act as a source of stimulus current for the resting membrane that lies just ahead of the advancing electrical impulse. This **local circuit current** flow from the active patch supplies an outward capacitive current across the resting membrane to depolarize it toward threshold. The process continuously and smoothly repeats itself during propagation.

Figure 7-12 shows the membrane potential as a function of distance along a nonmyelinated axon at a specific point in time during the propagation of an action potential from right to left. The local circuit currents are shown with arrows. Ahead of and behind the advancing action potential, the membrane potential is near the negative resting level. At the active patch of membrane, where the upstroke of the action potential is occurring, the current is dominated by inward I_{Na}. This inward ionic current

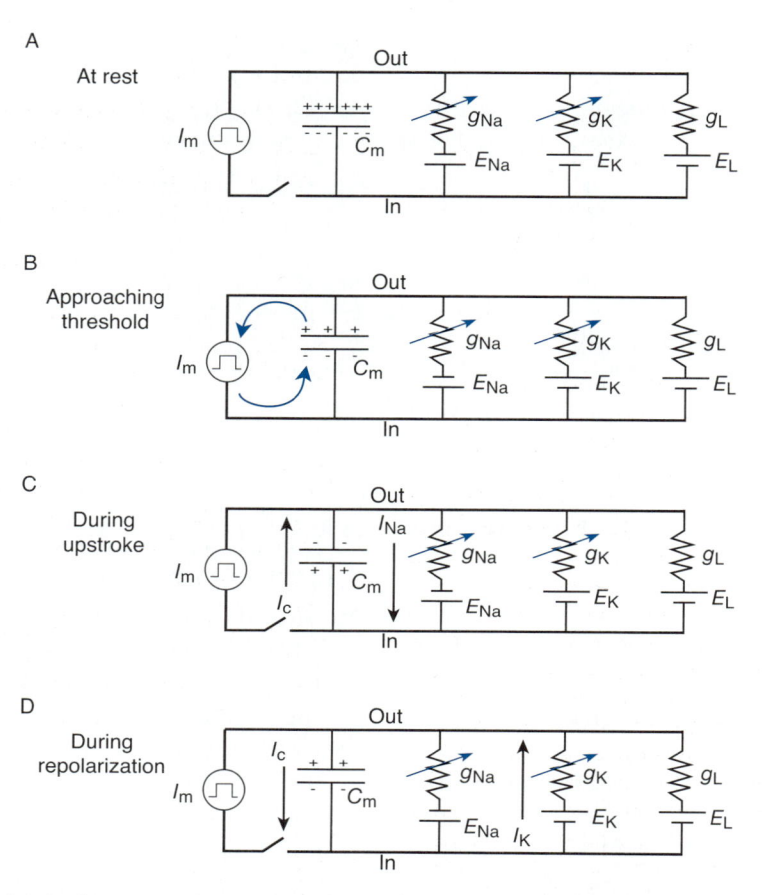

Figure 7-9 ■ The equivalent circuit of a patch of axon membrane (A) illustrates the mechanism of action potential generation. A constant current source (I_m) is connected to the membrane through a switch. The resistors g_{Na} and g_K are the voltage-gated conductances of the membrane to Na⁺ and K⁺, respectively, and g_L is the "leakage" conductance. E_{Na} and E_K are the equilibrium potentials for Na⁺ and K⁺, respectively, and E_L is the "equilibrium" potential for the leakage channels. B, A stimulus from an external current source (or an adjacent patch of membrane) supplies outward current that depolarizes the membrane toward threshold. C, The depolarization opens Na⁺ channels, and the resulting inward Na⁺ current produces outward capacitive current that further depolarizes the membrane and causes the upstroke of the action potential. D, Later, the Na⁺ channels inactivate and K⁺ channels open. Outward current through the K⁺ channels generates inward capacitive current that repolarizes the membrane.

---

further depolarizes the membrane in the vicinity of the open Na⁺ channels, and it is *also* a current source that depolarizes the resting membrane lying ahead of the action potential (this is the electrotonic spread of current described in Chapter 6; see Figure 6-7). Initially, the outward current ahead of the spike is mostly capacitive current that depolarizes the membrane toward

Generation and Propagation of the Action Potential

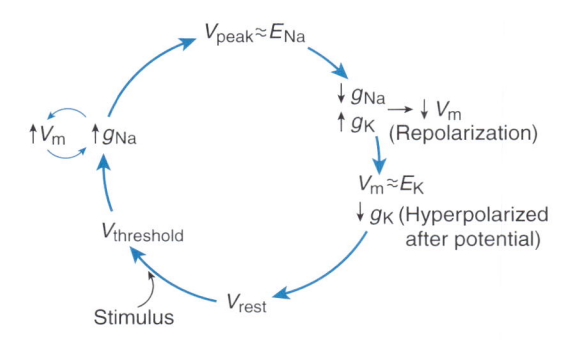

Figure 7-10 ■ The cycle of events in the generation of an action potential in a patch of membrane. Starting at the bottom (V_{rest}) and going clockwise, a stimulus depolarizes the membrane from the resting potential (V_{rest}) toward threshold ($V_{threshold}$). If threshold is exceeded, g_{Na} increases rapidly and an inward Na^+ current develops that depolarizes V_m further. This reflects positive feedback of V_m on g_{Na}: an increase in g_{Na} causes depolarization, which further increases g_{Na}, resulting in the very rapid upstroke of the action potential. Next, Na^+ channels begin to inactivate and voltage-gated K^+ channels open. An outward K^+ current develops, causing repolarization. The membrane potential becomes more negative than V_{rest} (closer to E_K) because the voltage-gated K^+ channels take time to close completely. As the K^+ channels close, V_m returns to V_{rest}.

BOX 7-5

Tetrodotoxin and Saxitoxin Are Examples of Numerous Toxins of Animal Origin That Alter Ion Channel Gating or Conduction

Tetrodotoxin (TTX) and saxitoxin (STX) are chemically different small molecules (MW 319 and 299, respectively) that are highly selective blockers of voltage-gated Na^+ channels. Only nanomolar (10^{-9} M) concentrations are required to block the channels. TTX is a paralytic poison found in the ovaries, liver, and skin of puffer fish. The puffer fish ("fugu") is a delicacy in Japan, but occasional fatalities result from eating this fish. STX is synthesized by marine dinoflagellates (algae of the genus *Gonyaulax*). Population explosions, or "blooms," of these dinoflagellates can be recognized by their reddish color (the "red tide"). Filter-feeding shellfish can accumulate toxin to such a level that eating a single shellfish can be fatal.

---

threshold. Behind the active region of membrane the outward current is mostly ionic, carried by K^+, which repolarizes the membrane. A few milliseconds later, the entire membrane potential profile is shifted along the axon in the direction of propagation (dashed line in Figure 7-12). The action potential propagates smoothly in this fashion, with an active region of membrane providing the current to stimulate the adjacent region to the threshold for spike initiation.

Under physiological conditions propagation is *unidirectional* for two reasons. First, behind the advancing wave of depolarization, the membrane is refractory because of Na^+ channel inactivation. Second, local circuit current, supplied from the active patch to membrane behind the active region, is primarily an outward ionic K^+ current that repolarizes the membrane.

Conduction Velocity Is Influenced by τ, by λ, and by I_{Na} Amplitude and Kinetics

The **conduction velocity** of the action potential can be affected by several parameters. In principle, conduction velocity can be increased either by increasing the length constant or by decreasing the time constant. In nonmyelinated axons the length constant,

$$\lambda = \sqrt{\frac{r_m}{r_i}} \qquad [7]$$

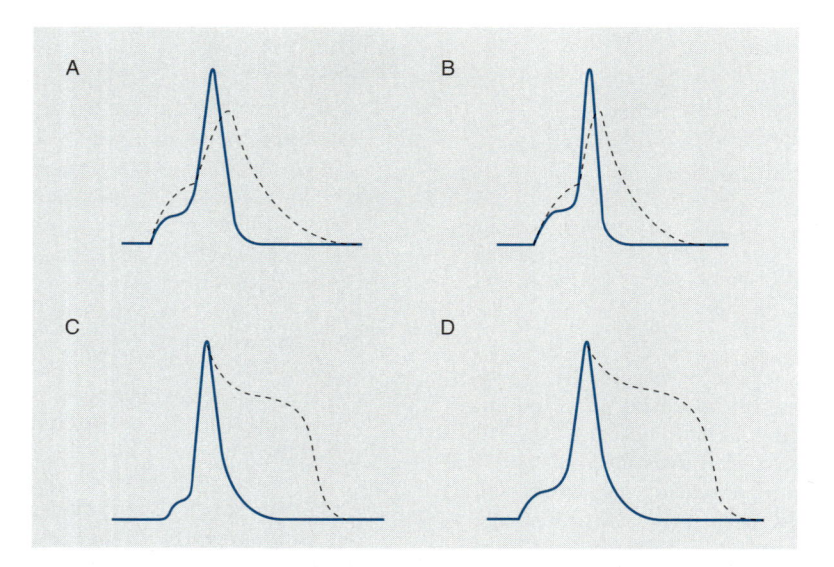

Figure 7-11 ■ Pharmacological agents that block Na⁺ or K⁺ channels, or interfere with Na⁺ channel inactivation, change the shape of the action potential. In each panel the solid trace is the control and the dashed trace is the action potential in the presence of the chemical agent. **A,** Partial block of Na⁺ channels with tetrodotoxin (TTX) increases the threshold for generating an action potential and decreases the amplitude and the rate of rise of the action potential. **B,** Partial block of the Na⁺ channels with a local anesthetic produces an effect similar to that observed with TTX. **C,** A peptide toxin isolated from sea anemones reduces the rate of Na⁺ channel inactivation and prolongs the duration of the action potential. **D,** Tetraethylammonium ions block voltage-gated K⁺ channels and prolong the duration of the action potential. (A and B redrawn from Narahashi T, Deguchi T, Urakawa N, Ohkubo Y: *Am J Physiol* 198:934, 1959. C redrawn from Rathmayer W: *Adv Cytopharmacol* 3:335, 1979. D redrawn from Armstrong CM, Binstock L: *J Gen Physiol* 48:859, 1965.)

increases as axon diameter (d) increases because $r_m \propto 1/d$, and $r_i \propto 1/d^2$ (Box 7-6). Therefore λ is proportional to $\sqrt{d}$. Then, because λ determines the electrotonic spread of the local circuit current that initiates the action potential, conduction velocity in *non*myelinated axons is proportional to $\sqrt{d}$. Increasing the length constant increases the conduction velocity because an active area of membrane will be able to depolarize more distant areas of the membrane to threshold.

The membrane time constant ($\tau_m = r_m \times c_m$) is not, on the other hand, an important determinant of variations in action potential conduction velocity. During action potential propagation along an axon, the stimulating current must flow through the axoplasmic resistance, r_i, before flowing out across the membrane capacitance, c_m. Therefore conduction velocity varies inversely with a different time constant, the **propagation time constant** ($\tau_p = R_i \times C_m$ where R_i is the axoplasmic resistance in ohms and C_m is the membrane capacitance in farads). A smaller τ_p results in faster conduction because the membrane potential changes more rapidly. This factor contributes to the increase in conduction speed in myelinated axons (see next section).

Anything that changes the kinetics or mag-

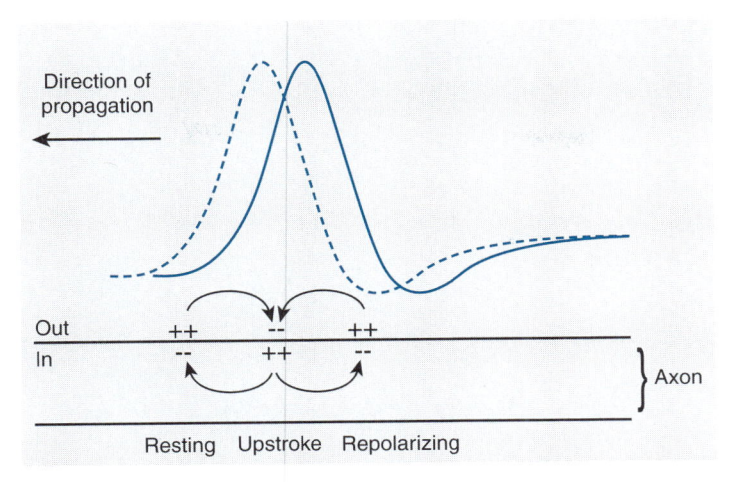

Figure 7-12 ■ The action potential propagates as a result of local circuit current flow. The traces at the top of the figure show V_m as a function of distance along the axon at a specific point in time during the propagation of the action potential. The dashed trace is at a slightly later point in time during propagation. The arrows in the diagram of the axon at the bottom illustrate the flow of local circuit currents.

BOX 7-6

The Parameters r_m, r_i, and λ Are a Function of Axon Diameter

In Chapter 6, r_m was defined as R_m/circumference. Since the circumference of a cylinder of diameter d is $\pi \times d$,

$$r_m = \frac{R_m}{\pi \times d}$$

(i.e., $r_m \propto 1/d$). We also noted that $r_i = \rho$/cross-sectional-area. The cross-sectional area of a cylinder (i.e., the area of a circle) is $\pi \times d^2/4$, so

$$r_i = \frac{4\rho}{\pi \times d^2}$$

(i.e., $r_i \propto 1/d^2$). Thus the relationship between the length constant and axon diameter is

$$\lambda = \sqrt{\frac{r_m}{r_i}} = \sqrt{\frac{R_m/(\pi \times d)}{4\rho/(\pi \times d^2)}} = \sqrt{\frac{R_m \times d)}{4\rho}}$$

In other words, the length constant is proportional to the square root of the axon diameter.

---

nitude of the voltage-dependent inward current will affect the conduction velocity. For example, reduction in the magnitude of the Na$^+$ conductance by local anesthetics, or reduction in the rate of activation of the Na$^+$ conductance by a decrease in temperature, will reduce the conduction velocity.

Myelination Increases Action Potential Conduction Velocity

The larger nerve fibers in vertebrate nervous systems are specialized for rapid conduction and are myelinated. In peripheral nerves the myelin is formed by Schwann cells, which wrap themselves around the axon several times, forming

TABLE 7-1

Conduction velocities for three different types of nerve fibers

Fiber type	Diameter (μm)	Conduction velocity (m/sec)
Aα (myelinated)	15.0	120
Nonmyelinated C fibers	0.5	1
Squid giant axon (nonmyelinated)	500.0	25

an insulating sheath. The myelin sheath is interrupted periodically by **nodes of Ranvier** where nearly all of the Na⁺ channels are located. The internode distance varies from 200 μm to 2 mm. Table 7-1 shows representative values for conduction velocities in three different types of nerve fibers. Clearly, myelination enables much more rapid conduction. Moreover, the conduction velocity of *myelinated* fibers is directly proportional to the fiber diameter (in contrast to the dependence on $\sqrt{d}$ for *non*myelinated axons). Therefore increases in the fiber diameter, above about 1 μm, give proportionately greater increases in conduction velocity in a myelinated than in a nonmyelinated fiber (Figure 7-13). Figure 7-13 also indicates that myelination may be disadvantageous for fibers with diameters less than about 1 μm. Nature seems to know this, too, because very small fibers in the mammalian nervous system are not myelinated (Table 7-1). Myelination enables vertebrates to pack large numbers of *rapid* communication lines into relatively small nerve tracts, increasing the information-processing capability.

The high conduction velocity of myelinated fibers is the result of a very large increase in length constant and a decrease in propagation time constant caused by the wrapping of fatty, insulating myelin around the fiber. This drama-

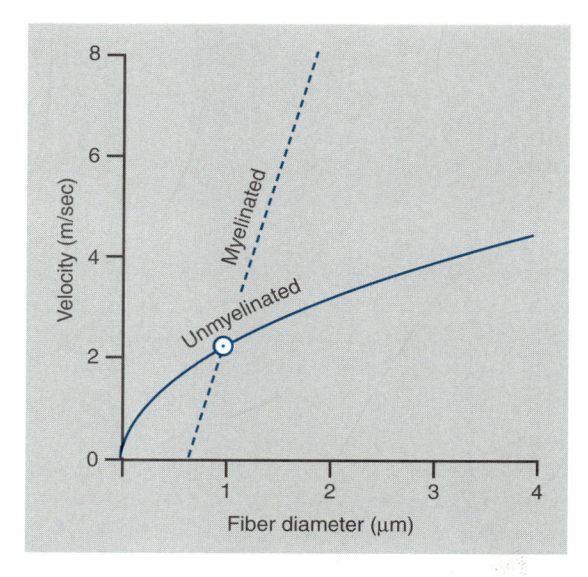

Figure 7-13 ■ **Theoretical relationship between conduction velocity and axon diameter for both myelinated and unmyelinated axons.** (From Rushton WAH: *J Physiol [Lond]* 115:101, 1951.)

tically *increases* r_m in the myelinated (internode) regions because the current has to pass across the myelin sheath as well as the axon plasma membrane (Figure 7-14). In addition, c_m is *reduced* by myelination: the thicker insulation results in less charge separation per unit membrane area. The lower c_m results in a smaller propagation time constant. Then, because Na⁺ channels are confined to the nodes of Ranvier, the action potential effectively skips from node to node along the fiber. A spike at one node rapidly depolarizes the adjacent node(s) to threshold by electrotonic spread of local circuit currents, giving a *saltatory* (from the Latin *saltare*, meaning to dance) conduction along the fiber.

The restriction of Na⁺ channels to the nodes has advantages and liabilities. Less total influx of Na⁺ occurs during impulse propagation along the fiber and thereby reduces metabolic demands on the recovery mechanism (the Na⁺/K⁺ pump).

Generation and Propagation of the Action Potential

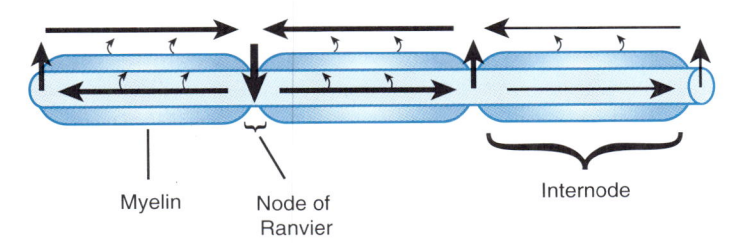

Figure 7-14 ■ Propagation of the action potential in a myelinated axon. Most of the current that enters the axon as Na⁺ current at an active node of Ranvier flows out the axon at adjacent nodes. Very little current flows out of the axon through myelin, in the internodes. As a result, propagation is very fast in the internodal region and the action potential appears to skip, or jump, from node to node.

BOX 7-7

Action Potential Propagation Is Impaired in Multiple Sclerosis

Multiple sclerosis is one of a number of common neurological diseases that are characterized by demyelination, or the loss of the myelin sheath. Demyelination causes a range of abnormalities in action potential propagation in myelinated axons. In some partially demyelinated axons the conduction velocity is decreased and different degrees of slowing can occur among axons within the same nerve tract. In more severely demyelinated axons, complete block of action potential propagation occurs.

What physiological factors contribute to the conduction abnormalities? In regions of demyelination the high-resistance, low-capacitance myelin sheath is disrupted or lost completely. This reduces conduction velocity for two reasons: the reduction in membrane resistance reduces the length constant, and the increased membrane capacitance increases the propagation time constant. These factors can account for the slowing of conduction through demyelinated regions. There is, however, an additional factor: the differences in the distribution of voltage-gated ion channels in nodal and internodal regions of axonal membrane. Voltage-gated Na⁺ channels are present at very high density (about 10,000 per μm^2) in axon membrane at the nodes, in contrast to a very low density (none to 25 per μm^2) in the internodal regions. There is an opposite distribution of voltage-gated K⁺ channels: they are nearly absent at the nodes and present in relatively high density at the internodes. This ion channel distribution helps to explain the loss of action potential propagation through severely demyelinated regions. The Na⁺ channels are not present in high enough density in the internodes to support action potential propagation following demyelination. In addition, the presence of K⁺ channels in the internodes tends to hold the membrane potential close to E_K.

This means, however, that in severe **demyelinating diseases,** such as *multiple sclerosis* (Box 7-7), conduction may not simply slow, but can fail completely. The reason is that the number of Na⁺ channels in the normally myelinated internode regions of the axon is insufficient to maintain action potential propagation when demyelination reduces the length constant and increases the action potential propagation time constant.

■ SUMMARY

1. An action potential is a rapid and transient depolarization of the membrane potential.
2. During an action potential in neurons and other excitable cells, the membrane rapidly increases its permeability to Na^+ ions. This permits Na^+ to flow into the cell and make the inside potential more positive. The Na^+ permeability then falls and the K^+ permeability rises. This allows K^+ to flow out of the cell and return the membrane potential to the resting level. The membrane permeabilities to Na^+ and K^+ are controlled by voltage-gated Na^+ and K^+ channels, respectively.
3. Ion channel properties are studied with a voltage clamp, which allows ionic current to be measured as a function of time at a constant membrane potential. Because ionic currents flow through open ion channels, many of the functional properties of channels can be investigated by analysis of the ionic current.
4. Depolarizing voltage clamp steps generate three separable components of current in nerve axons:
   a. A voltage-independent component, which contains capacitive current and linear ionic current.
   b. Na^+ current flowing through voltage-gated Na^+ channels.
   c. K^+ current flowing through voltage-gated K^+ channels.
5. Voltage-gated Na^+ channels open early during depolarization and then close by inactivating later during depolarization. Voltage-gated K^+ channels open more slowly than Na^+ channels and stay open during the depolarization.
6. The open probability for voltage-gated Na^+ and K^+ channels is both voltage and time dependent.
7. Single ion channels are studied with a patch clamp, which is a variation of the voltage clamp technique. Many single ion channels have two conductance levels: zero when the channel is closed and a constant conductance, γ, when the channel is open.
8. Voltage-gated Na^+ channels have two gates: an activation and an inactivation gate. During depolarization, rapid opening of the activation gate opens the channel. Closure of the more slowly moving inactivation gate then closes the channel by inactivation. Both gates must be open for the channel to conduct Na^+ ions. Closure of either gate closes the channel.
9. Action potential propagation along a nonmyelinated axon occurs by local circuit current flow. Conduction velocity is influenced by the length constant, λ, the time constant, τ, and the Na^+ current, I_{Na}.
10. In myelinated axons, Na^+ channels are located at the nodes of Ranvier. Propagation occurs by local circuit current flow, but the conduction velocity is much faster than in nonmyelinated axons for two reasons. The internodal region has a large length constant because of the large membrane resistance and has a short propagation time constant because of the low membrane capacitance.

■ KEY WORDS AND CONCEPTS

- Action potential
- Threshold
- All-or-none
- Absolute and relative refractory periods
- Voltage clamp
- Ionic currents
- Voltage-gated Na^+ channels
- Voltage-gated K^+ channels
- Inactivation
- Conductance
- Activation and deactivation
- Channel open probability
- Patch clamp

Generation and Propagation of the Action Potential

- Propagation
- Local circuit current
- Conduction velocity
- Propagation time constant (τ_p)
- Nodes of Ranvier
- Demyelinating diseases (e.g., multiple sclerosis)

STUDY PROBLEMS

1. Voltage-gated Na^+ channels in a nerve axon are being studied by recording macroscopic Na^+ currents with a voltage clamp. Assume that all of the Na^+ channels in the membrane are opened with a voltage clamp step to +20 mV, that the peak magnitude of the Na^+ current is -2 mA/cm^2 during this step to +20 mV, and that E_{Na} = +60 mV.
   a. Estimate the maximum Na^+ conductance ($g_{Na,max}$) of this membrane.
   b. Describe $g_{Na,max}$ in terms of single Na^+ channels.
   c. During a voltage clamp step to -20 mV we also measure a Na^+ current with a peak magnitude of -2 mA/cm^2. Estimate the probability that a Na^+ channel is open at -20 mV.
   d. What voltage-dependent property of Na^+ channels is illustrated by the calculations in a to c?
2. a. An action potential is initiated in an axon by passing outward current across the membrane using an external current source. Describe the sequence of events that occurs at the site of initiation of the action potential. Include the role of voltage-gated Na^+ channels, voltage-gated K^+ channels, I_{Na}, I_K, I_C, and inactivation.
   b. The total membrane current (I_m) flowing across the axonal membrane is monitored at a point on the axon several centimeters away from the site of initiation as the action potential propagates past that point. The current consists of an initial phase of outward current, followed by an inward current and finally another phase of outward current. Explain the origin of these currents.
   c. Does the action potential propagate in both directions away from the initiation site? Why?
3. List three factors that can alter the conduction velocity of an action potential in a nerve axon. Describe the change caused by each factor, and explain how it occurs.

■ BIBLIOGRAPHY

Armstrong CM: Voltage-dependent ion channels and their gating, *Physiol Rev* 72:S5, 1992.

Armstrong CM, Bezanilla F: Charge movement associated with the opening and closing of the activation gates of the Na channels, *J Gen Physiol* 63:533, 1974.

Armstrong CM, Binstock L: Anomalous rectification in the squid giant axon injected with tetraethylammonium chloride, *J Gen Physiol* 48:859, 1965.

Armstrong CM, Hille B: Voltage-gated ion channels and electrical excitability, *Neuron* 20:371, 1998.

Cannon SC, Brown RH Jr, Corey DP: A sodium channel defect in hyperkalemic periodic paralysis: potassium-induced failure of inactivation, *Neuron* 6:619, 1991.

Hille B: *Ionic channels of excitable membranes,* ed 3, Sunderland, Mass, 2001, Sinauer.

Hodgkin AL: Chapter 4. In *The conduction of the nervous impulse*, Springfield, Ill, 1964, Charles C Thomas.

Hodgkin AL, Huxley AF: A quantitative description of membrane current and its application to conduction and excitation in nerve, *J Physiol (Lond)* 117:500, 1952.

Hodgkin AL, Huxley AF, Katz B: Measurements of current-voltage relations in the membrane of the giant axon of *Loligo, J Physiol (Lond)* 116:424, 1952.

Narahashi T, Deguchi T, Urakawa N, Ohkubo Y: Stabilization and rectification of muscle fiber membrane by tetrodotoxin, *Am J Physiol* 198:934, 1959.

Rathmayer W: Sea anemone toxins: tools in the study of excitable membranes, *Adv Cytopharmacol* 3:335, 1979.

Rushton WAH: A theory of the effects of fibre size in medulated nerve, *J Physiol (Lond)* 115:101, 1951.

Sigworth FJ, Neher E: Single Na^+ channel currents observed in cultured rat muscle cells, *Nature* 287:447, 1980.

CHAPTER 8

Ion Channel Diversity

Objectives:

1. Compare and contrast the properties of voltage-gated Ca^{2+} and Na^+ channels.
2. Understand the mechanism of action of Ca^{2+} antagonist drugs, and describe their use as therapeutic agents.
3. Describe the role of A-type K^+ channels and Ca^{2+}-activated K^+ channels in regulating the action potential firing pattern in a bursting neuron.
4. Describe the properties of ATP-sensitive K^+ channels, and explain their role in glucose-induced insulin release from pancreatic β-cells.
5. Describe the function of nicotinic acetylcholine (ACh)-gated channels at the neuromuscular junction.
6. Understand how the activation of β-adrenergic receptors modulates Ca^{2+} channel activity and how this modulation enhances force development in the heart.

■ VARIOUS TYPES OF ION CHANNELS HELP TO REGULATE CELLULAR PROCESSES

Ion channels are found in all cells. The properties of voltage-gated Na^+ and K^+ channels in squid giant axons are described in Chapter 7. These channels are essential for generating the action potential in nerve axons and skeletal muscle cells. Many other types of ion channels also play important roles in regulating membrane electrical activity. Table 8-1 lists some examples. Each of the ion channel types is defined by a combination of specific physiological, pharmacological, and structural characteristics. As an example, the characteristics of voltage-gated Na^+ channels in nerve axons include, in part, Na^+ selectivity, voltage-dependent activation, fast inactivation, and high-affinity block by tetrodotoxin. In this chapter we focus on the properties of several physiologically important channels. These examples illustrate the diversity of ion channel types, the variety of roles they play in normal cell function, and their pathophysiology.

■ VOLTAGE-GATED Ca^{2+} CHANNELS CONTRIBUTE TO ELECTRICAL ACTIVITY AND MEDIATE Ca^{2+} ENTRY INTO CELLS

Ion channels that selectively allow Ca^{2+} ions to permeate are of vital importance in the normal

TABLE 8-1
Examples of three classes of ion channels

Channel type	Location	Functions
Voltage-Gated Channels		
Na$^+$ channel	Axon, skeletal muscle	Upstroke of the action potential
K$^+$ channels	Axon, skeletal muscle	Action potential repolarization
Ca^{2+} channels (many types exist)	Heart, nerve terminals, endocrine cells	Inject Ca^{2+} into cells
Ligand-Gated Channels		
Nicotinic acetylcholine (ACh)-receptor channel	Neuromuscular junction, neurons	Synaptic transmission
Glutamate receptor channels	Neurons	Synaptic transmission
γ-Aminobutyric acid (GABA) receptor channel	Neurons	Synaptic transmission
Ca-activated K$^+$ channel	Almost all excitable cells	Regulate burst length
Other Channels		
ATP-sensitive K$^+$ channel	Pancreas, heart, smooth muscle	Glucose sensor in β-cells
Inward rectifier K$^+$ channel	Heart, brain, skeletal muscle	Permit long depolarizations
Two-pore K$^+$ channel	All cells	Regulate resting potential

functioning of nearly all cells. All excitable cells have Ca^{2+} channels. In some cells, **voltage-gated Ca^{2+} channels** can generate action potentials in the absence of Na$^+$ channels. However, in many cells that express both voltage-gated Na$^+$ and Ca^{2+} channels, Ca^{2+} channel activity modifies the shape of the action potential. Ca^{2+} channels contribute to the action potentials generated in the heart (Figure 8-1), some endocrine cells (e.g., pancreatic β-cells), and specific regions of neurons (e.g., dendrites and nerve terminals).

Ca^{2+} channels influence a wide range of cellular activities by allowing Ca^{2+} ions to enter the cell. The extracellular free Ca^{2+} concentration is about 1 mM (10^{-3} M), while the intracellular free Ca^{2+} concentration ([Ca^{2+}]$_i$) is normally about 0.0001 mM (10^{-7} M). This means that the Ca^{2+} equilibrium potential (E_{Ca}) is approximately +120 mV. Therefore, when a Ca^{2+} channel opens, Ca^{2+} ions flow into the cell down their electrochemical gradient. Because [Ca^{2+}]$_i$ is normally very low, a relatively small influx of Ca^{2+} can produce a significant increase in [Ca^{2+}]$_i$. Intracellular Ca^{2+} ions directly regulate secretion, contraction, energy metabolism, ion channel activity, and numerous other processes.

Several distinct types of Ca^{2+} channels have been identified based on their physiological and pharmacological properties (Box 8-1 and Table 8-2). Indeed, several Ca^{2+} channel mutations have been identified that are associated with hereditary diseases. One example is X-linked congenital stationary night blindness. This is caused by loss-of-function mutations in the L-type **Ca^{2+} channel subtype** that is expressed in photoreceptors (Box 8-2).

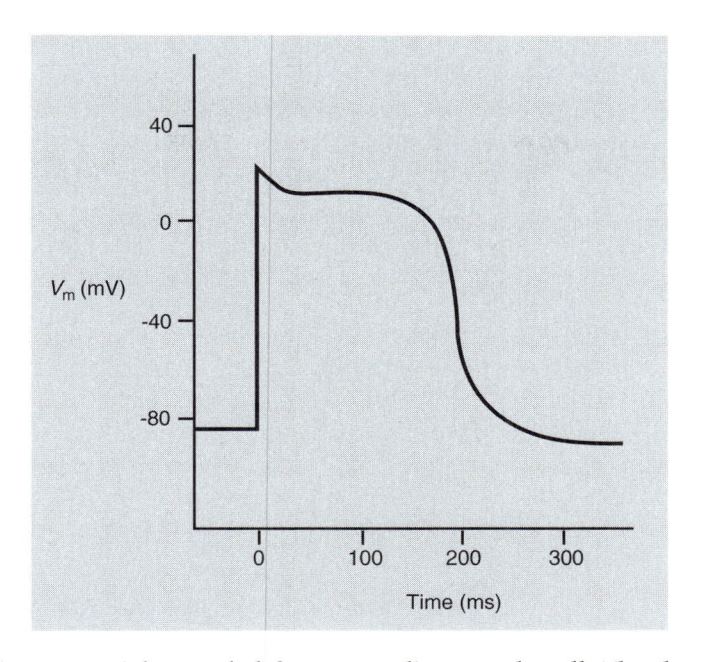

Figure 8-1 ■ An action potential recorded from a cardiac muscle cell. The duration of the action potential in ventricular muscle cells is hundreds of times longer than the action potential in a nerve axon (see Figure 7-1). Calcium influx through voltage-gated Ca^{2+} channels contributes to the long duration of these action potentials. (Modified from Berne RM, Levy MN: *Cardiovascular physiology*, ed 8, St Louis, 2001, Mosby.)

Calcium Currents Can Be Recorded with a Voltage Clamp

Voltage-gated Ca^{2+} channels can be studied with the voltage clamp. Whole-cell currents recorded from a neuronal cell body with a voltage clamp are shown in Figure 8-2. With K^+ channels blocked, a depolarizing voltage clamp step evokes an inward current that has both a fast transient component and a more sustained component. The fast, transient component of the current is generated by Na^+ channels. When external Na^+ is removed, the Na^+ channels no longer conduct inward current (because there are no Na^+ ions to flow into the cell), and the remaining inward current is carried by Ca^{2+} ions flowing into the cell through voltage-gated Ca^{2+} channels (Figure 8-2). The Ca^{2+} channels activate more slowly than Na^+ channels. Furthermore, the magnitude of the Ca^{2+} current decreases very slowly over tens of milliseconds. This indicates that Ca^{2+} channels inactivate slowly (much more slowly than Na^+ channels). Inactivation also is incomplete, so that Ca^{2+} current can continue to flow during maintained depolarization. The maximum amplitude of the Ca^{2+} current (about 100 $\mu A/cm^2$ of membrane area) is usually smaller than the Na^+ or K^+ currents in axons.

The relationship between Ca^{2+} channel open probability and membrane potential is similar to that for voltage-gated Na^+ channels, except that the channels activate over a more depolarized voltage range. In some cell types, voltage-gated

> ### BOX 8-1
>
> #### Types of Voltage-Gated Ca^{2+} Channels
>
> Multiple types of voltage-gated Ca^{2+} channels have been identified on the basis of physiological and pharmacological criteria. These include the following.
>
> #### L Type
>
> The L type is the major type of Ca^{2+} channel in muscle cells (cardiac, smooth, and skeletal). L-type Ca^{2+} current is characterized by a relatively high voltage for activation, fast deactivation, slow voltage-dependent inactivation, a large single-channel conductance, modulation by cAMP-dependent phosphorylation, and inhibition by dihydropyridines, phenylalkylamines, and benzothiazepines. These Ca^{2+} channels are called L-type channels because of their *l*arge conductance (25 pS) and *l*ong-lasting single-channel open times.
>
> #### T Type
>
> In comparison with L-type Ca^{2+} currents, T-type currents activate at more negative voltages, have fast voltage-dependent inactivation, have slow deactivation, have a small single-channel conductance (8 pS), and are insensitive to the drugs that block L-type channels. They are named T type for their *t*iny single channel conductance and their *t*ransient kinetics.
>
> #### N Type
>
> N-type Ca^{2+} currents were first identified by their intermediate voltage-dependence and intermediate inactivation kinetics. The channels are insensitive to the L-type Ca^{2+} channel blockers but are blocked selectively by a cone snail peptide toxin, ω-conotoxin GVIA. They were called N type because they were *n*either L type nor T type.
>
> #### P/Q Type
>
> P-type Ca^{2+} currents were first recorded in cerebellar Purkinje cells and are blocked selectively by the spider toxin, ω-agatoxin IVA. Q-type Ca^{2+} currents were first recorded in cerebellar granule cells and have a lower affinity for ω-agatoxin IVA.

TABLE 8-2

Voltage-gated Ca^{2+} channel subtypes

Ca^{2+} current type	Location	Specific blocker	Function
L	Cardiac muscle, endocrine cells	Dihydropyridines	Excitation-contraction coupling, hormone secretion
P/Q	Nerve terminals	ω-Agatoxin IVA	Neurotransmitter release
N	Nerve terminals	ω-Conotoxin-GVIA	Neurotransmitter release
R	Neurons	SNX482	Neurotransmitter release
T	Heart, neurons	Mibefradil	Pacemaker currents

Ca^{2+} channels can generate action potentials in a manner similar to Na^+ channels. A depolarizing stimulus opens Ca^{2+} channels, and Ca^{2+} ions flow into the cell down their electrochemical gradient. This Ca^{2+} current further depolarizes the cell and opens more channels. The positive feedback of membrane depolarization on channel opening produces the action potential upstroke. Compared with axonal action potentials generated by Na^+ channels, pure Ca^{2+} action

BOX 8-2

X-Linked Congenital Stationary Night Blindness Is Caused by a Loss of Function Mutation in the Photoreceptor L-Type Ca^{2+} Channel

X-linked congenital stationary night blindness (CSNB) is a recessive retinal abnormality characterized by night blindness, decreased visual acuity, and myopia. Two distinct clinical types are observed, and they exhibit different photoreceptor (rod and cone) abnormalities. With *complete* CSNB the rods are completely nonfunctional and the cones are normal. With *incomplete* CSNB, function of both rods and cones is depressed but measurable. The disorder is caused by mutations in retina-specific L-type Ca^{2+} channels (different isoforms of the L-type Ca^{2+} channel are expressed in different cell types). In incomplete CSNB, mutations in the L-type Ca^{2+} channels in both rods and cones result in reduced activity of Ca^{2+} channels. The consequent reduction in Ca^{2+} entry decreases the tonic release of the neurotransmitter glutamate from photoreceptor nerve terminals. As a result, synaptic transmission from the photoreceptors to the second-order bipolar cells is inhibited. The bipolar cell is an interneuron that transmits information from photoreceptors to ganglion cells, and axons of the ganglion cells form the optic nerve. Thus the reduction in glutamate release from photoreceptors results in decreased output from the optic nerve, which helps to explain the visual defects that characterize CSNB.

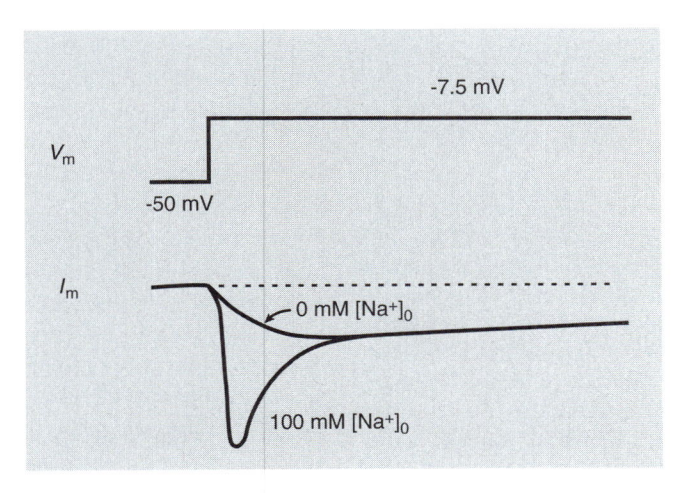

Figure 8-2 ■ Calcium and sodium currents recorded from the same neuron during a voltage clamp step (V_m) from −50 mV to −7.5 mV. With 100 mM $[Na^+]_o$ there are two current components: (1) a fast, transient inward current that is generated by voltage-gated Na^+ channels, and (2) a steady inward current that remains after removal of the external Na^+ (0 mM $[Na^+]_o$). Voltage-gated Ca^{2+} channels generate the second component. (From Kostyuk PG, Kristhal OA, Shakhovalov YA: *J Physiol [Lond]* 270:545, 1977.)

potentials have slower upstrokes and longer durations because the Ca^{2+} channels activate more slowly than Na^+ channels and inactivation is slow and incomplete.

Ca^{2+} Channel Blockers Are Useful Therapeutic Agents

Various drugs reduce Ca^{2+} currents by blocking voltage-gated Ca^{2+} channels. These **Ca^{2+} antagonist drugs** include phenylalkylamines (e.g., verapamil and its methoxy derivative known as D600 or gallopamil), benzothiazepines (e.g., diltiazem), and the dihydropyridine derivatives (e.g., nifedipine, nimodipine, and nicardipine). At physiological pH, D600 and diltiazem are protonated and therefore positively charged, whereas nifedipine is uncharged. These drugs selectively block L-type Ca^{2+} channels (Box 8-1).

Ca^{2+} channel blockers are widely used as therapeutic agents in the management of coronary artery disease, hypertension, and cardiac arrhythmias (Box 8-3). Some properties of the block produced by Ca^{2+} antagonist drugs are shown in Figure 8-3. The data in Figure 8-3, *A*, illustrate the effect of repetitive depolarizations on the development of block by the charged compound D600. Very little reduction in I_{Ca} occurs in response to the first stimulus after D600 is added (Figure 8-3, *A*). Subsequent depolarizations, however, produce smaller and smaller Ca^{2+} currents. This behavior is called **use-dependent block** of the Ca^{2+} channels. In contrast, uncharged drugs, such as nifedipine, block Ca^{2+} channels without requiring depolarization; that is, they produce a significant degree of *tonic* block and very little use-dependent block. Diltiazem is intermediate between D600 and nifedipine in its use dependence. Use-dependent block by charged drugs is explained by the idea that the activation gate in the channel must open before charged drug molecules can gain access to the blocking site (Figure 8-3, *B*).

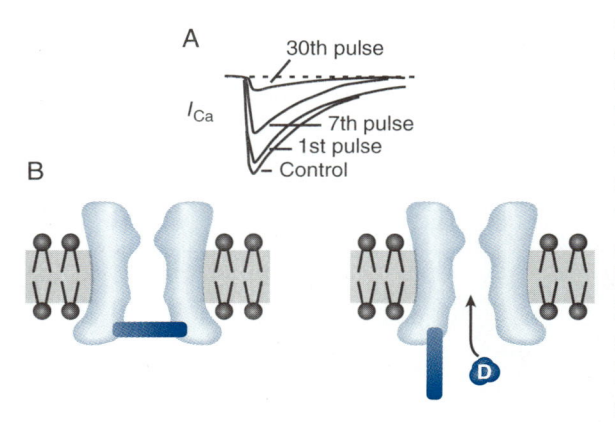

Figure 8-3 ■ Ca^{2+} channel block by D600. A, Ca^{2+} currents were recorded during 120-msec voltage clamp steps to +20 mV. The trace-labeled control was recorded before the addition of D600. The remaining traces were obtained in the presence of D600 by use of a series of voltage clamp pulses (to +20 mV) delivered at the rate of three pulses per minute. Little block occurs in the absence of pulses, but blockade becomes progressively larger with repeated depolarizations. This type of channel inhibition is called use-dependent block. B, Use-dependent block by D600 will occur if the drug cannot gain access to its binding site when the channel activation gate is closed. When the gate opens, D600 *(D)* can enter the inner vestibule of the channel, bind to its receptor, and block the channel. (**A** modified from Lee KS, Tsien RW: *Nature* 302:790, 1983.)

■ POTASSIUM-SELECTIVE CHANNELS ARE THE MOST DIVERSE TYPE OF CHANNEL

Potassium-selective ion channels are found in all cells. They are very diverse in their activity, structure, and distribution. For example, potassium channels are important in regulating cell volume, insulin secretion, heart rate, neuronal excitability, neuronal firing patterns, and epithelial transport (see Chapter 11).

The first K^+ channel gene was cloned from the *Shaker* mutant of the fruit fly, *Drosophila*, in 1987. Since then, more than 200 genes

BOX 8-3

Ca^{2+} Antagonist Drugs Are Used as Therapeutic Agents

The force generated by contracting cardiac or vascular smooth muscle cells depends on [Ca^{2+}]$_i$. A major pathway for Ca^{2+} entry into these cells is through voltage-gated Ca^{2+} channels. Thus block of Ca^{2+} channels with a Ca^{2+} antagonist drug decreases Ca^{2+} entry into the cell and thereby decreases the force of contraction. The relaxation of vascular smooth muscle results in arterial vasodilation. This effect underlies the rationale for using Ca^{2+} channel blockers to treat hypertension (high blood pressure). Chronic hypertension is the result of increased vascular resistance. Ca^{2+} channel blockers reduce blood pressure by relaxing arteriolar smooth muscle and decreasing vascular resistance. Ca^{2+} antagonists are also used in the treatment of angina pectoris (chest pain arising from inadequate blood supply to heart muscle). The benefits may result from coronary artery dilation (and consequently increased blood supply) or from decreased myocardial oxygen consumption that is secondary to decreased cardiac contractility.

TABLE 8-3

Potassium channel types and associated heritable diseases

Type	Nomenclature	Genetic disorder
Voltage-gated (Shaker)	Kv1.1-1.7	Episodic ataxia*
Shab, Shaw, Shal	Kv2.1-Kv6.1	
Human *ether-a-go-go*	hERG	Long QT syndrome†
KvLQT1	KCNQ1	Long QT syndrome
Inward rectifier	Kir1.1-Kir7.1	Bartter's syndrome (see Chapter 11)
Large conductance Ca^{2+} activated	Slo, BK$_{Ca}$	
Small conductance Ca^{2+} activated	SK1-SK3	
Two pore	TWIK1, TREK, TASK, TRAAK	
Sulfonylurea receptor	SUR1	Persistent hyperinsulinemic hypoglycemia of infancy

*Episodic ataxia is an autosomal dominant disease characterized by hyperexcitability in motor neurons. Exercise may provoke attacks of atactic (uncoordinated) walking and jerking movements that can last minutes.
†Long QT syndrome is a group of disorders characterized by a long QT interval in the electrocardiogram, indicating delayed repolarization of the ventricles. It can be associated with lightheadedness or sudden death caused by cardiac arrhythmias.

(including more than 50 human genes) have been identified that encode various types of K$^+$ channels (Table 8-3 and Box 8-4). Recent genetic advances have led to the identification of naturally occurring K$^+$ channel mutations that are associated with a variety of diseases.

Neuronal K+ Channel Diversity Contributes to the Regulation of Action Potential Firing Patterns

One of the most important ways that information is encoded in the nervous system is in the temporal pattern of action potentials. The

BOX 8-4

Potassium Channels Are Structurally and Functionally Diverse

More than 200 genes have been cloned that encode the pore-forming subunit of various types of K$^+$ channels. Each functional K$^+$ channel is composed of four such subunits. All of the channels have a homologous pore-forming region that selectively allows passage of K$^+$ ions. As a result of other structural homologies, the channels can be classified into three families based on the number of hydrophobic transmembrane α-helical segments that are present (see Chapter 5):

1. Channels with six transmembrane α-helical segments. Included in this family are the voltage-gated K$^+$ channels (the Kv channels in Table 8-2), human *ether-a-go-go* (hERG), Ca^{2+}-activated K$^+$ channels, and KCNQ channels. Voltage-gated K$^+$ channels in nerve axons contribute to the repolarization of the action potential (see Chapter 7).

2. Channels with two transmembrane α-helical segments. The inward rectifier K$^+$ channels (Kir1.1-Kir7.1) all have two transmembrane segments with a pore-forming loop between them. The inward rectifiers have a much larger conductance for inward current than for outward current. An example is the K$_{ATP}$ channel in pancreatic β-cells. This channel is composed of four Kir6.2 inward rectifier subunits and four SUR1 sulfonylurea receptors.

3. Channels with four transmembrane α-helical segments and two pore domains. TWIK, TREK, TASK, and TRAAK are recently discovered genes that form channels containing two pore regions. These channels are believed to play a role in setting the resting membrane potential.

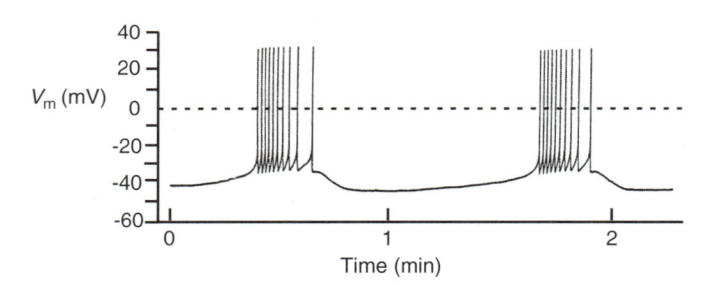

Figure 8-4 ■ Spontaneous bursts of action potentials generated by a neuron. The membrane potential in this cell alternates between a quiet period near −40 mV and an active period containing a high-frequency burst of about 10 action potentials. During the quiet period the cell slowly depolarizes toward the threshold for initiation of an action potential. (From Hille B: *Ionic channels of excitable membranes,* ed 2, Sunderland, Mass, 1991, Sinauer.)

simplest form of encoding involves variations in action potential frequency. Indeed, some cells generate complex patterns of action potentials, such as the *high-frequency bursts* shown in Figure 8-4. In most neurons the cell body is responsible for initiating the action potential.

The cell body and dendrites integrate a large number of electrical inputs that either depolarize or hyperpolarize the cell; when threshold is reached, an action potential is generated. Two populations of ion channels in axons, voltage-gated Na$^+$ channels and one type of voltage-gated

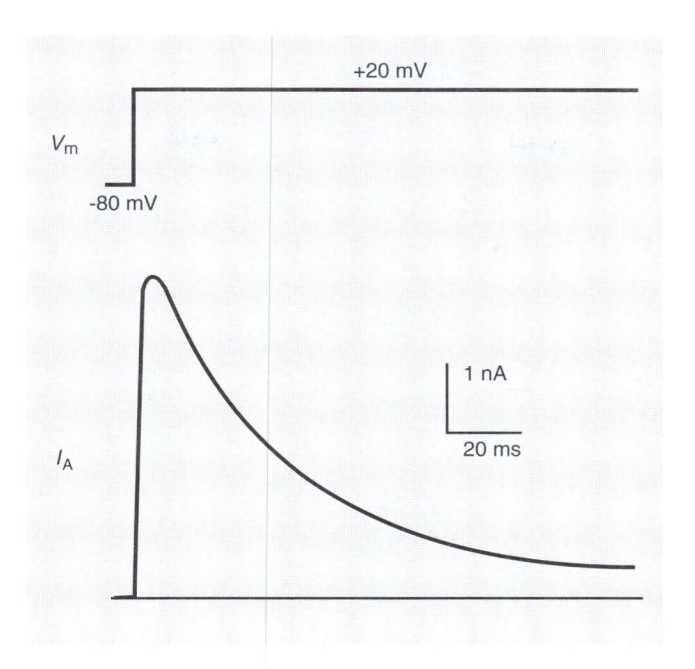

Ion Channel Diversity

Figure 8-5 ■ An outward K$^+$ current through K$_A$ channels (I_A) during a depolarizing voltage clamp step. The channels open, or activate, in a few milliseconds following the depolarization. Over the next 100 to 200 msec, the current decreases in size as the K$_A$ channels inactivate.

K$^+$ channel, are responsible for action potential propagation (see Chapter 7). Through these channels the axon can faithfully transmit to the nerve terminals an action potential initiated at the cell body. In contrast, the cell body often contains many other types of ion channels that contribute significantly to the regulation of action potential firing patterns. We now consider two such channels: rapidly inactivating voltage-gated K$^+$ channels and Ca^{2+}-activated K$^+$ channels.

Rapidly Inactivating Voltage-Gated K$^+$ Channels Cause Delays in Action Potential Generation

Many neurons contain a population of K$^+$ channels that generate *transient* outward K$^+$ currents (Figure 8-5). For historical reasons these currents are called A-currents (I_A); we will therefore refer to the channels that produce these currents as **K$_A$ channels.** In response to a depolarizing voltage clamp step, K$_A$ channels activate relatively rapidly, in a few milliseconds, and then inactivate over tens of milliseconds during the maintained depolarization (Figure 8-5). The overall time course of these transient K$^+$ currents resembles that of voltage-dependent Na$^+$ currents, although the absolute rate of K$_A$ channel gating is about 10 times slower than Na$^+$ channel gating.

Steady-state activation and inactivation curves for K$_A$ channels are shown in Figure 8-6. K$_A$ channels inactivate over a relatively negative range of membrane potentials. The resting potential of many neurons can vary from about –50 to –75 mV. Over this range of membrane

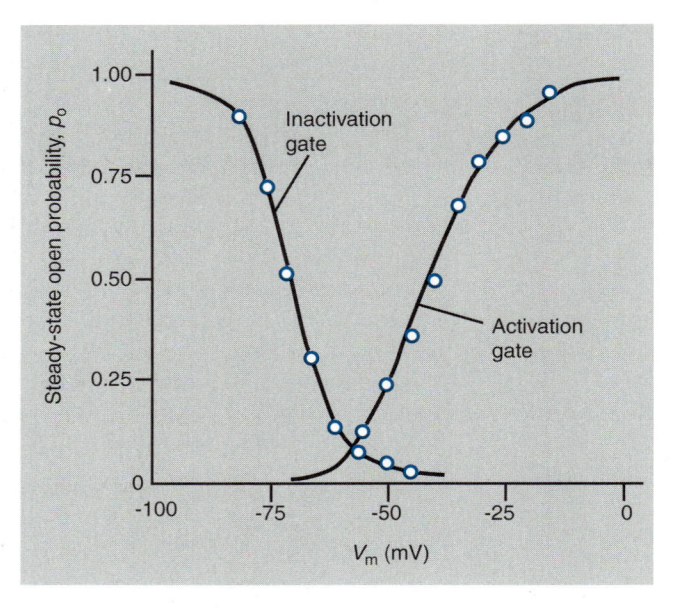

Figure 8-6 ■ Steady-state activation and inactivation curves for K_A channels. The curves show the probability that the activation or inactivation gate is open in the steady state. K_A channels activate and inactivate over a relatively negative voltage range when compared with the Na^+ and K^+ channels in nerve axons (see Figure 7-6). (Modified from Hille B: *Ionic channels of excitable membranes,* ed 2, Sunderland, Mass, 1991, Sinauer.)

---

potentials, there is a significant change in the number of K_A channels that are inactivated (Figure 8-6). If the cell's resting potential is −50 mV, most K_A channels are inactivated. If the resting potential is more negative, fewer K_A channels are inactivated, so more noninactivated channels are available to regulate subsequent electrical activity.

Neurons often fire action potentials repetitively, and by doing so they can encode information in the spike frequency. K_A channels are found in neuronal cell bodies where they help to regulate the rate of repetitive action potential firing. The outward current through open K_A channels produces a delay in the approach toward action potential threshold. This can be demonstrated by pharmacological blocking of K_A channels. Figure 8-7 illustrates the effect of blocking K_A channels on action potential generation. The neuron is stimulated by injection of a constant depolarizing current. The depolarization causes the cell to fire an action potential. After the action potential, the maintained stimulation again causes the cell to depolarize. K_A channels now open in response to this depolarization. The increase in outward I_A opposes the inward stimulus current, and the rate of depolarization is slowed. Only a single action potential is generated during the 50-msec stimulus under control conditions (Figure 8-7). When the K_A channels are blocked with 4-aminopyridine (4-AP), the reduced I_A is less effective in opposing the inward stimulus current. As a result, depolarization is faster and

Ion Channel Diversity

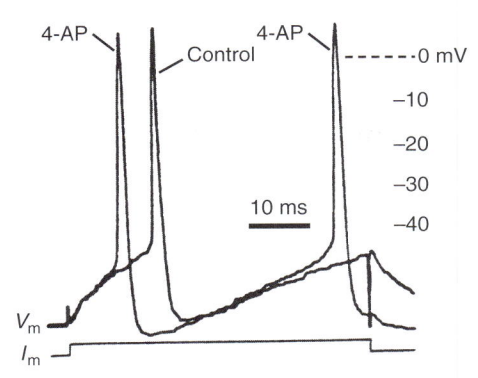

Figure 8-7 ■ K_A channels regulate the frequency of action potentials in some neurons. This figure shows the response of a hippocampal neuron to a 50-msec depolarizing current pulse. The control response shows a single action potential generated during the stimulus. In the presence of 5 mM 4-aminopyridine, which blocks K_A channels, the threshold is reached earlier, the latency to the first action potential is reduced, and a second action potential is generated during the stimulus. (From Segal M, Rogawski MA, Barker JL: *J Neurosci* 4:604, 1984.)

a second action potential is generated before the end of the stimulus. Thus K_A channel activity can regulate the interval between action potentials in a burst.

Ca^{2+}-Activated K^+ Channels Are Opened by Intracellular Ca^{2+}

K^+-selective channels that are opened, at least in part, by intracellular Ca^{2+} are found in almost all excitable cells. There are three subtypes of **Ca^{2+}-activated K^+ channels:** large, intermediate, and small conductance channels. Here we consider only the large conductance (**BK_{Ca}**) **channel**, whose single-channel conductance is one of the largest (>200 pS). The probability that a BK_{Ca} channel is open depends not only on $[Ca^{2+}]_i$, but also on the membrane potential (Figure 8-8). At −50 mV, in the presence of 1 μM $[Ca^{2+}]_i$, the channels are closed almost all of the time. If $[Ca^{2+}]_i$ is raised to 100 μM and the membrane potential is held constant at −50 mV, channel openings increase dramatically (Figure 8-8, *B*). If $[Ca^{2+}]_i$ is held at 1 μM, changing the membrane potential from −50 mV to +50 mV opens nearly all of the BK_{Ca} channels (Figure 8-8, *A*). Thus the open probability of BK_{Ca} channels depends on both the membrane potential and $[Ca^{2+}]_i$. The increase in $[Ca^{2+}]_i$ that potentiates or triggers the opening of BK_{Ca} channels could result from Ca^{2+} entry through Ca^{2+} channels near the BK_{Ca} channels or from Ca^{2+} release by intracellular stores. In arteriolar smooth muscle cells, Ca^{2+} release from the sarcoplasmic reticulum opens BK_{Ca} channels in the plasma membrane and causes membrane hyperpolarization, relaxation of the smooth muscle, and dilation of the arteriole (see Chapter 13).

In cells that generate bursts of action potentials such as certain neurons and pancreatic β-cells, K_{Ca} channels play a role in regulating the burst pattern. During a burst of action potentials, Ca^{2+} ions enter the cell through voltage-gated Ca^{2+} channels that open during the action potentials. This Ca^{2+} influx can produce a significant increase in $[Ca^{2+}]_i$. The increase in $[Ca^{2+}]_i$ activates K_{Ca} channels, and the outward K^+ current through these channels hyperpolarizes the cell and terminates the burst.

ATP-Sensitive K^+ Channels Are Involved in Glucose-Induced Insulin Secretion from Pancreatic β-Cells

The β-cells in the islets of Langerhans in the endocrine pancreas play a critical role in the regulation of the plasma glucose concentration. The β-cell secretes the hormone insulin in response to increased plasma levels of glucose. This normally occurs immediately after a meal, when glucose and other nutrients are absorbed from the gastrointestinal tract. Insulin stimulates the uptake, metabolism, and storage of glucose in muscle and fat cells. Thus glucose and insulin

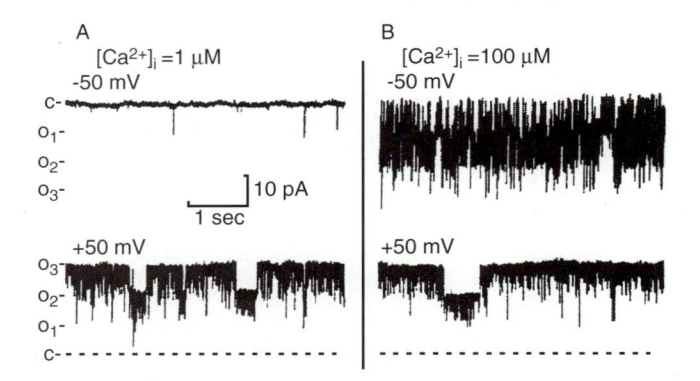

Figure 8-8 ■ BK_{Ca} channels are opened by elevation of $[Ca^{2+}]$ and by depolarization. These single-channel patch clamp recordings were obtained from an isolated patch of skeletal muscle membrane in which the former inside (cytosolic) surface of the membrane is exposed to the bathing solution. The K^+ concentrations on the two sides of the membrane are the same (so that $E_K = 0$ mV). This patch contained 3 BK_{Ca} channels, and the current levels corresponding to all channels closed (c) or to one, two, or three channels open (o_1, o_2, and o_3 respectively) are indicated at the left-hand side of the figure. A, With 1 μM Ca^{2+} at the cytosolic surface of the membrane, the BK_{Ca} channels are closed most of the time at −50 mV and are open most of the time at +50 mV. B, With 100 μM Ca^{2+} at the cytosolic surface of the membrane, channel openings are frequent even at −50 mV. Note that the current is inward at −50 mV and outward at +50 mV because of the difference in the driving force ($V_m - E_K$) at these two membrane potentials. (From Barrett JN, Magleby KL, Pallotta BS: *J Physiol [Lond]* 331:211, 1982.)

are involved in a negative feedback system that regulates the plasma glucose concentration. When the plasma glucose level rises, insulin is secreted by the pancreas. Insulin then stimulates the uptake and storage of glucose, and as a result, the plasma glucose level falls.

The ATP-sensitive K^+ (K_{ATP}) channel in the pancreatic β-cell plays an important role in linking the glucose concentration, via cellular metabolism, to β-cell electrical activity and insulin secretion. The K_{ATP} channel is blocked by a high concentration of intracellular ATP ($[ATP]_i$). When the plasma glucose concentration rises, glucose is transported into the β-cell (by the GLUT-2 transporter; see Chapter 10), and glucose metabolism results in an increase in $[ATP]_i$. This closes K_{ATP} channels and thus reduces membrane K^+ permeability. As a result of the reduced K^+ permeability, the β-cell depolarizes and generates bursts of action potentials (Figure 8-9). Voltage-gated Ca^{2+} channels are activated during this glucose-induced electrical activity, and Ca^{2+} ions enter the cell through the open Ca^{2+} channels. The resulting increase in $[Ca^{2+}]_i$ activates insulin secretion. Thus the β-cell K_{ATP} channel plays a critical role in glucose-induced insulin secretion and consequently the regulation of the plasma glucose concentration. Sulfonylureas, such as glibenclamide, selectively block K_{ATP} channels and thereby enhance insulin secretion. For this reason sulfonylureas are used in the treatment of **type II diabetes mellitus** (Box 8-5). Loss-of-function mutations of the K_{ATP} channel cause a metabolic disease, familial persistent hyperinsulinemic hypoglycemia of infancy (Box 8-6).

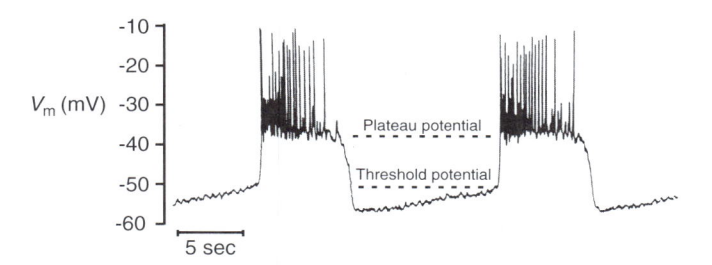

Figure 8-9 ■ Glucose-induced bursts of action potentials in a pancreatic β-cell. In the presence of elevated extracellular glucose levels ([glucose]$_o$ >7 mM), β-cells generate bursts of action potentials. Starting from a negative membrane potential of about −55 mV, the membrane potential slowly depolarizes. When threshold is reached, the cell rapidly depolarizes to a plateau at about −35 mV. At the plateau a burst of small-amplitude action potentials is generated. After a few seconds the burst terminates, the membrane repolarizes, and the cycle repeats. The rate of depolarization (from the resting potential) and the frequency and duration of the bursts, which trigger insulin secretion, are directly related to [glucose]$_o$. (From Ashcroft FM, Rorsman P: *Prog Biophys Molec Biol* 54:87, 1989.)

BOX 8-5

Non-Insulin-Dependent Diabetes Mellitus (Type II Diabetes) Can Be Treated with Sulfonylurea Drugs

Diabetes mellitus is a disease characterized by insulin deficiency or by decreased receptor sensitivity to insulin. Diabetes is a heterogeneous disease, but all forms have in common the diagnostic features hyperglycemia, polyuria, and polydipsia. Hyperglycemia, or high plasma glucose concentration, occurs because glucose uptake and metabolism in peripheral tissues are reduced. Polyuria, or excessive urine production, occurs because the kidneys cannot reabsorb all of the filtered glucose and the glucose in the urine acts as an osmotic diuretic. This diuresis causes dehydration and increased thirst, or polydipsia.

The two main types of diabetes are insulin-dependent diabetes mellitus (IDDM) and non-insulin-dependent diabetes mellitus (NIDDM).

NIDDM, which is also called type II diabetes, affects about 14 million people in the United States and is usually associated with obesity. In contrast to patients with IDDM, those with NIDDM do not usually require exogenous insulin. This form of the disease is often associated with a decreased receptor sensitivity to insulin and a decreased insulin secretion from β-cells. Sulfonylurea drugs (e.g., tolbutamide, glibenclamide) stimulate insulin secretion and are commonly used in the treatment of NIDDM. The sulfonylurea receptor is part of the K$_{ATP}$ channel, and binding of the drug closes the channel. This leads to depolarization, bursts of action potentials, and enhanced insulin secretion.

■ LIGAND-GATED CHANNELS ARE GATED BY AGONIST BINDING

Neurons transfer information to other cells at specialized junctions called *synapses*. At chemical synapses the two cells are separated by a narrow extracellular space, the synaptic cleft. (At electrical synapses there is electrical continuity from one cell to the other through gap junction channels that connect the two cells.)

> **BOX 8-6**
>
> ### Familial Persistent Hyperinsulinemic Hypoglycemia of Infancy Is Due to Loss-of-Function Mutations in K_{ATP} Channels
>
> Familial hyperinsulinism is a rare autosomal recessive disorder characterized by severe hypoglycemia caused by continuous, unregulated insulin secretion. Symptoms of the disease, which is referred to as persistent hyperinsulinemic hypoglycemia of infancy (PHHI), include lethargy, poor feeding, high-pitched cry, irritability, and convulsions. If the disease is untreated, neurological damage and mental retardation can occur. Milder forms of the disease are often successfully treated with intravenous glucose or with drugs that inhibit insulin secretion (e.g., diazoxide, which opens K_{ATP} channels). More severe forms necessitate near-total pancreatectomy to control the hypoglycemia. After pancreatectomy, growth and development are normal but insulin-dependent diabetes sometimes develops because of the loss of too many β-cells.
>
> Mutations of the K_{ATP} channel are implicated in PHHI. A number of distinct mutations have been reported, all of which result in loss of function of the K_{ATP} channels in pancreatic β-cells. As a result, the β-cells generate bursts of action potentials continuously, even when the plasma glucose concentration is very low (hypoglycemia). Thus insulin is secreted continuously.

An action potential in the *presynaptic* neuron causes neurotransmitter molecules to be released. The neurotransmitter diffuses across the synaptic cleft and binds to specific receptors on the *postsynaptic* cell. This causes ion channels in the postsynaptic membrane to open and change the excitability of the postsynaptic cell.

Ion channels that open after the binding of a neurotransmitter or other chemical activator are called **ligand-gated ion channels.** Different channels can be opened by acetylcholine (ACh), γ-aminobutyric acid (GABA), glutamate, or glycine. Glutamate and ACh channels pass inward currents that move the membrane potential toward the action potential threshold and are therefore *excitatory* channels. In contrast, GABA and glycine open channels that are selectively permeable to Cl⁻. These are *inhibitory* ion channels because E_{Cl} is close to the resting potential (V_{rest}) in most neurons. In this case the increased membrane conductance (a Cl⁻ conductance, g_{Cl}) helps to "clamp" the membrane potential close to V_{rest}, making it more difficult for inward current to depolarize the cell.

Acetylcholine Opens Channels at the Neuromuscular Junction

The synapse formed between a spinal motor neuron and a skeletal muscle fiber is called the *neuromuscular junction*. Studies of neuromuscular transmission have provided much information about the operation of chemical synapses. When an action potential in the motor neuron reaches the nerve terminals, voltage-gated Ca^{2+} channels open and Ca^{2+} ions enter the presynaptic nerve terminals. The increase in $[Ca^{2+}]_i$ causes *quanta*, or packets, of ACh, each containing about 10,000 molecules of ACh, to be released into the synaptic cleft. The ACh diffuses to the postsynaptic membrane where it binds to receptors on **ACh-gated ion channels.** These channels are normally closed in the absence of ACh. Channel opening is a multistep process. First, the neurotransmitter binds to a receptor site on the channel (actually, two molecules of ACh must bind). Ligand binding is followed by a conformational change in the channel protein that opens the channel. The open ion channel allows ionic current to flow into the cell. This current depolarizes the skeletal muscle cell toward threshold for action potential generation. Stimulation of a single motor axon normally releases enough ACh to evoke an action potential in all the muscle cells it innervates. The skeletal muscle action potential is generated by increases first in g_{Na} and then in g_K, just as in the nerve axon (see Chapter 7). A number of heritable diseases involve defects in neuromuscular transmission. Some of the inherited diseases result from defects in the ACh channel (Box 8-7).

■ ION CHANNEL ACTIVITY CAN BE REGULATED BY SECOND-MESSENGER PATHWAYS

The activity of many ion channels can be modulated by a variety of intracellular second messengers. Second messengers are diffusible intracellular molecules that undergo a concentration change as a result of neurotransmitter or hormone action. The cyclic adenosine monophosphate (cAMP) system is a typical second-messenger pathway. The membrane-bound enzyme adenylyl cyclase converts ATP to cAMP and is activated by transmitter binding to a coupled receptor (e.g., the β-adrenergic receptor activates adenylyl cyclase). The main effect of cAMP in most cells is to activate the cAMP-dependent protein kinase (PKA). The activated kinase can then phosphorylate ion channels or other proteins and thereby change their activity to produce a cellular response.

β-Adrenergic Receptor Activation Modulates L-Type Ca^{2+} Channels in Cardiac Muscle

Heart muscle cell membranes contain a number of hormone and neurotransmitter receptors that play a role in regulating the activity of the heart. One such receptor, the β-adrenergic receptor, is activated by circulating epinephrine or by norepinephrine released from sympathetic nerve endings. Activation of cardiac β-adrenergic receptors causes an increase in the duration of the cardiac action potential and increased cardiac contractility (i.e., an increase in the force generated by contracting heart muscle; see Chapter 13). These effects result from enhanced Ca^{2+} entry into the cell through voltage-gated L-type Ca^{2+} channels. Voltage clamp experiments show that the amplitude of cardiac Ca^{2+} currents is increased in the presence of β-adrenergic agonists. The enhanced I_{Ca} prolongs the duration of the cardiac action potential. This, in turn, allows the Ca^{2+} channels to stay open longer, resulting in a larger influx of Ca^{2+} ions. The increase in [Ca^{2+}]$_i$ causes a more complete activation of the contractile machinery and a larger resultant force (see Chapter 13).

The β-adrenergic enhancement of I_{Ca} in the heart is mediated by the second messenger cAMP. The β-adrenergic receptor is coupled to the membrane-bound enzyme adenylate cyclase, which catalyzes the conversion of ATP to cAMP. β-Adrenergic receptor activation increases the activity of adenylyl cyclase, and this results in an increase in the cytosolic cAMP concentration, [cAMP]$_i$. The increase in [cAMP]$_i$ activates cAMP-dependent protein kinase, which then phosphorylates the Ca^{2+} channel. Two factors contribute to the increase in I_{Ca} that results from channel phosphorylation: (1) the number of *functional* Ca^{2+} channels that can be activated by depolarization increases, and (2) the probability of channel opening at a given voltage increases. Thus, after activation of β-adrenergic receptors, the number of functional Ca^{2+} channels in the cardiac cell membrane is greater and, when the membrane is depolarized (e.g., during an action potential), a larger fraction of the functional channels is activated. This allows a larger influx of Ca^{2+} ions, which triggers a stronger activation of the contractile apparatus and greater force development. This increased development of force is called a **positive inotropic effect**.

BOX 8-7

Congenital Myasthenic Syndromes Result from Defective Neuromuscular Transmission

Congenital myasthenic syndromes (CMS) are heterogeneous disorders caused by presynaptic, synaptic, or postsynaptic defects at the neuromuscular junction. Only the postsynaptic defects involving mutations in the ACh channel are considered here. The clinical picture in all forms of this syndrome consists of respiratory and feeding difficulties at birth or weakness of the ocular and bulbar muscles (muscles of the tongue, lips, and pharynx) during the first 2 years of life. Postsynaptic CMS can be associated with changes in the gating kinetics of ACh channels or with a reduction in the density of ACh channels in the postsynaptic membrane. In the "fast channel syndrome" a mutation in the ACh channel results in a greatly reduced postsynaptic response to ACh. Patch clamp recordings of single ACh channels reveal that the mutation causes the channel open time to be much shorter than that of wild-type channels (Figure B-1). Because of the reduced inward current through ACh-gated channels, many skeletal muscle cells fail to reach threshold and thus fail to contract. This results in muscle weakness.

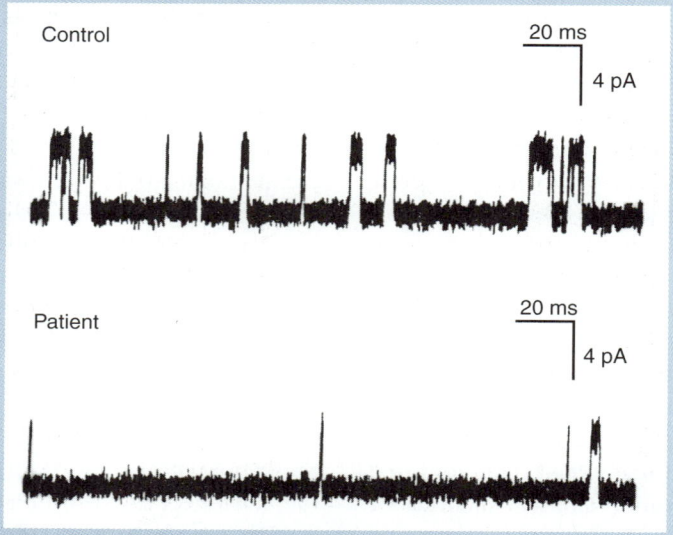

Figure B-1 ■ Acetylcholine (ACh)-gated channel openings in a patient with congenital myasthenic syndrome (CMS) are briefer than normal. Single ACh-gated channel openings (shown as upward deflections) were recorded at a neuromuscular junction from a normal individual *(control)* and from a patient with CMS *(patient)*. The single channel openings in the patient are briefer and less frequent than in the control subject. (From Ohno K, Wang H-L, Milone M, et al: *Neuron* 17:157, 1996.)

SUMMARY

1. Ion channel types are characterized by their selectivity and by their structures and pharmacology.
2. The various types of ion channels play specific, critical roles in normal cell function, and channel defects can have serious pathophysiological consequences.
3. Voltage-gated Ca^{2+} channels can generate the upstroke of action potentials. In addition, Ca^{2+} channels can influence a large variety of cellular activities because Ca^{2+} ions regulate many cellular processes.
4. Several distinct types of Ca^{2+} channels can be distinguished on the basis of their physiological and pharmacological properties.
5. Ca antagonist drugs reduce Ca^{2+} entry into the cell by blocking voltage-gated Ca^{2+} channels. These Ca^{2+} channel blockers are widely used as therapeutic agents in the management of cardiac arrhythmias, coronary artery disease, and hypertension.
6. Potassium-selective ion channels, which are found in all cells, are diverse in their activity, structure, and distribution. Neuronal K^+ channel diversity contributes to the regulation of action potential firing patterns.
7. Many neurons express K_A channels, which generate transient outward currents. These channels activate relatively rapidly, in a few milliseconds, during depolarization and then inactivate over tens of milliseconds. In neurons that generate bursts of action potentials, the length of the interval between action potentials in the burst is regulated by the activity of K_A channels.
8. The three subtypes of Ca^{2+}-activated K^+ (K_{Ca}) channels (large, intermediate, and small conductance) are all opened by intracellular Ca^{2+}. The BK_{Ca} channels have one of the largest single-channel conductances. The current through K_{Ca} channels helps to repolarize individual action potentials and can also play a role in terminating a burst of action potentials.
9. ATP-sensitive K^+ (K_{ATP}) channels in the pancreatic β-cell, which are blocked by high $[ATP]_i$, are involved in glucose-induced insulin secretion. In response to a rise in plasma glucose concentration, glucose metabolism by the β-cell leads to an increase in $[ATP]_i$, which blocks K_{ATP} channels. Consequently, the β-cell depolarizes, thereby opening voltage-gated Ca^{2+} channels, allowing Ca^{2+} ions to enter the cell and activate insulin secretion.
10. Sulfonylureas, which block K_{ATP} channels and thereby enhance insulin secretion, are used in the treatment of type II diabetes.
11. Ligand-gated channels are opened following the binding of an appropriate neurotransmitter or other chemical activator.
12. Acetylcholine (ACh)-gated ion channels are opened by the binding of ACh to its receptor on the channel. These channels are found in the surface membrane of skeletal muscle at the neuromuscular junction, where they mediate communication between nerve and muscle.
13. Ion channel activity can be regulated by second-messenger pathways. For example, L-type Ca^{2+} channel activity in cardiac muscle is regulated by β-adrenergic receptors. The activation of these β-adrenergic receptors by epinephrine or norepinephrine causes phosphorylation of the Ca^{2+} channels. This increases the activity of the L-type Ca^{2+} channels, enhances Ca^{2+} entry, and increases force development in the heart.

KEY WORDS AND CONCEPTS

- Voltage-gated Ca^{2+} channels
- Ca^{2+} channel subtypes (e.g., L-type, T-type)
- Ca^{2+} antagonist drugs (Ca^{2+} channel blockers)
- Use-dependent block
- K_A channels

- Ca^{2+}-activated K^+ channels
- BK_{Ca} channels
- K_{ATP} channels
- Sulfonylureas
- Type II diabetes mellitus
- Ligand-gated ion channels
- Acetylcholine-gated ion channels
- Positive inotropic effect

STUDY PROBLEMS

1. In Chapter 4 we discussed the fact that the ionic flux that occurs during a nerve action potential does not *significantly* alter the ion concentration in the cell (Box 4-3). Why, then, can Ca^{2+} entry through Ca^{2+} channels significantly increase the intracellular Ca^{2+} concentration? Support your answer with a calculation of the change in $[Ca^{2+}]_i$ that would occur under the following conditions: an average I_{Ca} of 20×10^{-12} amps flows for 100 msec into a spherical cell that has a diameter of 10 μm.
2. A certain type of neuron has a resting membrane potential of –75 mV, and it generates a single burst of action potentials in response to a brief depolarizing stimulus. The time interval between action potentials in the burst is regulated in part by the activity of K_A channels. If the resting potential of the cell becomes depolarized (e.g., to –65 mV), what would you expect to happen to the frequency of action potentials in the burst? Explain your answer.
3. The bursting pattern of electrical activity in pancreatic β-cells is controlled by the following populations of ion channels: L-type Ca^{2+} channels, BK_{Ca} channels, K_{ATP} channels, and voltage-gated K^+ channels. Propose some mechanisms involving ion channels (in addition to sulfonylurea block of K_{ATP} channels) that might be used to enhance insulin secretion from β-cells in type II diabetics.

■ BIBLIOGRAPHY

Ashcroft FM, Rorsman P: Electrophysiology of the pancreatic β-cell, *Prog Biophys Molec Biol* 54:87, 1989.

Barrett EF, Magleby KL, Pallotta BS: Properties of single calcium-activated potassium channels in cultured rat muscle, *J Physiol (Lond)* 331:211, 1982.

Berne RM, Levy MN: *Cardiovascular physiology,* ed 8, St Louis, 2001, Mosby.

Catterall WA: Structure and regulation of voltage-gated Ca^{2+} channels, *Annu Rev Cell Dev Biol* 16:521, 2000.

Connor JA, Stevens CF: Prediction of repetitive firing behaviour from voltage clamp data on an isolated neurone soma, *J Physiol (Lond)* 213:31, 1971.

Hille B: *Ionic channels of excitable membranes,* ed 2, Sunderland, Mass, 1991, Sinauer.

Kostyuk PG, Kristhal OA, Shakhovalov YA: Separation of sodium and calcium currents in the somatic membrane of mollusc neurones, *J Physiol (Lond)* 270:545, 1977.

Lee KS, Tsien RW: Mechanism of calcium channel blockade by verapamil, D600, diltiazem and nitrendipine in single dialysed heart cells, *Nature* 302:790, 1983.

Lehmann-Horn F, Jurkat-Rott K: Voltage-gated ion channels and hereditary disease, *Physiol Rev* 79:1317, 1999.

Ohno K, Wang H-L, Milone M, et al: Congenital myasthenic syndrome caused by decreased agonist binding affinity due to a mutation in the acetylcholine receptor e subunit, *Neuron* 17:157, 1996.

Segal M, Rogawski MA, Barker JL: A transient potassium conductance regulates the excitability of cultured hippocampal and spinal neurons, *J Neurosci* 4:604, 1984.

Shieh C-C, Coghlan M, Sullivan JP, Gopalakrishnan M: Potassium channels: molecular defects, diseases, and therapeutic opportunities, *Pharm Rev* 52:557, 2000.

CHAPTER 9

SECTION III Solute Transport
Electrochemical Potential Energy and Transport Processes

Objectives:

1. Understand that concentration gradients and electrical potential gradients store chemical and electrical potential energy, respectively.
2. Understand that electrochemical potential energy drives all transport processes.
3. Use the concept of electrochemical potential energy to analyze transport processes.

■ ELECTROCHEMICAL POTENTIAL ENERGY DRIVES ALL TRANSPORT PROCESSES

In Chapter 2, by examining the permeability of biological membranes to various solutes, we concluded that, with the exception of simple, small, and typically lipid-soluble molecules (e.g., O_2, CO_2, ethanol), most biologically important solutes (e.g., sugars, amino acids, inorganic ions) cannot readily traverse cellular membranes. Therefore special transport mechanisms are required to move these impermeant solutes from one side of a membrane to the other. An important class of special transport mechanisms—the ion channels—has already been discussed in Chapters 5 to 8. There we observed that differences in ion concentrations and electrical potential across a membrane can drive the movement of ions through channels. In this chapter we introduce the concepts of chemical and electrical potential energy, which are stored in concentration gradients and electrical potential gradients, respectively. We also demonstrate that electrochemical potential energy drives all solute transport processes.

The Relationship Between Potential Energy and Force Is Revealed by an Examination of Gravity

Experience tells us that the gravitational **force** acts on an object at any height so that, when the object is released, it is pulled toward the ground. Since force is mass (m) times acceleration (a), the gravitational force (F_G) must be

$$F_G = -ma_G \quad [1]$$

where a_G is the acceleration caused by gravity and the minus sign indicates that the force is directed downward (in the negative y direction).

Lifting an object of mass, m, from the ground to some height, y, is a process that requires an investment of energy. The amount of energy invested in lifting an object is directly proportional to the mass of the object, as well as the height to which the object is lifted. One way to conceptualize this is to say that the object has greater **potential energy** when it is at a greater height from the surface of the earth. These considerations are neatly summarized in the definition of gravitational potential energy (PE_G):

$$PE_G = ma_G\, y \qquad [2]$$

Implicit in this equation is the fact that ground level is the reference point against which gravitational potential energy is measured; that is, at ground level ($y = 0$), $PE_G = 0$. From this definition, it is clear that a change in height, Δy, causes a corresponding change in gravitational potential energy, $\Delta PE_G = ma_G \Delta y$. In other words, a gradient of gravitational potential energy exists in the y direction. The gravitational potential energy gradient is $\Delta PE_G / \Delta y$, or, when written as a derivative, dPE_G/dy:

$$\frac{dPE_G}{dy} = ma_G = -F_G \qquad [3]$$

We interpret this equation as saying that a gradient in gravitational potential energy gives rise to the gravitational force, which moves an object *down* the potential energy gradient, that is, from some height toward ground level. This example provides an important and general insight: a **gradient of potential energy** gives rise to a force that will tend to move material *down* the potential energy gradient.

A Gradient in Chemical Potential Energy Gives Rise to a Chemical Force That Drives the Movement of Molecules

In Chapter 2 we introduced Fick's First Law of Diffusion, which describes how a concentration gradient drives the diffusion of molecules down the concentration gradient. This diffusive movement of molecules may be viewed as being driven by a "chemical force." Because we now know that a potential energy gradient gives rise to a force, if a concentration gradient can give rise to a chemical force, the concentration gradient must also embody a gradient of **chemical potential energy.** The chemical potential energy is commonly represented by the symbol μ (Greek letter *mu*). For one mole of any solute, S, at concentration [S], the chemical potential energy has the form (Box 9-1)

$$\mu_s = \mu_s^0 + RT \ln[S] \qquad [4]$$

where μ_s^0 is the chemical potential energy of the solute at the reference concentration of 1 M; thus, at $[S] = 1$ M, $\mu_s = \mu_s^0$. Equation [4] tells us that solute molecules located in a region of high concentration are at a higher chemical potential energy than the same molecules located in a region of low concentration.

An Ion Can Have Both Electrical and Chemical Potential Energy

All molecules have chemical potential energy. Ions, because they carry electric charge, can also have **electrical potential energy.** At any electrical potential, V, the potential energy associated with a single ion carrying z charges (e.g., $z = +2$ for Ca^{2+}; $z = -1$ for Cl^-) is $z \times e \times V$, where e is the magnitude of a single electric charge ($e = 1.602 \times 10^{-19}$ coulomb). For a mole of such ions, the electrical potential energy should be multiplied by Avogadro's number ($N_A = 6.022 \times 10^{23}$ per mole). The magnitude of one mole of elementary charges is given a special name, the *Faraday* (symbol F), and has the value 96,485 coulombs/mole. Thus the electrical potential energy for one mole of ions, each carrying z charges, is $z \times F \times V$.

Because an ionic solute, S^z, can be at a particular concentration and electrical potential, its potential energy is the sum of both chemical

Electrochemical Potential Energy and Transport Processes

BOX 9-1

A Concentration Gradient Stores Chemical Potential Energy, Which Drives the Movement of Molecules

In diffusion, a gradient in the concentration of a solute ([S]), drives a net flux, J, of the solute, as described by Fick's First Law (see Chapter 2):

$$J = -D\frac{d[S]}{dx} \quad [\text{B1}]$$

Alternatively, we can view the diffusive movement as the result of a chemical force pushing on the solute molecules. It is quite reasonable that the velocity of the molecule, v, should be proportional to the magnitude of the chemical force, F_c:

$$v = uF_c \quad [\text{B2}]$$

where u is the *mobility coefficient* of the molecule. We can determine how the flux is related to the molecular velocity by examining Figure B-1, which shows molecules moving at velocity, v, along a cylinder of solution. The flux, J, is simply the number of moles of molecules passing through the cross-sectional area, A, per unit time. Since the molecules are moving at velocity, v, in a time period, Δt, they would move a distance $v\Delta t$, which is the distance between the two shaded areas. Thus any molecule initially located between these two areas would pass through the area, A, during the time interval, Δt. The volume contained between the two shaded areas is $A \times (v\Delta t)$. The number of moles of solute in this volume is just $[S] \times A \times (v\Delta t)$. But the flux is just this number of moles of solute passing through the area, A, in the time interval, Δt, or

$$J = \frac{\text{moles of S}/A}{\Delta t} = \frac{[S] \times A \times (v\Delta t)/A}{\Delta t}$$
$$= [S]v = [S]uF_c \quad [\text{B3}]$$

We can verify that the concentration, [S], times the velocity, v, is indeed a flux by checking the units. Since [S] has units of moles per volume (e.g., moles/cm^3), and v is expressed as distance per unit time (e.g., cm/s), $[S] \times v$ must have units of moles per unit area per unit time [e.g., (moles/cm^2)/s]. These units imply the movement of a certain amount of material through a certain area in a certain amount of time, which is indeed the definition of flux.

The flux driven by the chemical force is the same flux as that specified by Fick's First Law, so the expressions for J in Equations [B1] and [B3] can be equated. Making use of the relationship between the mobility, u, and the diffusion coefficient, D, $u = D/RT$, and solving for the chemical force yields

$$F_c = -RT\frac{1}{[S]}\frac{d[S]}{dx} = -RT\frac{d\ln[S]}{dx} \quad [\text{B4}]$$

The last step of Equation [B4] required us to recognize the derivative of the natural logarithm function (see Appendix A).

We already know that the chemical force arises from a gradient in chemical potential energy, μ_S,

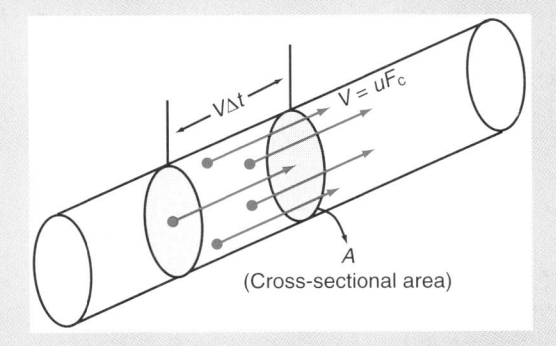

Figure B-1 ■ Movement of molecules being driven by a "chemical force." Molecules are moving at average velocity, v, under the influence of a chemical force, F_c. In a time period, Δt, each molecule will move a distance equal to $v \times \Delta t$. Two surfaces of cross-sectional area, A, and separated by a distance, $v \times \Delta t$, are shown. All molecules located between these two surfaces are expected to move past the back surface after a time period, Δt, has elapsed.

> **BOX 9-1**
>
> ### A Concentration Gradient Stores Chemical Potential Energy, Which Drives the Movement of Molecules—Cont'd
>
> and tends to push molecules *down* the gradient. In other words,
>
> $$\frac{d\mu_s}{dx} = -F_c = RT\frac{d\ln[S]}{dx} \quad [B5]$$
>
> By applying the integration techniques of Appendix A, we find that the chemical potential energy must have the form
>
> $$\mu_s = \text{constant} + RT\ln[S] \quad [B6]$$
>
> where *constant* is the integration constant, which must be determined independently. Examining Equation [B6] shows that when $[S] = 1$ M, $\mu_s =$ *constant*. In other words, the constant is the chemical potential energy when the solute is at a concentration of 1 M. This special value is given the special symbol, μ_s^0. Therefore the complete expression for the chemical potential energy of a mole of solute, S, at concentration, [S], is
>
> $$\mu_s = \mu_s^0 + RT\ln[S] \quad [B7]$$
>
> Although μ_s has the units of energy, it is more commonly referred to as the *chemical potential*.

and electrical components. The complete expression for the **electrochemical potential energy** of one mole of an ionic solute, S^z, at concentration, $[S^z]$, and at an electrical potential, V, is

$$\mu_{S^z} = (\mu_{S^z}^0 + RT\ln[S^z]) + zFV \quad [5]$$

Again, it should be pointed out that although μ_{S^z} has the units of energy, it is more commonly referred to as the **electrochemical potential.** Shown in Box 9-2 are examples of expressions for the electrochemical potential energy of two common solutes.

The Nernst Equation Is a Simple Manifestation of the Electrochemical Potential Energy

To illustrate the usefulness of the concept of electrochemical potential energy, we first revisit a scenario we analyzed in Chapter 4. We take a cell whose intracellular and extracellular concentrations are $[K^+]_i = 140$ mM and $[K^+]_o = 5$ mM, respectively, and whose plasma membrane is permeable *only* to K^+ (Figure 9-1). We know that the K^+ concentration gradient would initially drive a net movement of K^+ ions out of the cell, causing the electrical potential inside the cell to become negative relative to the outside. The developing negative membrane potential of the cell tends to resist further efflux of K^+ ions. When equilibrium is reached, a stable unchanging membrane potential will be established and no net flux of K^+, either into or out of the cell, will occur. In Chapter 4, by analyzing the fluxes, we reached the conclusion that the membrane potential attained at equilibrium is given by the Nernst equation.

We now analyze the same situation by focusing on the meaning of *equilibrium*, without giving any attention to dynamic processes such as fluxes. When equilibrium is reached, no net movement of K^+ ions occurs between the inside and the outside of the cell. We know that it is a difference in electrochemical potential energy between two locations (i.e., a gradient) that gives rise to the electrochemical force driving the movement of ions. Therefore the only way to have zero net K^+ flux is to have no net

Electrochemical Potential Energy and Transport Processes

> **BOX 9-2**
>
> ### Mathematical Expressions for the Electrochemical Potential Energy of Solutes Inside and Outside a Cell
>
> The general expression for the electrochemical potential energy of a solute is given by Equation [B1]:
>
> $$\mu_{S^z} = (\mu^0_{S^z} + RT \ln[S^z]) + zFV \qquad [B1]$$
>
> For a neutral solute like glucose (G), which carries no electrical charge ($z = 0$), its potential energy should not depend on the membrane potential, V_m, of the cell. Therefore the electrochemical potential energies of glucose inside and outside the cell are given by the simple expressions
>
> $$\mu_{G,i} = \mu^0_G + RT \ln[G]_i \qquad [B2]$$
>
> and
>
> $$\mu_{G,o} = \mu^0_G + RT \ln[G]_o \qquad [B3]$$
>
> respectively.
>
> For an ionic solute like the sulfate ion, SO_4^{2-}, which carries a charge ($z = -2$), its potential energy is expected to depend on the membrane potential. We recall from Chapter 4 that the membrane potential, V_m, is defined to be the electrical potential inside, measured relative to the electrical potential outside, which can be conveniently defined to be zero. Therefore the electrochemical potential energy for sulfate inside the cell ($\mu_{SO_4^{2-},i}$) is given by
>
> $$\mu_{SO_4^{2-},i} = (\mu^0_{SO_4^{2-}} + RT \ln[SO_4^{2-}]_i) + (-2)FV_m$$
> $$= \mu^0_{SO_4^{2-}} + RT \ln[SO_4^{2-}]_i - 2FV_m \qquad [B4]$$
>
> while for sulfate outside the cell $\mu_{SO_4^{2-},o}$ is given by
>
> $$\mu_{SO_4^{2-},o} = (\mu^0_{SO_4^{2-}} + RT \ln[SO_4^{2-}]_o) + (-2)F(0) \qquad [B5]$$
> $$= \mu^0_{SO_4^{2-}} + RT \ln[SO_4^{2-}]_o$$

electrochemical force. This is possible only if there is no longer any difference in electrochemical potential energy for K^+ between the inside and outside of the cell. In other words, at equilibrium, $\mu_{K^+,i}$ must be equal to $\mu_{K^+,o}$. The expression for $\mu_{K^+,i}$ is

$$\mu_{K^+,i} = \mu^0_{K^+} + RT \ln[K^+]_i + (+1)FV_m \qquad [6]$$

and the expression for $\mu_{K^+,o}$ is

$$\mu_{K^+,o} = \mu^0_{K^+} + RT \ln[K^+]_o + (+1)F(0) \qquad [7]$$
$$= \mu^0_{K^+} + RT \ln[K^+]_o$$

In writing these two expressions, we have used the same convention that was introduced in Chapter 4. That is, the intracellular electrical potential, V_m, is measured relative to the outside electrical potential, which is defined to be zero. Setting $\mu_{K^+,i} = \mu_{K^+,o}$ and rearranging algebraically (Box 9-3) gives

$$V_{m,eq} = \frac{RT}{(+1)F} \ln \frac{[K^+]_o}{[K^+]_i} = E_K \qquad [8]$$

which we recognize as the Nernst equation. The membrane potential reached at equilibrium is indeed the K^+ equilibrium potential, E_K. This example illustrates the simplicity of using the electrochemical potential in analyzing equilibrium situations.

How to Use the Electrochemical Potential Energy to Analyze Transport Processes

The scenario we just discussed, involving K^+ efflux and attainment of the K^+ equilibrium potential, is the simplest example of a cellular *transport process*, that is, a process whereby solute on one side of a membrane is moved to

A slightly more complex transport process is chloride-bicarbonate (Cl^-/HCO_3^-) exchange, which is mediated by an integral membrane protein in the plasma membrane of erythrocytes. The process involves the coordinated movement of one Cl^- ion into the cell and one HCO_3^- ion out of the cell, or vice-versa. The Cl^-/HCO_3^- exchange process can be represented by the reaction scheme

$$Cl^-_{out} + HCO_3^-{}_{in} \rightleftharpoons Cl^-_{in} + HCO_3^-{}_{out}$$

To obtain the mathematical equation that describes how all the concentrations and the membrane potential are related *at equilibrium,* we equate the total electrochemical potential energy on the two sides of the reaction scheme:

$$\mu_{Cl^-,o} + \mu_{HCO_3^-,i} = \mu_{Cl^-,i} + \mu_{HCO_3^-,o} \qquad [9]$$

Then, substitution of the full expressions for the electrochemical potentials and algebraic rearrangement yield (see Box 9-4 for details):

$$\frac{[HCO_3^-]_i}{[HCO_3^-]_o} = \frac{[Cl^-]_i}{[Cl^-]_o} \qquad [10]$$

We see that the membrane potential, V_m, does not appear in this equation. This is not unexpected, because for every Cl^- ion transported in one direction, an HCO_3^- is transported in the opposite direction by the exchanger protein. The net transport of electrical charges is zero; that is, Cl^-/HCO_3^- exchange is *electroneutral*. Therefore the transport process should affect only the concentrations of Cl^- and HCO_3^-, without affecting the membrane potential. It is thus entirely reasonable that the equilibrium concentrations of Cl^- and HCO_3^- are *not* related to the membrane potential. Although the operation of the Cl^-/HCO_3^- exchanger is relatively simple, it has fundamental physiological importance in allowing the circulatory system to transport carbon dioxide generated metabolically in the body tissues to the lungs, where the gas can be expelled from the body (Box 9-5).

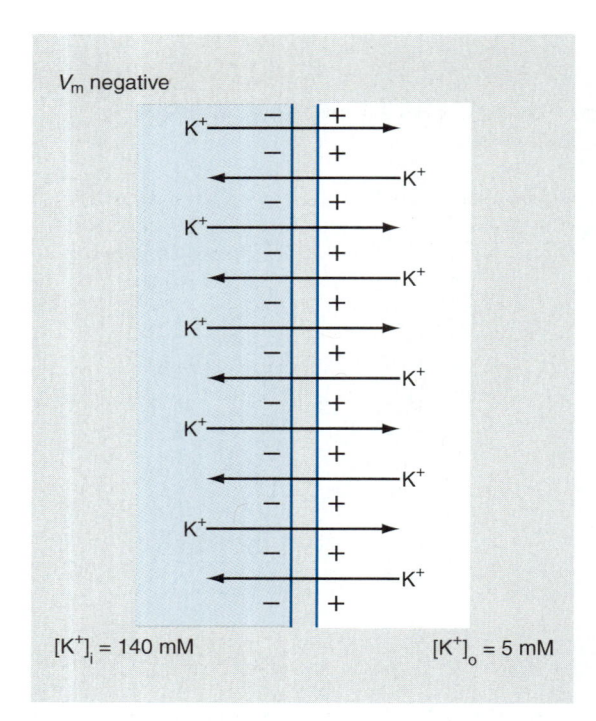

Figure 9-1 ■ Equilibration of K^+ across a plasma membrane that is permeable only to K^+. A plasma membrane separates the cytosolic compartment, with $[K^+]_i$ = 140 mM, from the extracellular solution, where $[K^+]_o$ = 5 mM. If the plasma membrane is permeable only to K^+, the K^+ concentration gradient will drive net movement of K^+ out of the cell, causing the electrical potential inside the cell to become negative relative to the outside. When equilibrium is reached, the negative membrane potential (V_m) established is just sufficient to prevent further net flux of K^+ across the plasma membrane.

the other side. The transport of K^+ can be represented as the "reaction" scheme,

$$K^+_{in} \rightleftharpoons K^+_{out}$$

To obtain the mathematical equation that describes the process *at equilibrium*, we simply equated the K^+ electrochemical potentials on the two sides of the reaction scheme.

Electrochemical Potential Energy and Transport Processes

BOX 9-3

The Nernst Equation Is a Natural Consequence of the Concept of Electrochemical Potential Energy

At equilibrium, the electrochemical potential energy of K^+ is equalized across the plasma membrane; that is,

$$\mu_{K^+,i} = \mu_{K^+,o} \quad [B1]$$

We can thus equate the expressions for $\mu_{K^+,i}$ and $\mu_{K^+,o}$ (Equations [6] and [7] in text).

$$\mu^0_{K^+} + RT \ln[K^+]_i + (+1)FV_m = \mu^0_{K^+} + RT \ln[K^+]_o \quad [B2]$$

The standard electrochemical potential energy of K^+, $\mu^0_{K^+}$, occurring on both sides of the equation, can be eliminated to give

$$RT \ln[K^+]_i + (+1)FV_m = RT \ln[K^+]_o \quad [B3]$$

Rearranging yields

$$V_m = \frac{RT}{F}(\ln[K^+]_o - \ln[K^+]_i) \quad [B4]$$

Knowing that the difference of two logarithms is the same as the logarithm of a quotient (see Appendix A), we can rewrite Equation [B4] as

$$V_m = \frac{RT}{F} \ln \frac{[K^+]_o}{[K^+]_i} \quad [B5]$$

which is the Nernst equation for K^+.

BOX 9-4

The Equilibrium Transport Equation for Chloride-Bicarbonate (Cl^-/HCO_3^-) Exchange

The Cl^-/HCO_3^- exchange process can be represented as

$$Cl^-_{out} + HCO_3^-{}_{in} \rightleftharpoons Cl^-_{in} + HCO_3^-{}_{out}$$

At equilibrium the following balance in electrochemical potential energy must be achieved:

$$\mu_{Cl^-,o} + \mu_{HCO_3^-,i} = \mu_{Cl^-,i} + \mu_{HCO_3^-,o} \quad [B1]$$

The electrochemical potential energies for Cl^- and HCO_3^- inside and outside the cells are given by the following equations:

$$\mu_{Cl^-,i} = \mu^0_{Cl^-} + RT \ln[Cl^-]_i + (-1)FV_m \quad [B2]$$

$$\mu_{Cl^-,o} = \mu^0_{Cl^-} + RT \ln[Cl^-]_o \quad [B3]$$

$$\mu_{HCO_3^-,i} = \mu^0_{HCO_3^-} + RT \ln[HCO_3^-]_i + (-1)FV_m \quad [B4]$$

$$\mu_{HCO_3^-,o} = \mu^0_{HCO_3^-} + RT \ln[HCO_3^-]_o \quad [B5]$$

Substituting the expressions [B2] to [B5] into Equation [B1] gives

$$(\mu^0_{Cl^-} + RT \ln[Cl^-]_o) + (\mu^0_{HCO_3^-} + RT \ln[HCO_3^-]_i + (-1)FV_m) = (\mu^0_{Cl^-} + RT \ln[Cl^-]_i + (-1)FV_m) + (\mu^0_{HCO_3^-} + RT \ln[HCO_3^-]_o) \quad [B6]$$

All terms involving μ^0 and V_m cancel to give

$$RT \ln[Cl^-]_o + RT \ln[HCO_3^-]_i = RT \ln[Cl^-]_i + RT \ln[HCO_3^-]_o \quad [B7]$$

Dividing both sides by RT and rearranging gives

$$\ln[HCO_3^-]_i - \ln[HCO_3^-]_o = \ln[Cl^-]_i - \ln[Cl^-]_o \quad [B8]$$

Noting that a difference of two logarithms is the same as the logarithm of the quotient, we can rewrite Equation [B8]:

$$\frac{[HCO_3^-]_i}{[HCO_3^-]_o} = \frac{[Cl^-]_i}{[C^-]_o} \quad [B9]$$

Equation [B9] relates the intracellular and extracellular Cl^- and HCO_3^- concentrations when the Cl^-/HCO_3^- exchange process has reached equilibrium (i.e., when no further net movement of Cl^- and HCO_3^- can occur).

BOX 9-5

The Chloride-Bicarbonate Exchanger Is Essential for Removing Carbon Dioxide from the Body

In the course of 24 hours an average person expires more than 800 liters of carbon dioxide (CO_2) gas. This represents more than 30 moles of CO_2 (~1400 g, or ~3 lb, by weight). This amount of CO_2, generated metabolically within tissues of the body, must be transported by the circulation to the lungs to be expelled. Although CO_2 is approximately 20 times more soluble than O_2 in plasma, its solubility is still far too low to allow its efficient transport as a simple dissolved gas in plasma. Just as hemoglobin is an evolutionary adaptation for transporting sparingly soluble O_2, a special mechanism has evolved to enable the transport of large amounts of CO_2 through the circulation.

CO_2 produced in the tissues travels by diffusion into capillaries and into the red blood cells (RBCs) that course through the capillaries (Figure B-1). RBCs contain high concentrations of carbonic anhydrase, an enzyme that catalyzes (accelerates) the reversible reaction of CO_2 with water to form carbonic acid:

$$CO_2 + H_2O \xrightleftharpoons[]{\text{Carbonic anhydrase}} H_2CO_3$$

Without catalysis, hydration of CO_2 is a very slow process; each CO_2 molecule takes many seconds to react with water. As one of the fastest enzymes on earth, carbonic anhydrase greatly speeds up the hydration process. Each molecule of enzyme can catalyze the reaction of 1 million CO_2 molecules per second.

As soon as the carbonic acid molecules are formed, they dissociate into protons and bicarbonate ions:

$$H_2CO_3 \rightleftharpoons H^+ + HCO_3^-$$

Most of the H^+ ions are immediately bound to hemoglobin, whose concentration within an RBC is in excess of 5 mM (i.e., hemoglobin is an effective buffer for H^+ ions). Abundant Cl^-/HCO_3^- exchangers in the RBC plasma membrane rapidly transport HCO_3^- ions out of the RBC into the plasma with the concomitant transport of Cl^- ions into the RBC. In the tissues the net result of the coordinated action of carbonic anhydrase and the Cl^-/HCO_3^- exchanger is to convert poorly soluble CO_2 into two highly soluble ions, H^+ and HCO_3^-, which are then kept in physically separate compartments (H^+ in the RBC and HCO_3^- out in the plasma), so that they cannot recombine to regenerate CO_2. These separated moieties are transported as an ensemble by the circulation toward the lungs.

As blood reaches the lungs, the processes that occurred in the tissues are now reversed (Figure B-1). The Cl^-/HCO_3^- exchanger now mediates movement of Cl^- out of, and HCO_3^- back into, the RBC. The HCO_3^- ions can thus combine with H^+ ions in the RBC to reform H_2CO_3, which is rapidly *de*hydrated by carbonic anhydrase to yield simple, dissolved CO_2. The CO_2 formed in the RBC then diffuses from the alveolar capillaries into the alveolar air space, where the CO_2 concentration (or partial pressure, p_{CO_2}) is low.

In summary, in the tissues the higher concentration of CO_2 drives CO_2 entry into RBCs, and the subsequent increase in $[HCO_3^-]_i$ drives the Cl^-/HCO_3^- exchanger to operate in the bicarbonate-out–chloride-in mode. In the alveolar capillaries the CO_2 concentration gradient is reversed (low CO_2 concentration in the alveolar space) and drives CO_2 from the RBCs into the alveolus. This leads to carbonic anhydrase catalyzing net dehydration of H_2CO_3. The consequent decrease in $[HCO_3^-]_i$ drives the Cl^-/HCO_3^- exchanger to operate in the bicarbonate-in–chloride-out mode.

The importance of the coordinated action of carbonic anhydrase and the Cl^-/HCO_3^- exchanger in CO_2 transport is reflected by the fact that 70% of the CO_2 produced in the body is moved into the lungs by this mechanism, while only 10% is carried in the plasma as simple dissolved CO_2. The remaining 20% is transported in protein-bound forms, which are commonly referred to as carbamino compounds (Figure B-1).

BOX 9-5

The Chloride-Bicarbonate Exchanger Is Essential for Removing Carbon Dioxide from the Body—Cont'd

In the Tissues

In the Lungs

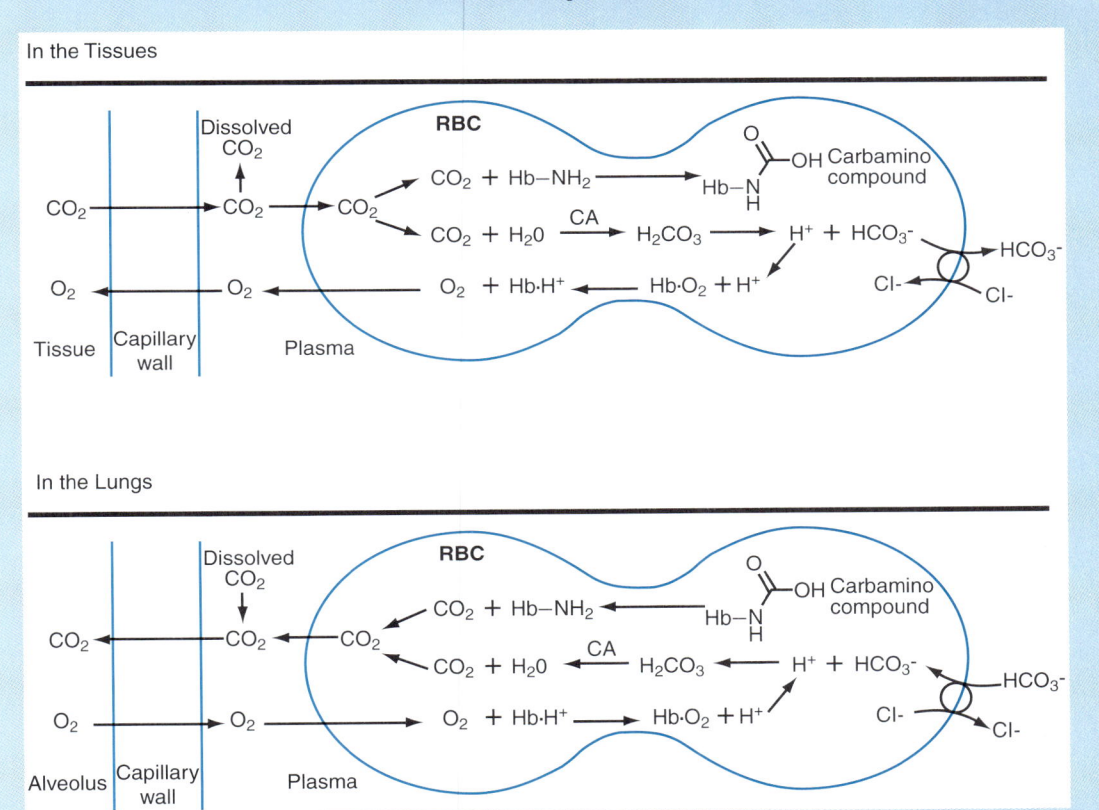

Figure B-1 ■ Transport of carbon dioxide by the circulation. Carbon dioxide (CO_2) generated by metabolism in tissues is transported in three forms in the circulation: as bicarbonate ions (HCO_3^-) in the plasma, as bound "carbamino compounds" formed with hemoglobin, and as dissolved CO_2 gas. CO_2 diffusing into the red blood cell (RBC) is rapidly converted to H^+ and HCO_3^- ions. Through the action of the chloride-bicarbonate exchanger, the HCO_3^- is extruded out of the RBC in exchange for Cl^- from the plasma. The H^+ ions bind to oxyhemoglobin ($Hb \cdot O_2$); this favors release of oxygen from hemoglobin and makes O_2 available to the tissues. Of the CO_2 produced in tissues, the greatest fraction (~70%) is transported as HCO_3^-. A smaller fraction (~20%) is carried by proteins in the blood (principally hemoglobin) in the form of carbamino compounds. Relatively little (~10%) is transported as simple dissolved CO_2. In the lungs the processes that occur in the tissues are reversed, allowing CO_2 to be released to, and O_2 to be taken up from, the alveolar air space. $Hb \cdot H^+$ is protonated hemoglobin; $Hb-NH_2$ represents a side-chain amino group on hemoglobin; CA is carbonic anhydrase.

We have seen that the electrochemical potential energy is a useful concept for analyzing processes that transport solutes across membranes. In Chapter 10 we use the same approach to analyze several physiologically important transport processes of greater complexity.

■ SUMMARY

1. The *chemical potential energy* of a substance is a function of its concentration. A molecule in a region of high concentration is at a higher chemical potential energy than the same molecule in a region of low concentration.
2. A difference in chemical potential energy between two regions gives rise to a "chemical force" that drives the movement of molecules down the potential energy gradient, that is, from a location of higher potential energy toward a location of lower potential energy.
3. An ion, being electrically charged, can also have *electrical potential energy*. The combined chemical and electrical potential energy is referred to as the *electrochemical potential energy*.
4. A difference in electrochemical potential energy between two regions drives the transport of ions and molecules down the electrochemical potential energy gradient.

■ KEY WORDS AND CONCEPTS

- Force
- Potential energy
- Gradient of potential energy
- Chemical potential energy
- Electrical potential energy
- Electrochemical potential energy (electrochemical potential)

STUDY PROBLEMS

1. A cell has a membrane potential V_m.
    a. The glucose concentration inside the cell is $[G]_i$. Write the mathematical expression representing the electrochemical potential energy of glucose inside the cell.
    b. The Ca^{2+} concentrations inside and outside the cell are $[Ca^{2+}]_i$ and $[Ca^{2+}]_o$, respectively. Write the mathematical expressions for the electrochemical potential energy of Ca^{2+} inside and outside the cell.

■ BIBLIOGRAPHY

Atkins PW: *Physical chemistry,* ed 5, New York, 1994, WH Freeman.

CHAPTER 10

Passive Solute Transport

Objectives:

1. Explain how the distribution of lipids and proteins in the cell membrane influences the membrane permeability to hydrophobic and hydrophilic solutes and ions.

2. Differentiate the following mechanisms based on the source of energy driving the process and the necessity for an integral cell membrane protein: diffusion, mediated (facilitated) transport, and secondary active transport.

3. Explain how the transport rates of certain molecules and ions are accelerated by specific integral membrane proteins ("carrier" and "channel" molecules).

4. Understand how coupling of solute transport enables one solute to be transported against its electrochemical gradient by using energy stored in the electrochemical gradient of the coupled solute.

5. Explain the two-step process involved in the net transport of certain solutes across epithelia.

■ DIFFUSION ACROSS BIOLOGICAL MEMBRANES IS LIMITED BY LIPID SOLUBILITY

We have just learned that all transport processes are driven by electrical or chemical gradients (see Chapter 9). The question is, "How are substances (solutes and the solvent, water) actually transported across biological membranes?" Bear in mind that some substances must be concentrated in cells, or rapidly taken up, because they are essential for cell function. Other substances must be excluded or extruded from cells. For example, too much Na^+ (or any other solute) in cells would be an excessive osmotic burden and cause cells to swell (see the discussion of the Donnan effect in Chapter 4).

Biological membranes are primarily lipid bilayers (see Chapter 1). Therefore let's begin by considering how substances move across pure lipid bilayers. Such experiments can be readily performed, and the results demonstrate that lipid bilayers are permeable to **nonpolar** or hydrophobic substances, including many gases such as oxygen and carbon dioxide. Indeed, the permeability of a substance across a lipid bilayer is, in general, directly proportional to the solubility of that substance in the lipid (see Chapter 2).

In marked contrast, lipid bilayers are poorly permeable to **polar** and hydrophilic solutes; these substances bear a net charge or have internal charge separation (i.e., uncharged molecules that behave like electric dipoles in which the positive and negative charge are separated). The ability of polar substances to pass across lipid membranes tends to be inversely proportional to molecular weight: the larger the molecule, the lower the permeability. Moreover, although pure phospholipid bilayers are modestly permeable to water, which is a polar solvent (see Chapter 2), the presence of cholesterol, as in the case of the plasma membrane, greatly reduces water permeability. Consequently, the phospholipid-cholesterol bilayers that constitute the plasma membranes in many types of cells are not sufficiently permeable to water for physiological needs.

Consider the problem of moving a polar solute, such as glucose, across biological membranes. Glucose crosses lipid bilayers extremely slowly (see Chapter 2). In other words, the bilayer is an effective barrier to the transport of these substances. Yet glucose is an essential fuel for cells.

■ CHANNEL, CARRIER, AND PUMP PROTEINS MEDIATE TRANSPORT ACROSS BIOLOGICAL MEMBRANES

To mediate and regulate the transfer of water and polar solutes, biological membranes contain integral proteins called channels, carriers, and "pumps" (Figure 10-1). More than one third of

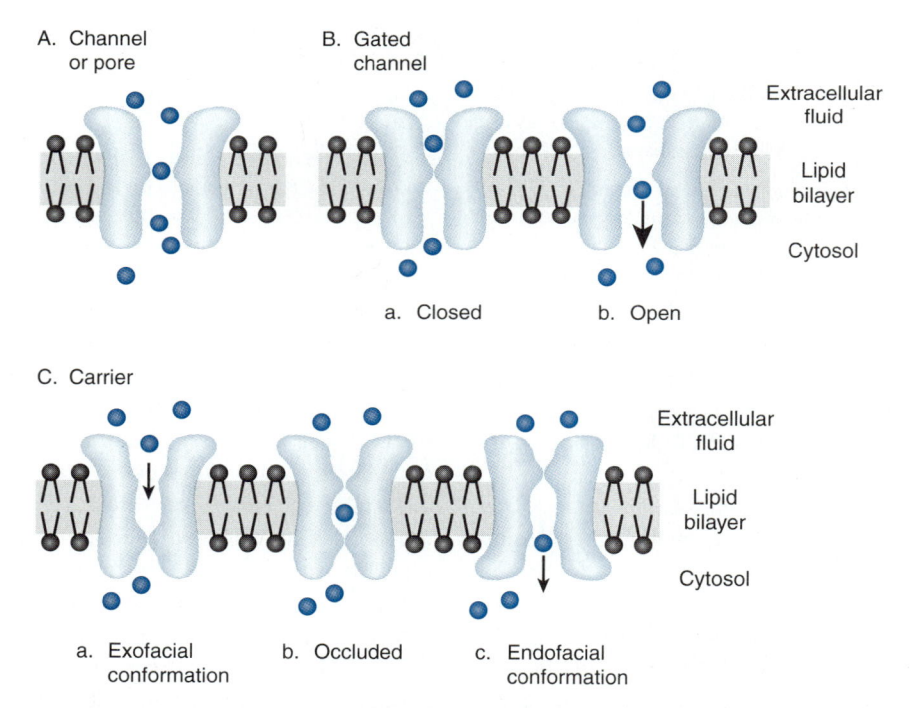

Figure 10-1 ■ Models of, A, a channel or pore; B, a gated channel; and, C, a carrier. The channel is shown in, *a*, closed and, *b*, open configurations. The carrier is shown in, *a*, the exofacial configuration, with the solute binding site open to the extracellular fluid; *b*, the "occluded" configuration, with the bound solute inaccessible to either fluid; and, *c*, the endofacial configuration, with the solute binding site open to the cytosol. Note that the "simple" carrier must also be able to switch between the exofacial and endofacial configurations in the absence of bound solute in order to effect net transport of the solute down its electrochemical gradient.

Passive Solute Transport

all the genes in the human genome code for membrane proteins, and about half of these genes (i.e., one sixth of the genome) code for transport proteins.

Transport Through Channels Is Relatively Fast

The topic of channels was introduced in Chapter 7, where the role of ion-selective channels in excitable cells was discussed. Thus we now know that the channels in biological membranes are proteins with central pores that open to both the extracellular fluid and the cytoplasm simultaneously (Figure 10-1, *A*). The narrowest region within the pore, called the selectivity filter, determines which substance(s) (ions, water, etc.) may pass through the channel. For example, channels in the family called **aquaporins*** are selectively permeable to water. Some other channels (see Chapters 7 and 8) are highly selective for Na^+ ions, for K^+ ions, or for Ca^{2+} ions, whereas still others are less selective and may, for example, be permeable to both Na^+ and K^+ (e.g., the nicotinic acetylcholine channel; see Chapter 8).

A characteristic feature of channels is their relatively high permeability. Typical **turnover numbers** for ion channels (i.e., the maximum number of ions that can pass through a channel in 1 second) are about 10^6 to 10^8. For example, about 30 million K^+ ions can pass through a single K^+ channel in 1 second (Table 10-1).

Permeability Through Channels Depends on the Density of Channels in the Membrane

Aquaporins facilitate water flow between the extracellular fluid and the cytoplasm to maintain osmotic balance (equilibrium) in cells that

TABLE 10-1
Relative transport rates for various types of transporters

Transporter	Turnover number* (per sec)
K^+ channel	30,000,000
Valinomycin (carrier)	30,000
Glucose carrier (GLUT-1)	3,000
Na^+/Ca^{2+} exchanger	2,000
Ca^{2+} pump (SERCA)	200
Na^+ pump	150

*Rate of cycling of the transporter molecule, except for ion channels such as the K^+ channel, where the turnover number indicates the maximum number of ions transported in 1 sec under physiological conditions. Thus each Na^+ pump molecule cycles 150 times per sec and transports 450 Na^+ (and 300 K^+) per sec.

require a high water permeability (e.g., skeletal muscle and some epithelia). The relative permeability to water depends on the number of channels (aquaporin tetramers) present, per unit area, in the plasma membrane (i.e., the channel density), and hormones may regulate this. For example, the hormone vasopressin increases water permeability in the principal cells of the renal cortical collecting duct by stimulating the production of cyclic adenosine monophosphate (cyclic AMP). In turn, cyclic AMP promotes the insertion of aquaporin-2 (AQP-2) molecules into the apical membrane of the epithelial cells. As a result, the osmotic driving force can promote the rapid reabsorption of water from the renal tubule lumen. Defects in this hormonal mechanism such as loss-of-function mutations in the vasopressin receptor or the AQP-2 molecule lead to *diabetes insipidus* (excretion of a high volume of dilute urine). This occurs because AQP-2 molecules cannot be inserted into the apical membrane of the renal cortical collecting duct. Therefore,

---

*The American biochemist Peter Agre shared the 2003 Nobel Prize in Chemistry for the discovery of aquaporins and the determination of their structure and function.

even though the osmotic force may favor water reabsorption, the intrinsically low water permeability in the kidney cortical collecting ducts prevents water reabsorption.

The Rate of Transport Through Open Channels Depends on the Net Driving Force

In contrast to the aforementioned situation, impaired insulin secretion or reduced sensitivity to insulin leads to a high glucose content in the proximal renal tubule fluid. The resulting osmotic force reduces the reabsorption of water even though the epithelial cell apical membranes may contain a large number of AQP-2 molecules. This results in *diabetes mellitus* (excretion of a high volume of sweet urine with an osmolality approaching that of plasma). In this case the abnormally high osmotic pressure in the lumen, and consequently small osmotic driving force, reduces water reabsorption from the kidney tubule lumen even though apical membrane water permeability may be high (see Chapter 11).

Transport of Substances Through Some Channels Is Controlled by "Gating" the Opening and Closing of the Channels

Another mechanism of regulating channel permeability is through various types of channel gating (Figure 10-1, *B*). As discussed in Chapters 7 and 8, gating may be regulated by voltage or by ligands such as Ca^{2+} or ATP.

Still other channels are gated by pressure and membrane deformation, as exemplified by the mechanosensitive monovalent cation channels in some sensory nerve terminals.

■ CARRIERS ARE INTEGRAL MEMBRANE PROTEINS THAT OPEN TO ONLY ONE SIDE OF THE MEMBRANE AT A TIME

In contrast to channels, the solute binding sites in carriers undergo spontaneous *conformational changes* and thus have *alternating access* to the two sides of the membrane. A solute binds to the carrier at one side of the membrane; then, as a result of a conformational change, a "gate" closes and the solute is transiently **occluded** (the **transition state**; Figure 10-1, *C*). Then, via a further conformational change in the protein, the "gate" on the opposite side opens so that the solute can dissociate from the carrier at this (second) side of the membrane (Figure 10-1, *C*). We use the terms "exofacial" and "endofacial" to denote the transporter conformations in which the solute binding sites face the extracellular fluid and cytoplasm, respectively.

Carriers Facilitate Transport Through Membranes

Simple **carriers** are integral membrane proteins that bind and transport a single solute species across a membrane. They move the bound solute down its electrochemical gradient (i.e., down concentration gradients and, in the case of charged solutes, voltage gradients). The rate of transport is substantially slower than that mediated by channels (Table 10-1) because substrate binding and carrier conformation changes take time. Nevertheless, transport is much faster than would be expected for diffusion in the absence of such carriers. In other words, carriers simply speed up (facilitate) processes that would normally occur, albeit much more slowly, by diffusion; hence this process is sometimes called **facilitated diffusion** (Box 10-1). Thus *transport via the simple carrier cannot be used to generate a* **steady-state** *electrochemical gradient* because the generation of such a gradient requires the expenditure of energy. This distinguishes **passive transport** from *active transport*, which is discussed below and in Chapter 11.

Sugars are transported by carriers A number of solutes are transported by solute-selective simple carriers. A good example is

BOX 10-1

The Mechanism of Carrier-Mediated Transport as Exemplified by the GLUT-1 Glucose Transporter

Carriers such as the GLUT-1 sugar transporter spontaneously change conformation, whether or not glucose is bound, so that the glucose binding site is open (accessible) either to the extracellular fluid or to the cytoplasm. Consider, as an example, the situation in which the glucose concentration in the extracellular fluid is high and the concentration in the cytoplasm is low. Glucose molecules will then tend to bind to the transporter's binding sites with higher probability (because of the higher glucose concentration) when the sites are facing the extracellular fluid than when the sites are facing the cytoplasm. Glucose that is bound at the outside will tend to dissociate when the carrier conformation changes and the sites face the cytoplasm with its low glucose concentration. The result will be a net transport of glucose from the extracellular fluid to the cytoplasm. When the concentrations of glucose are equal on the two sides of the membrane, no *net* transport will occur because the probability of glucose binding at the internal and at the external faces of the membrane will then be the same. Large movements of glucose (fluxes) in both directions may take place under the latter circumstances, but they will be equal in magnitude. Thus, in the steady state, the simple carrier cannot be used to transport a solute against a concentration gradient.

---

the **simple glucose carrier,** which mediates glucose transport across the human red blood cell (RBC) plasma membrane. This protein (the glucose transporter GLUT-1, which is a member of a family of sugar transporters; see Box 10-2) has a molecular weight of 46,000. The amino acid sequence predicts that this transporter has 12 membrane-spanning helices. Of these helices, 5 are *amphiphilic*: each has a hydrophobic surface and a hydrophilic surface. The hydrophobic regions are believed to interact with the surrounding lipids in the bilayer. In contrast, the hydrophilic surfaces of the 5 helices apparently face one another and form a central, water-filled transmembrane channel or pore (Figure 10-2). This is the general structure of many transporter molecules.

The need for carrier-mediated glucose transport is exemplified by the consequences of a mutation in the human GLUT-1 gene. GLUT-1 protein is expressed in the brain, where it

BOX 10-2

The Family of Sugar Transporters

GLUT-1 is one of five homologous human sugar transporters (GLUT-1 to GLUT-5). Each is the product of a different gene, and each has a different tissue distribution and is regulated differently. Moreover, these transporters are members of one family of a superfamily of solute transporters, the *major facilitator superfamily*, with more than 1000 members and some well-conserved sequence motifs. The superfamily already includes as many as 34 separate families. Each family has a family-specific signature sequence and specificity for a single class of substrates. Some other families within this superfamily include the monocarboxylic acid transporters that transport pyruvate and lactate, for example, and the anion/cation cotransporters that transport Na^+ and phosphate simultaneously.

mediates glucose transport across the blood-brain barrier and glucose uptake by glial cells. Individuals with a mutated GLUT-1 gene have an abnormally low cerebrospinal fluid glucose concentration (about half normal) despite a normal blood glucose level. The reduced brain glucose causes a devastating neurological syndrome (Box 10-3).

Transport by Carriers Exhibits Kinetic Properties Similar to Those of Enzyme Catalysis

Carrier-mediated transport is saturable and vectorial Because a limited number of carrier molecules are present in the membrane, raising the solute (e.g., sugar) concentration sufficiently will saturate all the carrier molecules so that no more sugar can be bound. This limits the maximal rate of transport (Figure 10-3). The transport follows *Michaelis-Menten (saturation) kinetics*, which also governs the rate of enzymatic reactions. Indeed, carriers are comparable

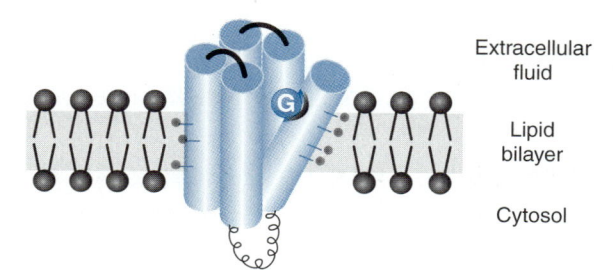

Figure 10-2 ■ Proposed structure of the core region of a simple glucose carrier (e.g., GLUT-1). The model shows the five transmembrane helices that surround the hydrophilic central pore, to which the glucose binds. One of the helices is tilted so that the glucose binding site (which is thereby made visible in this rendition) is accessible to the extracellular fluid only. Also diagrammed in this model are some of the hydrophobic residues on the amphipathic helices that face the surrounding phospholipids.

BOX 10-3

The Defective Glucose Transporter Protein Syndrome

About 17 persons with a defective GLUT-1 glucose transporter have been identified. Individuals with this rare defect have infantile seizures (convulsions), starting at age 3 to 4 months. They also have microcephaly (small head size) and developmental delays. Laboratory examination reveals *hypoglycorrhachia* (i.e., a very low glucose concentration, about half normal) in the cerebrospinal fluid (CSF) and a low CSF/blood glucose ratio (<0.5). The rate of glucose uptake by the red blood cells (RBCs) from these patients is also less than 50% of normal; this can be used as a diagnostic test. These manifestations can be explained by mutations in the GLUT-1 gene that cause malfunction of the expressed protein (a reduced turnover rate or maximum velocity of transport). GLUT-1 normally is expressed in many cells, including RBCs and epithelial cells of the choroid plexus and ependyma, as well as in blood vessel endothelial cells; it facilitates the transport of glucose from the blood to the CSF. GLUT-1 is also expressed in glia, where the transporter is concentrated in foot processes that surround neuronal synapses. Thus, in patients with defective GLUT-1, the glucose concentration within glial cells may be particularly low. This may be rate limiting for cellular energy metabolism and brain function.

Passive Solute Transport

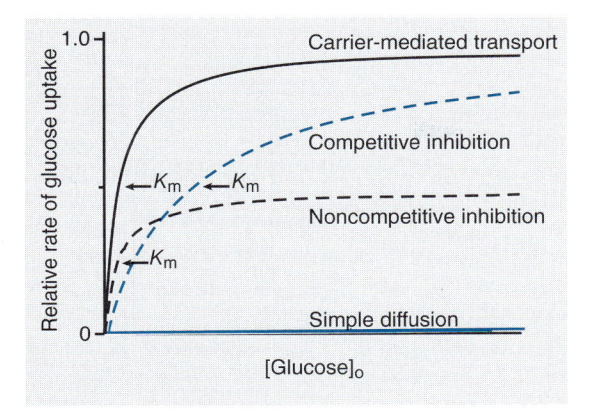

Figure 10-3 ■ Relative rate of glucose uptake into human red blood cells (mediated by GLUT-1) graphed as a function of the glucose concentration in the medium ([glucose]$_o$). The curves show the uptake under control conditions ("carrier-mediated transport") and in the presence of a competitive inhibitor (e.g., galactose) and a noncompetitive inhibitor (e.g., phloretin). GLUT-1 uptake is half-maximally activated by 1.6 mM glucose (= "K_m"; indicated by arrows on the control carrier-mediated transport and noncompetitive inhibitor curves). The competitive inhibitor increased the apparent K_m for glucose 4-fold. The maximum rate of glucose uptake is 0.6 mmole/sec at 20° C. A saturating concentration of noncompetitive inhibitor reduces the rate to that of simple diffusion, which is vanishingly low. (See Stein, 1986.)

to enzymes because both of them speed up spontaneous processes. The product of a carrier's reaction, however, is the *vectorial* (directional) movement of the substrate from one side of the membrane to the other, rather than the chemical alteration of the substrate.

Carrier-mediated transport exhibits substrate specificity The binding site on a transporter protein recognizes certain solutes, but not others. For example, the red blood cell glucose carrier GLUT-1 transports D-glucose and D-galactose, but not L-glucose (the transporter is *stereospecific*) or maltose or ribose.

Carrier-mediated transport can be inhibited either competitively or noncompetitively

Competitive inhibition GLUT-1 transports both D-galactose and D-glucose. Therefore, by competing for sugar binding sites on the carriers, D-galactose can be expected to inhibit the transport of D-glucose and vice-versa. The presence of galactose reduces the *apparent* affinity of GLUT-1 for glucose (K_m) but does not affect the maximum velocity of glucose transport at saturating glucose concentrations (Figure 10-3, *A*).

Noncompetitive inhibition Several molecules such as phloretin and dinitrofluorobenzene are noncompetitive inhibitors of GLUT-1. These inhibitors have no effect on the affinity of the carrier for glucose, but they reduce the maximum velocity of glucose transport (Figure 10-3, *B*).

Simple carriers exhibit reversibility and countertransport Carriers facilitate the movement of solutes in *both* directions across the membrane (i.e., they are "reversible"). The direction of *net* movement is, in general, determined by the electrochemical gradient of the transported substance. But now consider a situation in which RBCs are equilibrated with glucose (i.e., *equilibrium* is achieved, in which external and internal concentrations are equal and there is no net driving force). If a high concentration of galactose is added to the extracellular solution, the carriers will mediate a *net efflux* of glucose (i.e., they will move glucose outward). Initially, carriers in the endofacial conformation bind only glucose (the only solute available). When these carriers change to the exofacial conformation, some of the bound glucose will be displaced by galactose, which will then be transported inward—this is "glucose-galactose exchange." The glucose concentration inside the RBCs will *temporarily* fall below that outside the cells until the galactose concentration inside the cells rises to equal that outside (i.e., when the galactose concentration *gradient* falls to zero). During this brief period (i.e., under *non-steady-state conditions*), a countertransport of glucose in exchange for galactose takes place. This countertransport phenomenon is one type of evidence that the carriers alternately face the two sides of the membrane.

Carrier-mediated transport can be regulated The glucose carrier isoform found in adipocytes (fat cells) and in skeletal and cardiac muscle cells, GLUT-4, is regulated by insulin. In the absence of insulin stimulation the majority of GLUT-4 molecules reside in intracellular vesicular membranes. Insulin stimulation promotes the fusion of these vesicles with the plasma membrane, thereby increasing the density of GLUT-4 molecules in the plasma membrane and accelerating glucose transport. As a result, insulin shortens the time required for the intracellular glucose concentration to reach that in the extracellular fluid. This is advantageous after a meal, when the blood sugar concentration rises and insulin secretion is increased. The enhanced rate of glucose entry enables faster glycogen synthesis in muscle and adipocytes. Note, however, that although insulin facilitates the storage of glucose (as glycogen), it does *not* enable the GLUT-4 carriers to concentrate glucose in the cells.

β-Adrenergic agonists such as epinephrine and isoproterenol inhibit GLUT-4 mediated glucose uptake in skeletal muscle. The inhibition of glucose uptake apparently results from stimulation of glycogenolysis. This causes the glucose concentration within the cells to rise, inhibiting further net entry of glucose. In other words, this inhibition is the result of a change in the glucose concentration gradient rather than a change in the GLUT-4 turnover (or cycling rate).

■ COUPLING THE TRANSPORT OF ONE SOLUTE TO THE "DOWNHILL" TRANSPORT OF ANOTHER SOLUTE ENABLES CARRIERS TO MOVE THE COTRANSPORTED OR COUNTERTRANSPORTED SOLUTE "UPHILL" AGAINST AN ELECTROCHEMICAL GRADIENT

Coupled transport that does not directly utilize ATP hydrolysis is sometimes called **secondary active transport**. The reason is that the movement of one substance down its electrochemical energy gradient (i.e., "downhill" movement; see Chapter 9) can be used to concentrate another substance (i.e., move it "uphill" against a concentration or voltage gradient). For example, the carrier-mediated transport of a variety of solutes is coupled to Na^+ transport, using energy from the Na^+ electrochemical gradient that is maintained by the **sodium pump** (see Chapter 12). The Na^+ may be either cotransported or countertransported with the coupled solute. **Cotransport** is also referred to as **symport** because both solutes move simultaneously in the same direction; **countertransport** is also called **antiport** or **exchange** because the two coupled solutes move in opposite directions.

Sodium/Proton Exchange Is an Example of Na^+-Coupled Countertransport

Intracellular pH regulation in all cells depends on several transport mechanisms. Among these are the Cl^-/base (e.g., Cl^-/HCO_3^-, and Cl^-/OH^-) exchangers, which can mediate net proton (H^+) influx or efflux, and the Na^+-HCO_3^- cotransporter, which mediates acid efflux. One other type of H^+ transport system, present in virtually all cells, is the Na^+/H^+ exchanger **(sodium/proton exchanger** or NHE) that mediates the electroneutral exchange (i.e., there is no net charge transfer) of 1 Na^+ for 1 H^+. Five molecular isoforms of NHE are expressed in mammalian cells in a tissue-specific manner. NHE1, for example, is expressed in cardiac muscle and kidney epithelia. It has a molecular weight of 91,000 Daltons and a putative structure consisting of 12 transmembrane segments with a large C-terminal cytoplasmic tail. The tail contains several sites that are involved in regulating the exchanger activity (e.g., by phosphorylation and by Ca^{2+}-calmodulin).

The role of NHE is the rapid extrusion of protons from cells when intracellular pH (pH_i) falls below the normal value of about 7.2. Enough energy is available in the Na^+ electrochemical gradient to transport sufficient H^+ out of most cells to raise the intracellular pH (pH_i) to above 8.0 (Box 10-4), but this pH is nonphysiological. To prevent pH_i from rising too much, intracellular H^+ regulates the NHE at an H^+ binding site that is distinct from the H^+ transport site. This H^+ regulatory site has a steep pH dependence and activates transport when protons are produced and pH_i falls. Then, as protons are extruded and pH_i approaches 7.2, NHE activity is rapidly downregulated. This behavior is different from that of many other types of Na^+-coupled transport systems (discussed below), which operate close to electrochemical equilibrium.

BOX 10-4

The Na^+/H^+ Exchanger Mediates the Electroneutral Extrusion of Protons from Cells

The transport process mediated by the Na^+/H^+ exchanger (NHE) with a 1 Na^+:1 H^+ coupling ratio is described by the following equation:

$$Na^+_{out} + H^+_{in} \rightleftharpoons Na^+_{in} + H^+_{out} \quad [B1]$$

To determine how the Na^+ and H^+ concentrations and the membrane potential are related at equilibrium, we equate the total electrochemical potential energy on the two sides of the membrane (see Chapter 9):

$$\mu_{Na, out} + \mu_{H, in} = \mu_{Na, in} + \mu_{H, out}. \quad [B2]$$

Expansion of this equation (see Chapter 9) yields

$$\mu°_{Na} + RT \ln[Na^+]_o + (+1)(0)F + \mu°_H + RT \ln[H^+]_i + (+1)V_mF = \mu°_{Na} + RT \ln[Na^+]_i + (+1)V_mF + \mu°_H + RT \ln[H^+]_o + (+1)(0)F \quad [B3]$$

Note that the electrical terms drop out of this equation because the coupled exchange of 1 Na^+ for 1 H^+ is electroneutral, as is also the case for Cl^-/HCO_3^- exchange (see Chapter 9).

Algebraic rearrangement and division by RT (see Box 9-4) then yield the expression

$$RT \ln[H^+]_i - RT \ln[H^+]_o = RT \ln[Na^+]_i - RT \ln[Na^+]_o \quad [B4]$$

or (see Box 9-4):

$$\frac{[H^+]_i}{[H^+]_o} = \frac{[Na^+]_i}{[Na^+]_o} \quad [B5]$$

Now, solving for $[H^+]_i$, we have:

$$[H^+]_i = \frac{[Na^+]_i}{[Na^+]_o} \times [H^+]_o \quad [B6]$$

Then, if $[Na^+]_i$ = 15 mM and $[Na^+]_o$ = 150 mM, at equilibrium the $[H^+]_i$ concentration should be 10-fold lower than $[H^+]_o$ (= $10^{-7.4}$ M). Alternatively, if $[H^+]$ is expressed as pH (the negative logarithm of $[H^+]$), intracellular pH (pH_i) should be 1.0 pH unit larger than extracellular pH (pH_o = 7.4). In other words, there is sufficient potential energy in the Na^+ electrochemical energy gradient to lower $[H^+]_i$ by a factor of 10, to about $10^{-8.4}$ M (i.e., raise pH_i to 8.4), via NHE. However, the fact that pH_i is normally about 7.2 and not 8.4 indicates that NHE-mediated proton extrusion is inactivated (as a result of the dissociation of H^+ from the regulatory site) before pH_i reaches the equilibrium value predicted by Equation [B6].

■ SODIUM IS COTRANSPORTED WITH A VARIETY OF SOLUTES SUCH AS GLUCOSE AND AMINO ACIDS

The **Na⁺ and glucose cotransporters**, SGLTs, some isoforms of which are found in the brush border (apical or luminal) membranes of intestinal and renal epithelial cells, are good examples of carriers that are obliged to cotransport two solutes simultaneously. These transporters (Figure 10-4) are members of a family of more than 35 Na⁺-coupled cotransporters. Other members include several Na⁺–amino acid cotransporters (e.g., the Na⁺-alanine cotransporter), the Na⁺-K⁺-2Cl⁻ cotransporter, various neurotransmitter transporters (e.g., the Na⁺-norepinephrine, Na⁺-dopamine, and Na⁺-serotonin cotransporters), and the **Na⁺-I⁻ cotransporter**.

Several widely prescribed antidepressant drugs such as fluoxetine (Prozac) act by selectively inhibiting presynaptic serotonin (5-hydroxytryptamine, 5-HT) reuptake by Na⁺-serotonin cotransport. This enhances and prolongs the activation of postsynaptic serotonergic neurons by 5-HT.

The Na⁺-I⁻ cotransporter (sometimes called the Na⁺-I⁻ symporter, or NIS) plays a central role in thyroid gland physiology and pathophysio-

---

> **BOX 10-5**
>
> ### Na⁺-I⁻ Cotransport: Physiology and Pathophysiology
>
> The Na⁺-I⁻ cotransporter (NIC), which is expressed in thyroid follicular cells, the stomach, lactating mammary gland, and several other cell types, cotransports 1 I⁻ with 2 Na⁺ ions. Thus I⁻, an ion normally present in trace amounts, may be concentrated as much as 1000-fold within these cells (see Boxes 10-6 and 10-7). The I⁻ trapped in the thyroid is used for the synthesis of the thyroid hormones *thyroxine* and *triiodothyronine*, which are *iodothyronines* that are made by forming an ether link between two *iodotyrosines*. The ability of the NIC to concentrate I⁻ in the thyroid is used to concentrate radioactive ^{131}I in cancerous thyroid cells, both to detect the spread of the cancer and, after surgery, to destroy the remaining cancer cells by radiation. Moreover, inherited defects in the NIC result in defective I⁻ trapping and thus in congenital *hypothyroidism* (low thyroid hormone levels).

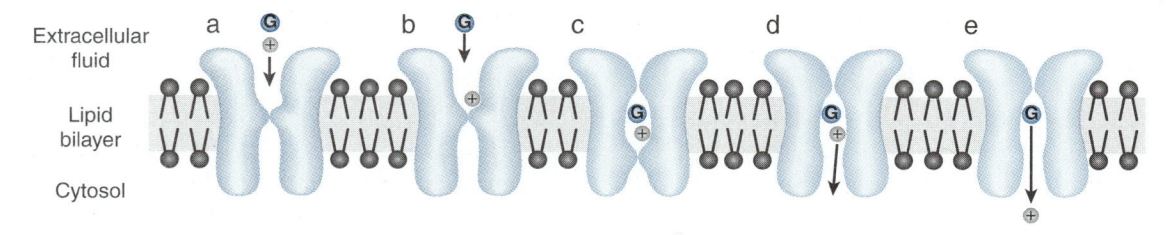

Figure 10-4 ■ Mechanism of glucose transport by an Na⁺-glucose cotransporter (SGLT-2) with a 1:1 coupling ratio. Note the ordered binding and release of the transported solutes: in the exofacial conformation (*a* and *b*), Na⁺ goes on first (*a*), followed by glucose (*b*). In the endofacial conformation (*d* and *e*), the sequence is reversed, and glucose comes off last (*e*). *c* is the occluded conformation with both substrates bound. Not shown is the occluded conformation in which neither substrate is bound; this is essential to effect *net* solute transport by the cotransporter (see text).

Passive Solute Transport

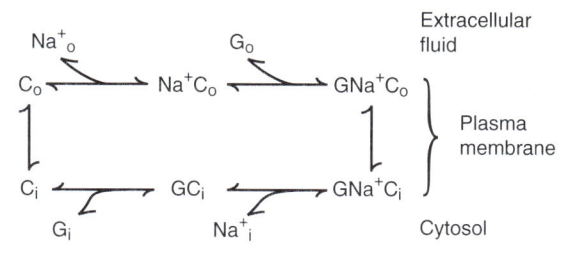

Figure 10-5 ■ State diagram of transport reactions mediated by the SGLT-2 Na$^+$-glucose cotransporter (C). Subscripts "o" and "i" refer to the extracellular fluid or exofacial configuration of the carrier and the cytosol or endofacial configuration of the carrier, respectively. Note that the carrier can switch between exofacial and endofacial conformations only when it is unloaded (C$_o$ and C$_i$) or when both Na$^+$ and glucose (G) are bound (GNa$^+$C$_o$ and GNa$^+$C$_i$).

logy. Thyroid glands use the coupled transport of Na$^+$ (see below) to concentrate I$^-$, a "trace" element (i.e., present at very low concentration). This promotes the iodination of tyrosine; iodinated tyrosine is then used to form the thyroid hormones, which are iodothyronines (Box 10-5).

How Does the Electrochemical Gradient for One Solute Affect the Gradient for a Cotransported Solute?

The answer to this question is based on the fact that both solutes must be bound to the carrier at the same side of the membrane before the carrier can alter its conformation so as to translocate either solute. We can visualize this by considering the steps involved in the SGLT-2 carrier cycle (Figure 10-5). This carrier isoform is expressed in the apical (brush border) membranes of kidney proximal tubule epithelial cells. It cotransports 1 Na$^+$ ion with 1 glucose molecule as summarized in Figure 10-6. With unloaded SGLT-2 in the exofacial conformation, the carrier readily binds Na$^+$ because of the high concentration of Na$^+$ in the renal tubular lumen.

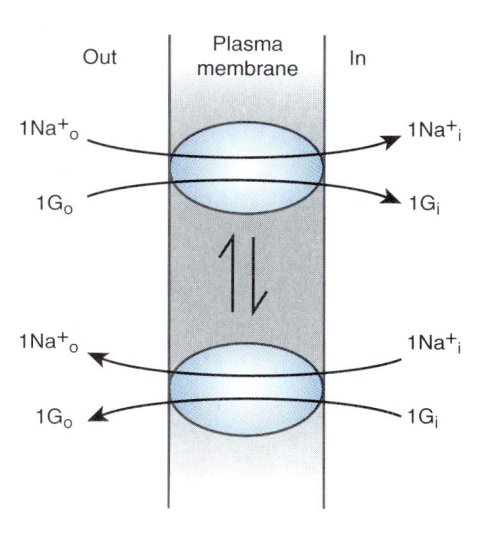

Figure 10-6 ■ Net transport reactions mediated by the SGLT-2 Na$^+$-glucose cotransporter. The transporter can move 1 Na$^+$ ion and 1 glucose molecule either into the cell *(top)* or out of the cell *(bottom)*.

The binding of Na$^+$ increases the affinity for luminal glucose, which also then binds to the carrier (Figure 10-5). The binding of both solutes permits a spontaneous conformational change to the endofacial configuration. Then, because of the low concentration of Na$^+$ in the cytoplasm, as well as the negative membrane potential (i.e., cytoplasm negative to tubule lumen), the bound Na$^+$ dissociates readily. This lowers the binding affinity for glucose so that it, too, is discharged into the cytoplasm. The conformational change between exofacial and endofacial configurations can take place only when *both* Na$^+$ and glucose are bound to the carrier or when *neither* solute is bound. Thus little glucose should exit from the cells via this carrier because the low [Na$^+$]$_i$ makes binding in the endofacial conformation highly unlikely.

Energetic consequences of cotransport If the transport of 1 molecule of glucose is tightly coupled to the transport of 1 Na$^+$ ion via SGLT-2 (Figure 10-6), the energy dissipated by the downhill movement of Na^+ can be stored in the glucose gradient. Of course, as Na^+ moves into the cell via SGLT-2 at the *apical membrane*, the Na^+ pump uses energy from the hydrolysis of ATP (see Chapter 11) to transport Na^+ out of the cell across the *basolateral membrane*. This maintains the Na^+ gradients across *both* the apical and basolateral membranes. In this coupled transport system no net gain or loss of energy can occur, so the energy built up in the glucose gradient must equal the energy that is available from the Na^+ gradient (Box 10-6). This type of transport is sometimes called secondary active transport because the energy from ATP is used only indirectly. In other words, the Na^+ pump (Chapter 11) uses the energy from ATP to build up and *maintain* the Na^+ electrochemical gradient, which is used, in turn, to drive the secondary transport of another solute.

BOX 10-6

The Energetics of Coupled Cotransport Is Exemplified by the 1 Na^+:1 Glucose Cotransporter (SGLT-2)

The transport of 1 molecule of glucose is tightly coupled to the transport of 1 Na^+ ion via the SGLT-2 cotransporter across the apical membrane of a renal proximal tubule cell. Accordingly, for this transporter, the coupled transport reaction is

$$G_{in} + Na^+_{in} \rightleftharpoons G_{out} + Na^+_{out} \quad [B1]$$

This transport reaction is somewhat more complex than NHE (Box 10-4) because Na^+-glucose cotransport involves the net movement of charge when 1 Na^+ and 1 G move across the membrane. The driving forces for this coupled transport are the electrochemical potential energies for Na^+ on the two sides of the membrane and the chemical potential energies for glucose (because $z = 0$; see Chapter 9). Equating the potential energies on the two sides of the membrane (i.e., at equilibrium), we have

$$\mu_{G,in} + \mu_{Na,in} = \mu_{G,out} + \mu_{Na,out} \quad [B2]$$

Expanding this equation (see Chapter 9), with $z = +1$ for Na^+, gives us

$$\mu^\circ_G + RT \ln[G]_i + \mu^\circ_{Na} + RT \ln[Na^+]_i + (+1)V_mF = $$
$$\mu^\circ_G + RT \ln[G]_o + \mu^\circ_{Na} + RT \ln[Na^+]_o + (+1)(0)F \quad [B3]$$

Rearrangement then yields

$$RT \ln[G]_i - RT \ln[G]_o = RT \ln[Na^+]_o - RT \ln[Na^+]_i - V_mF \quad [B4]$$

Dividing by RT, we have

$$\ln[G]_i - \ln[G]_o = \ln[Na^+]_o - \ln[Na^+]_i - V_mF/RT \quad [B5]$$

Then, recalling that, for any solute, S, $(\ln[S]_i - \ln[S]_o) = \ln([S]_i/[S]_o)$ (see Appendix A), we can rewrite the preceding equation as

$$\ln \frac{[G]_i}{[G]_o} = \ln \frac{[Na^+]_o}{[Na^+]_i} - zV_mF/RT \quad [B6]$$

Taking antilogarithms (see Appendix A), we get

$$\frac{[G]_i}{[G]_o} = \frac{[Na^+]_o}{[Na^+]_i} \exp(-V_mF/RT) \quad [B7]$$

where "exp (X)" is "e" (the base of the natural logarithms) raised to the power, X, the term in the parentheses [i.e., $\exp(X) = e^X$], and $e = 2.7$ (see Appendix A). Thus, if $[Na^+]_o = 150$ mM, $[Na^+]_i = 15$ mM, and $V_m = -62$ mV, since RT/F has a value of 26.7 mV at 37° C, the expected maximal glucose gradient, $[G]_i/[G]_o$, is

$$\frac{[G]_i}{[G]_o} = \frac{150}{15} \times e^{2.32} = 10 \times 10 = 100 \quad [B8]$$

In other words, with a typical Na^+ concentration gradient ($[Na^+]_o/[Na^+]_i = 10$), $[G]_i = 100 \times [G]_o$; that is, the SGLT-2 carrier should be able to concentrate glucose 100-fold within the cell. (Note the importance of V_m when net transfer of charge occurs during the transport cycle.)

A more quantitative, thermodynamic treatment is presented in Box 10-6. It shows that the SGLT-2 transporter should be able to concentrate glucose 100-fold within the cell when the Na^+ concentration ratio ($[Na^+]_o/[Na^+]_i$) is 10 and the membrane potential across the apical (brush border) membrane is –60 mV. This is important in the kidneys, where we need to reabsorb as much glucose from the lumen of the renal tubule as possible.

Glucose Uptake Efficiency Can Be Increased by a Change in the Na^+-Glucose Coupling Ratio

SGLT-2, with an Na^+-glucose coupling ratio of 1:1, is expressed in the early portion of kidney proximal convoluted tubules. The late portion of the proximal convoluted tubules contains a different Na^+-glucose cotransporter isoform, SGLT-1, with an Na^+-glucose coupling ratio of 2:1. SGLT-2 markedly lowers the glucose concentration in the renal tubular fluid. Then SGLT-1, which can concentrate glucose 100-fold more than can SGLT-2 (Box 10-7), further minimizes the loss of glucose in the urine by mediating uptake of most of the residual glucose in the late proximal tubule fluid.

■ NET TRANSPORT OF SOME SOLUTES ACROSS EPITHELIA IS EFFECTED BY COUPLING TWO TRANSPORT PROCESSES IN SERIES

We have just seen that SGLT-2 and SGLT-1 are capable of markedly concentrating glucose in epithelial cells. If the transported glucose actually accumulated in cells, however, the

---

BOX 10-7

The Energetics of a 2 Na^+:1 Glucose Carrier (SGLT-1) Illustrates the Power of the Exponents in the Transport Equation

Because the Na^+-glucose cotransporter, SGLT-1, has a coupling ratio of 2 Na^+:1 glucose, the transport process in this case is (contrast with Box 10-6):

$$G_{in} + 2\ Na^+_{in} \rightleftharpoons G_{out} + 2\ Na^+_{out} \quad [B1]$$

Rewriting this equation in terms of the electrochemical and chemical potential energies, we have:

$$\mu_{G, in} + 2\ \mu_{Na, in} = \mu_{G, out} + 2\ \mu_{Na, out} \quad [B2]$$

Note that, when more than one ion or molecule of a single species is transported during a transporter cycle, the electrochemical potential energy for that species must be multiplied by the number of ions or molecules transported. Expanding this equation (see Box 10-6) now gives us:

$$\mu^\circ_G + RT \ln[G]_i + 2\ \mu^\circ_{Na} + 2\ RT \ln[Na^+]_i +$$
$$2\ (+1)V_M F = \mu^\circ_G + RT \ln[G]_o + 2\ \mu^\circ_{Na} + \quad [B3]$$
$$2\ RT \ln[Na^+]_o + 2\ (+1)(0)F$$

Rearrangement, and division by RT, then yields:

$$\ln[G]_i - \ln[G]_o = 2 \ln[Na^+]_o - \\ 2 \ln[Na^+]_i - 2\ V_m F/RT \quad [B4]$$

Taking antilogarithms (see Box 10-6), and remembering that the antilogarithm of $n\ln X$ is X^n (see Appendix A), gives

$$\frac{[G]_i}{[G]_o} = \left(\frac{[Na^+]_o}{[Na^+]_i}\right)^2 \exp(-2V_m F/RT) \quad [B5]$$

Thus, if $[Na^+]_o = 150$ mM, $[Na^+]_i = 15$ mM, and $V_m = -62$ mV, since $RT/F = 26.7$ mV, the expected maximal glucose concentration gradient, $[G]_i/[G]_o$ is

$$\frac{[G]_i}{[G]_o} = \left(\frac{150}{15}\right)^2 \times e^{4.64} = 10^2 \times 100 = 10,000 \quad [B6]$$

In other words, with the same Na^+ electrochemical gradient as is used in the preceding example (Box 10-6), SGLT-1 should be able to concentrate glucose 10,000-fold within the cell.

osmotic stress would cause the cells to gain water and swell (see Chapter 3). Moreover, another issue to consider is that the object of glucose transport across the apical membranes of the epithelial cells is *not* to concentrate the glucose in these cells. Rather, the object is to transfer glucose from the renal tubule or intestinal lumen, *across the epithelium* to the interstitial space, so as to get the glucose into the blood to circulate to other cells in the body. To accomplish this net intestinal absorption (or renal reabsorption) of glucose, GLUT-2, a simple glucose carrier (and an isoform of GLUT-1), is expressed in the basolateral membranes of these epithelial cells. Thus the net transepithelial transport occurs in a two-step process, as illustrated in Figure 10-7: Glucose is transported into these epithelial cells, across their apical membranes, by SGLT-2 or SGLT-1. The glucose diffuses through the cytoplasm to the basolateral membrane and is then transported into the interstitial space by GLUT-2, so that it can be carried, in the blood plasma, to all the other cells in the body. Consequently, no large buildup of glucose occurs in the cytoplasm of the epithelial cells; thus osmotic pressure does not increase and the cells do not swell.

Osmotic problems do not arise in neurons as a result of Na$^+$-coupled neurotransmitter reuptake for a different reason: the *total* amount of neurotransmitter that must be reaccumulated at the end of an action potential is very small relative to the total cell volume. Cell volume changes therefore are negligible.

A Variety of Inherited Defects of Glucose Transport Have Been Identified

SGLT-1 is also expressed in intestinal tract (jejunum) epithelial cells, where it is responsible for glucose and galactose absorption. Mutations in SGLT-1 result in glucose-galactose malabsorption, a rare syndrome that is manifested as a severe, potentially fatal diarrhea (Box 10-8).

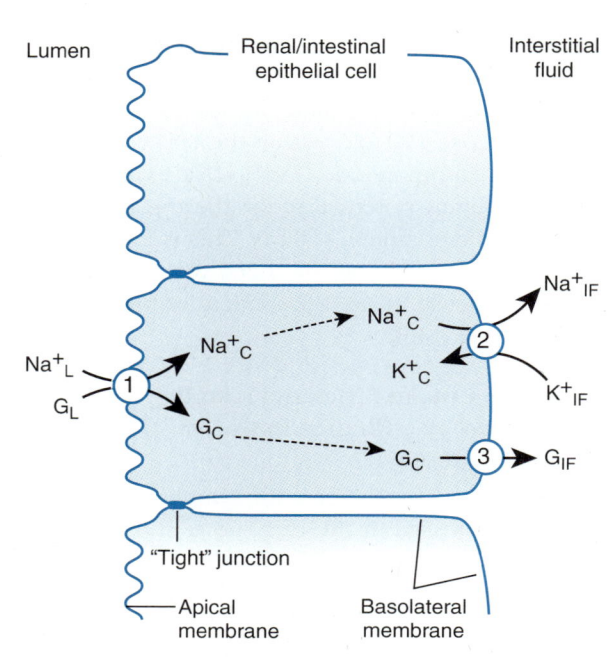

Figure 10-7 ■ **Renal proximal tubule or small intestine epithelial cell illustrating the two-step sequential transport of glucose across the apical and basolateral membranes. Glucose (G) is cotransported, with Na$^+$, across the epithelial cell apical membrane by SGLT-2 or SGLT-1 (1). Na$^+$ and G then diffuse, in the cytosol, to the basolateral membrane where Na$^+$ is extruded by the Na$^+$ pump (2) (see Chapter 11), and glucose is transported into the interstitial fluid by the simple glucose carrier, GLUT-2 (3). Subscripts "L", "C," and "IF" refer to lumen, cytosol, and interstitial fluid, respectively.**

These mutations in SGLT-1 cause only a mild *glycosuria* (glucose in the urine) because most of the renal glucose uptake in the proximal tubules is mediated by SGLT-2. Genetically defective SGLT-2 is associated with a much more marked glycosuria (in this situation, caused by a renal tubular defect rather than by a high blood glucose level and excessive glucose in the glomerular filtrate, as occurs in diabetes mellitus). Apparently SGLT-2 is the main carrier responsible

Passive Solute Transport

> **BOX 10-8**
>
> ### *Glucose-Galactose Malabsorption*
>
> Glucose-galactose malabsorption is a rare disorder of sugar transport. The disease is manifested, beginning in neonatal life, as a severe watery, acidic diarrhea that is brought on by ingestion of lactose [milk sugar, 4-(β-D-galactosido)-D-glucose], which is hydrolyzed to glucose and galactose in the intestinal lumen. The disease can be fatal within a few weeks if lactose and glucose (or sucrose, which is hydrolyzed to glucose and fructose) are not removed from the diet. The cause of the disease is a mutational defect in the intestinal brush border SGLT-1 Na⁺-glucose cotransporter that virtually abolishes the absorption of glucose and galactose in the intestine. The diarrhea results from retention of these sugars (and Na⁺) in the intestinal lumen. These solutes exert an osmotic effect; thus, not only is fluid absorption reduced, but also fluid is drawn from the plasma into the intestinal lumen. For this reason, this type of diarrhea is referred to as an osmotic diarrhea.

for glucose reabsorption in the kidney, but it has little role in intestinal glucose uptake, whereas SGLT-1 is most important in the intestine.

Fanconi-Bickel syndrome is a rare inherited disorder that results from loss-of-function mutations in GLUT-2, which is expressed in the intestine, kidney, liver, and pancreas. The syndrome is manifested by glucose intolerance, resting hypoglycemia (low blood glucose level), and renal, pancreatic, and hepatic abnormalities. Glucose absorption in the intestine and kidneys is impaired, and the liver exhibits excessive (pathological) glycogen storage because it cannot export the glucose it produces by *gluconeogenesis*.

■ SODIUM IS EXCHANGED FOR SOLUTES SUCH AS CALCIUM AND PROTONS BY COUNTERTRANSPORT MECHANISMS

Now let's consider carriers in which the inward (downhill) transport of Na⁺ is tightly coupled to the outward transport of other solutes. Two good examples of this second, countertransported solute are protons (Na⁺/H⁺ exchange) and calcium ions (**Na⁺/Ca²⁺ exchange**). As we have already learned, the Na⁺/H⁺ exchanger is one of several transporters (the Cl⁻/HCO₃⁻ exchanger is another) involved in maintaining intracellular pH in various types of cells. Na⁺/H⁺ exchange also plays a major role in the reabsorption of Na⁺ and excretion of protons in the kidney. The Na⁺/Ca²⁺ exchanger, another important countertransporter, helps to maintain intracellular Ca²⁺ balance. This is critical because of the central role of Ca²⁺ ions in cell signaling.

Na⁺/Ca²⁺ Exchange Is an Example of Coupled Countertransport

The Na⁺/Ca²⁺ exchanger is found in the plasma membranes of a large variety of cell types. These include all types of muscle (cardiac, skeletal, and smooth muscle), neurons, and intestinal and renal epithelial cells (where it is prevalent in the basolateral membranes of cells involved in Ca²⁺ absorption or resorption). In these cells the coupling ratio (stoichiometry) of the exchanger is 3 Na⁺:1 Ca²⁺ and there is a net movement of one positive charge during each cycle. In other words, the Na⁺/Ca²⁺ exchanger, which is reversible, can mediate the entry of 3 Na⁺ ions in exchange for 1 exiting Ca²⁺ ion or it can mediate the entry of 1 Ca²⁺ ion in exchange for 3 exiting Na⁺ ions (Figure 10-8; Figure 10-9 summarizes the net transport reactions). With this coupling ratio, and with an Na⁺ concentration ratio ($[Na^+]_o/[Na^+]_i$) of 10:1 and a membrane potential of −60 mV, the Na⁺ electrochemical potential gradient ($\mu_{Na, out} - \mu_{Na, in}$) provides sufficient energy to maintain a Ca²⁺ concentration ratio

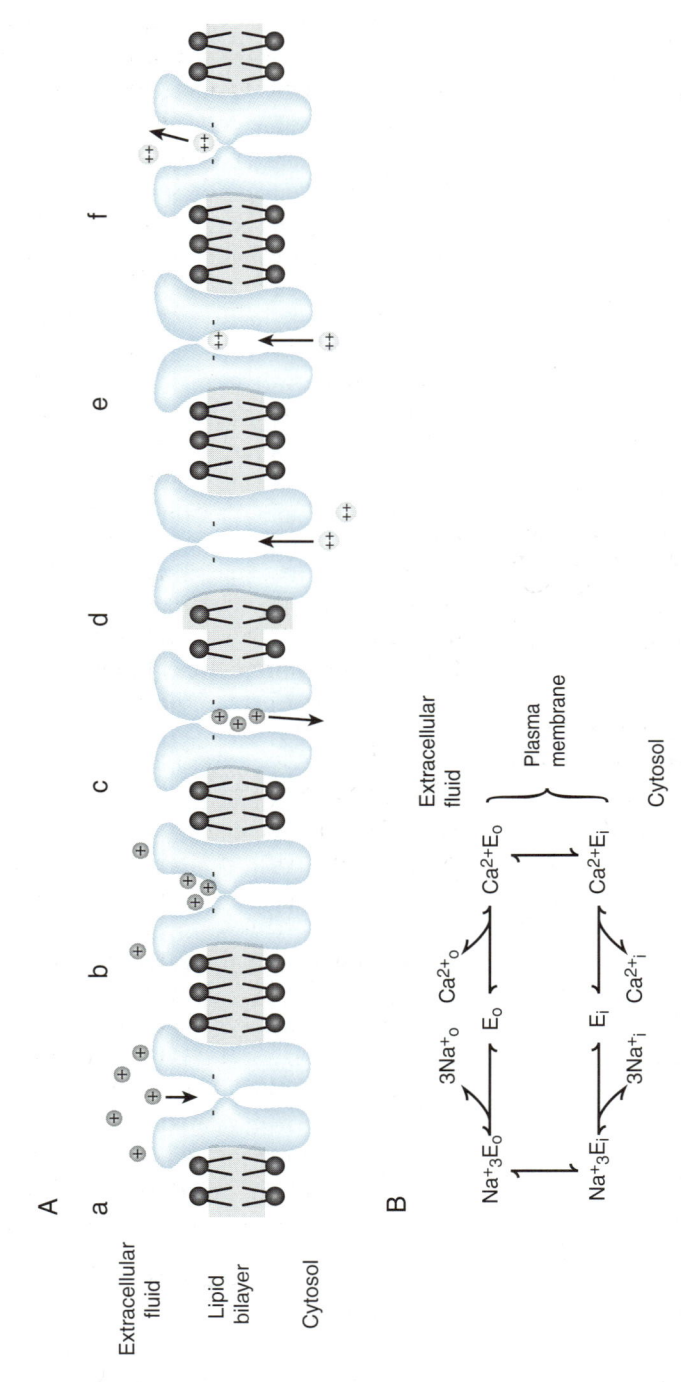

Figure 10-8 ■ **A,** Mechanism of Ca^{2+} transport by the Na^+/Ca^{2+} exchanger. In the exofacial configuration (*a*) the exchanger can bind either 3 Na^+ (*b*) or 1 Ca^{2+} (not shown). Then, after a transition through an occluded state (not shown) to the endofacial configuration (*c*), one solute species can dissociate (e.g., Na^+, as in the "*c*"-"*d*" transition) and either Na^+ (not shown) or Ca^{2+} (*e*) can bind. After another conformation change (via the occluded state) to the exofacial conformation, the bound solute (Ca^{2+} in this case) can be discharged to the extracellular fluid (*f*). **B,** State diagram of the transport reactions mediated by the Na^+/Ca^{2+} exchanger (E). Subscripts "o" and "i" refer to the extracellular fluid or exofacial configuration of the carrier and the cytosol or endofacial configuration of the carrier, respectively. Note that the carrier can switch between exofacial and endofacial conformations only when it is loaded ($Na^+{}_3E_o$, $Na^+{}_3E_i$, $Ca^{2+}E_o$, or $Ca^{2+}E_i$); the unloaded carrier does not undergo conformational change (i.e., between E_o and E_i).

Passive Solute Transport

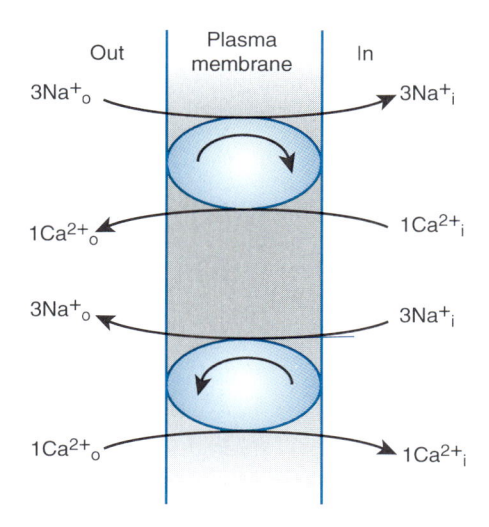

Figure 10-9 ■ Net transport reactions mediated by the Na$^+$/Ca^{2+} exchanger. The exchanger can either move 3 Na$^+$ ions into the cell in exchange for 1 exiting Ca^{2+} ion *(top)* or move 3 Na$^+$ ions out of the cell in exchange for 1 entering Ca^{2+} ion *(bottom)*.

($[Ca^{2+}]_o/[Ca^{2+}]_i$) of 10,000:1 (Box 10-9). Then, because the free (unbound, ionized) Ca^{2+} concentration in blood plasma ($[Ca^{2+}]_o$) is about 1 mM (0.001 M = 10^{-3} M), we would expect the free Ca^{2+} concentration in the cytoplasm ($[Ca^{2+}]_i$) to be about 10^{-7} M, or 100 nM (Box 10-9). In fact, this is essentially correct. In most resting cells, $[Ca^{2+}]_i$ is about 100 nM, or about 1/10,000th of the Ca^{2+} concentration in the extracellular fluid. Thus the exchanger operates close to electrochemical equilibrium (Box 10-9).

Na$^+$/Ca^{2+} Exchange Is Influenced by Changes in the Membrane Potential

As discussed in Chapters 7 and 8, excitable cell membrane potentials undergo marked changes when the cells are activated. This has special significance for Ca^{2+} transport mediated by the Na$^+$/Ca^{2+} exchanger in these cells because the exchanger is influenced by the membrane potential (Box 10-9). A noteworthy example is cardiac muscle, in which the action potential has a relatively long duration (see Figure 8-1). Since $[Na^+]_o$, $[Na^+]_i$, and $[Ca^{2+}]_o$ do not change during the action potential, the direction of the exchanger-mediated Ca^{2+} movement is determined by the change in membrane potential. As indicated in Box 10-9, with a resting membrane potential of V_m = –62 mV there is no net exchanger-mediated movement of Ca^{2+} under the (resting) conditions shown. During the cardiac action potential, however, when the membrane is markedly depolarized (Figure 8-1), Ca^{2+} is driven *into* the cells by the exchanger. This helps to initiate and maintain cardiac contraction. Conversely, early in diastole (the relaxation phase of the cardiac contraction cycle), when the membrane repolarizes and, even briefly hyperpolarizes (i.e., V_m is more negative than –62 mV), while $[Ca^{2+}]_i$ is elevated, Ca^{2+} is driven *out* of the cells by the exchanger. This promotes cardiac relaxation and recovery.

Na$^+$/Ca^{2+} Exchange Is Regulated by Several Different Mechanisms

As is the case for many transport systems, the kinetic properties of the Na$^+$/Ca^{2+} exchanger are regulated in a tissue-specific manner. This enables the exchanger to accommodate to physiological demands. For example, the exchanger activity may be increased when the exchanger is phosphorylated or when it is activated by phosphatidyl-inositol bis-phosphate (PIP$_2$) or even by intracellular Ca^{2+}, which acts at a site distinct from the one involved in transport. For example, even with a high $[Na^+]_i$, the exchanger will not transport Ca^{2+} *into* cells if the $[Ca^{2+}]_i$ concentration is low (i.e., about 100 nM).

Intracellular Ca^{2+} Plays Many Important Physiological Roles

A low resting $[Ca^{2+}]_i$ is important physiologically because small increases in $[Ca^{2+}]_i$ serve

BOX 10-9

The Energetics of Coupled Countertransport Is Exemplified by Na$^+$/Ca^{2+} Exchange

The cardiac/neuronal plasma membrane (PM) Na$^+$/Ca^{2+} exchanger transports 3 Na$^+$ ions in exchange for 1 Ca^{2+}. Thus the transport equation can be written as:

$$Ca^{2+}{}_{in} + 3\,Na^+{}_{out} \rightleftharpoons Ca^{2+}{}_{out} + 3\,Na^+{}_{in} \quad [B1]$$

Rewriting this equation in terms of the electrochemical potential energies on the two sides of the PM, we have (see Box 10-7):

$$\mu_{Ca,\,in} + 3\,\mu_{Na,\,out} = \mu_{Ca,\,out} + 3\,\mu_{Na,\,in} \quad [B2]$$

Expanding this equation (remembering that $z = +2$ for Ca^{2+}) gives:

$$\mu^\circ_{Ca} + RT\ln[Ca^{2+}]_i + (+2)V_mF + 3\,\mu^\circ_{Na} + 3\,RT\ln[Na^+]_o + 3(+1)0F = \mu^\circ_{Ca} + RT\ln[Ca^{2+}]_o \quad [B3]$$
$$+ (+2)0F + 3\,\mu^\circ_{Na} + 3\,RT\ln[Na^+]_i + 3(+1)V_mF$$

Rearrangement and division by RT yields:

$$\ln[Ca^{2+}]_i - \ln[Ca^{2+}]_o = 3\ln[Na^+]_i - 3\ln[Na^+]_o + V_mF/RT$$

Taking antilogarithms (and remembering that the antilogarithm of $3\ln X$ is X^3) yields:

$$\frac{[Ca^{2+}]_i}{[Ca^{2+}]_o} = \left(\frac{[Na^+]_i}{[Na^+]_o}\right)^3 \exp\left(\frac{V_mF}{RT}\right) \quad [B5]$$

Thus, with $[Na^+]_o = 150$ mM, $[Na^+]_i = 15$ mM, and $V_m = -62$ mV, since $RT/F = 26.7$ mV, we get:

$$\frac{[Ca^{2+}]_i}{[Ca^{2+}]_o} = \left(\frac{[Na^+]_i}{[Na^+]_o}\right)^3 \times e^{-2.32} = (0.1)^3 \times 0.1 = 0.0001 \quad [B6]$$

Solving for $[Ca^{2+}]_i$ gives:

$$[Ca^{2+}]_i = [Ca^{2+}]_o \times (15/150)^3 \times e^{-2.32}$$
$$= [Ca^{2+}]_o \times (0.1)^3 \times 0.1$$
$$= 0.0001[Ca^{2+}]_o$$

Then, since the free Ca^{2+} concentration in blood plasma ($[Ca^{2+}]_o$) is about 1.0 mM (0.001 M), we have:

$$[Ca^{2+}]_i = 0.001 \times 0.0001\,M = 0.0000001\,M$$
$$= 100 \times 10^{-9}\,M \text{ or } 100\,nM$$

The equation indicates that $[Ca^{2+}]_i$ should be approximately 100 nM, which is just about what is actually observed in most cells.

---

numerous essential second-messenger functions.* An increase in the $[Ca^{2+}]_i$ level triggers contraction in all types of muscle (skeletal, cardiac, and smooth; see Chapters 12 and 13); it activates neurotransmitter release at nerve endings and secretion in most secretory cells; it controls visual adaptation and auditory processes; and it also controls the fertilization of the ovum and cell division, as well as numerous other physiological processes. Moreover, many pathophysiological processes are associated with deranged Ca^{2+} homeostasis, and Ca^{2+} overload usually leads to cell death. Thus cellular regulation of $[Ca^{2+}]_i$ is extremely important, and Na$^+$/Ca^{2+} exchange is one of the critical mechanisms involved in this regulation (see Chapter 11).

■ MULTIPLE TRANSPORT SYSTEMS CAN BE FUNCTIONALLY COUPLED

The same principles of coupled transport (cotransport and countertransport) apply to the transport of numerous other solutes. As we have already seen in the discussion of Cl$^-$/HCO$_3^-$ exchange (Chapter 9), Na$^+$-coupled transport systems are not the only coupled solute transport systems. Moreover, like most Na$^+$-coupled transport systems, the red cell and kidney

---

*In the 1950s, the Austrian pharmacologist and Nobel Laureate Otto Loewi made the prescient and off-cited statement, "Ja, Kalzium, das ist alles!" (Calcium is everything!).

Cl$^-$/HCO$_3^-$ exchanger (also known as anion exchanger type 1, or AE1) operates near equilibrium so that it can use the gradient of either one of the transported ions to move the other.

AE1 mediates the exchange of the anion of a weak acid (H$_2$CO$_3$, carbonic acid) for the anion of a strong acid (HCl, hydrochloric acid). In the distal convoluted tubule of the kidney, AE1 is used to reabsorb HCO$_3^-$ and extrude Cl$^-$ into the tubular lumen, thereby acidifying the urine. Consequently, hereditary defects in AE1 are associated with *renal tubular acidosis* because the kidneys cannot excrete sufficient acid.

Tertiary Active Transport

Figure 10-10 shows how a metabolic intermediate, α-ketoglutarate (αKG^{2-}), is coupled to the countertransport of organic anions (OA$^-$) in the basolateral membrane of the kidney *proximal* tubule cells. This transporter, the "multispecific" organic anion transporter-1, or OAT-1, is a major route of drug excretion. Examples of OA$^-$ transported by this system are urate, *p*-aminohippurate (PAH$^-$, an agent used to measure renal plasma flow), the penicillins, and salicylates (e.g., acetylsalicylic acid, or aspirin, is excreted primarily as salicylurate). Mitochondrial metabolism provides the αKG^{2-} that is transported out of the cell in exchange for entering OA$^-$. OAT-1 is selective for αKG^{2-}: other dicarboxylic acids such as succinate, fumarate, and malate cannot replace the αKG^{2-}. So that αKG^{2-} will not be wasted (and cellular αKG^{2-} levels will be maintained), αKG^{2-} is transported back into the cells across the basolateral membrane by an Na$^+$/dicarboxylate cotransporter with a high affinity for dicarboxylates (NaDC-3); it couples the transport of 1 αKG^{2-} to 3 Na$^+$. Indeed, the Na$^+$ pump indirectly promotes the transport of OA$^-$ into the cells by inducing a gradient for αKG^{2-} (so-called **tertiary active transport**). The OA$^-$ does not accumulate in the cell but rather leaves the cell across the apical

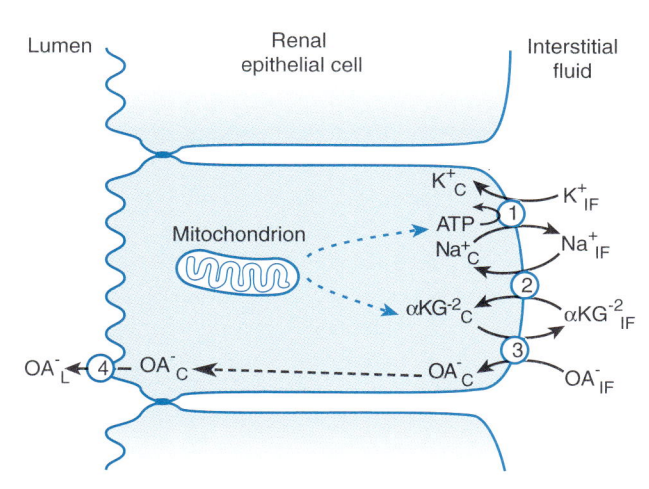

Figure 10-10 ■ Renal tubule epithelial cell illustrating the two-step sequential transport of organic anions (OA$^-$) across the basolateral and apical membranes. To move from the interstitial fluid (IF) into the cell cytosol, OA$^-$ is transported across the basolateral membrane by an OA$^-$/α-ketoglutarate (αKG^{-2}) exchanger, OAT-1 (3). The OA$^-$ then diffuses through the cytosol to the apical membrane; it is next transported into the renal tubular lumen (L) by another organic acid carrier (4). The αKG^{-2} is a Krebs cycle intermediate produced in mitochondria; it is reclaimed from the interstitial fluid by the basolateral Na$^+$/αKG^{-2} cotransporter, NaDC-3, which couples the transport of 3 Na$^+$ to 1 αKG^{2-} (2). The Na$^+$ electrochemical gradient that drives this cotransporter is maintained by the basolateral membrane Na$^+$ pump (1) (see Chapter 11). (Redrawn from Dantzler WH, Wright SH: *Comprehensive toxicology.* Vol 7. *Renal toxicology,* Oxford, Eng, 1997, Pergamon.)

(brush border) membrane by a different carrier-mediated transport system. The net effect is secretion of the OA$^-$ while the Na$^+$ and αKG^{2-} are recycled, as illustrated in Figure 10-10. This is particularly important for rapid clearance of xenobiotics ("foreign" chemicals) from the body. Indeed, this efficient transport system can "clear" (i.e., remove) 90% of some agents from plasma in a single passage through the kidneys, provided that the plasma concentration of the agents is not too high. This high clearance is the reason that PAH^- can be used to estimate renal blood flow.

Net secretion of organic cations such as creatine and morphine occurs by an analogous mechanism. In this case the facilitated diffusion step is at the basolateral membrane: independent carriers mediate monovalent cation and divalent cation transport into epithelial cells. The basolateral membrane voltage (≈ -50 to -70 mV) provides the energy to concentrate these solutes about 10- or 100-fold inside the cells. In the apical membrane an organic cation/proton (OC^+/H^+) exchanger that transports both OC^+ and OC^{2+} serves as the secondary active transport system to effect net secretion of the OCs into the renal tubular fluid. The protons are recycled across the apical membrane by an Na^+/H^+ exchanger (H^+ ions are extruded into the tubule lumen and Na^+ ions are taken up). The Na^+ is conserved: it is transported into the interstitial space by the Na^+ pump in the basolateral membrane.

■ SUMMARY

1. Biological membranes are poorly permeable to polar solutes. Specialized carrier and pump proteins are therefore needed to mediate the transfer of specific solutes across the plasma membrane and to maintain the intracellular concentrations of critical solutes.
2. Solute carriers are integral membrane proteins that have kinetic properties similar to those of enzymes, but carriers mediate *vectorial* transport across biological membranes.
3. Some carriers simply speed the rate at which their substrate solutes (e.g., glucose) diffuse down a transmembrane concentration or electrochemical gradient. These "simple carriers" mediate "facilitated diffusion." They cannot maintain a solute concentration or electrochemical gradient.
4. Some carriers couple the transport of two solutes. These cotransporters or countertransporters can generate a concentration or electrochemical gradient for one solute when the coupled solute, often Na^+, moves down its concentration or electrochemical gradient. This process is sometimes called secondary active transport.
5. The coupled exchange of 1 Na^+ for 1 H^+ (proton) is an example of electroneutral ion countertransport. It is used to extrude H^+ rapidly when pH_i falls below about 7.4. The entering Na^+ is then extruded against its electrochemical gradient by the plasma membrane Na^+ pump (see Chapter 11).
6. Na^+-glucose cotransporters, which are expressed in the brush border (apical) membranes of intestinal and renal epithelia, play important roles in the absorption and reabsorption of glucose from the intestinal and renal tubule lumen. These cotransporters mediate transport with a net movement of charge; therefore Na^+-glucose cotransport is sensitive to the membrane potential.
7. Among the numerous other cotransporters are the Na^+-I^- cotransporter, various Na^+-amino acid and Na^+/neurotransmitter cotransporters, and the Na^+-K^+-Cl^- cotransporter.
8. Na^+/Ca^{2+} exchangers are expressed in many types of cells, including all types of muscle and neurons. They mediate the voltage-sensitive exchange of 1 Ca^{2+} for 3 Na^+ ions. By using the energy stored in the Na^+ electrochemical gradient, these exchangers are able to help maintain a resting $[Ca^{2+}]_i$ of about 100 nM.
9. Among the many other types of countertransporters are the Cl^-/HCO_3^- exchanger and the multispecific organic anion transporter-1.
10. The properties (substrate affinities or turnover rate) of some carriers can be regulated

Passive Solute Transport

by mechanisms such as phosphorylation and dephosphorylation or the membrane insertion and retrieval of carriers. Thus the rate of solute transport can be markedly altered to accommodate physiological needs.

■ KEY WORDS AND CONCEPTS

- Polar versus nonpolar solutes
- Aquaporin
- Transporter turnover number
- Carrier-mediated transport
- Facilitated diffusion
- Passive transport
- Transition state
- Occluded solute
- Simple glucose carrier
- Secondary active transport
- Cotransport (symport)
- Sodium-glucose cotransport
- Sodium-iodide cotransport
- Countertransport (antiport or exchange)
- Sodium/calcium exchange
- Sodium/proton exchange
- Chloride/bicarbonate exchange
- Tertiary active transport

STUDY PROBLEMS

1. Why are Na^+-dependent cotransport systems generally limited to epithelial cells, whereas Na^+-dependent countertransport systems (and other exchangers such as the Cl^-/HCO_3^- exchanger) are expressed in all types of cells?
2. What $[Ca^{2+}]_i$ concentration would be expected in a cell with $V_m = -60$ mV and $[Ca^{2+}]_o = 1$ mM if intracellular Ca^{2+} is at electrochemical equilibrium? Why is this physiologically unrealistic?
3. Photoreceptor (retinal rods and cones) Na^+/Ca^{2+} exchangers mediate the exchange of 4 Na^+ for 1 Ca^{2+} + 1 K^+. This exchanger, like the cardiac/neuronal exchanger (which exchanges 3 Na^+ for 1 Ca^{2+}), operates close to equilibrium (i.e., $4\ \mu_{Na,out} + \mu_{Ca,in} + \mu_{K,in} = 4\ \mu_{Na,in} + \mu_{Ca,out} + \mu_{K,out}$). Can you explain why an exchanger with this coupling ratio is needed in the photoreceptors to maintain "resting" $[Ca^{2+}]_i$ concentration at about 100 nM? (Hint: Under dark conditions, retinal photoreceptor $[Na^+]_i \approx 30\text{-}40$ mM, $[K^+]_i \approx 120$ mM, and $V_m \approx -40$ mV.)
4. What is the possible advantage of using an Na^+/H^+ exchanger rather than another transport system to extrude protons if the exchanger does not operate close to equilibrium?
5. What is the significance of having Na^+-glucose cotransporters with different coupling ratios located at different levels of the kidney proximal tubule to minimize the spillover of glucose in the urine? Assume that the plasma glucose (MW 180) concentration is 5 mM. This is also the concentration in the glomerular filtrate (180 liters/day) that enters the proximal tubules; 67% of the fluid is reabsorbed (i.e., 120 liters/day) in the proximal tubules, the only renal tubule segment in which glucose is absorbed.

■ BIBLIOGRAPHY

Blaustein MP: Physiological effects of endogenous ouabain: control of intracellular Ca^{2+} stores and cell responsiveness, *Am J Physiol* 264:C1367, 1993.

Blaustein MP, Lederer WJ: Sodium/calcium exchange: its physiological implications, *Physiol Rev* 79:763, 1999.

De La Vieja A, Dohan O, Levy O, Carrasco N: Molecular analysis of the sodium/iodide symporter: impact on thyroid and extrathyroid pathophysiology, *Physiol Rev* 80:1083, 2000.

Karmazyn M, Gan XT, Humphreys RA, et al: The myocardial Na^+-H^+ exchange: structure, regulation, and its role in heart disease, *Circ Res* 85:777, 1999.

Klepper J, Wang D, Fischbarg J, et al: Defective glucose transport across brain tissue barriers: a newly recognized neurological syndrome, *Neurochem Res* 24:587, 1999.

Philipson KD, Nicoll DA: Sodium-calcium exchange: a molecular perspective, *Annu Rev Physiol* 62:111, 2000.

Riedel C, Dohan O, De la Vieja A, et al: Journey of the iodide transporter NIS: from its molecular identification to its clinical role in cancer, *Trends Biochem Sci* 26:490, 2001.

Seatter MJ, Gould GW: The mammalian facilitative glucose transporter (GLUT) family, *Pharm Biotechnol* 12:201, 1999.

Wright EM: Renal Na^+-glucose cotransporters, *Am J Physiol Renal Physiol* 280:F10, 2001.

Wright EM, Turk E, Martin MG: Molecular basis for glucose-galactose malabsorption, *Cell Biochem Biophys* 36:115, 2002.

CHAPTER 11

Active Transport

Objectives:

1. Understand how the Na^+ pump uses energy from ATP to keep $[Na^+]_i$ low and $[K^+]_i$ high by transporting Na^+ and K^+ against their electrochemical gradients.

2. Understand how Ca^{2+} is sequestered in the sarcoplasmic and endoplasmic reticulum and transported across the plasma membrane by ATP-dependent active transport systems.

3. Understand how intracellular Ca^{2+} is controlled and Ca^{2+} signaling is regulated by the cooperative action of many transport systems.

4. Understand the roles of ATP-dependent transport systems in the transport of such ions as protons and copper, as well as a variety of other solutes.

5. Understand how different transport systems in the apical and basolateral membranes of epithelia, which separate two different extracellular compartments, act cooperatively to effect net transfer of solutes and water across epithelial cells.

■ PRIMARY ACTIVE TRANSPORT CONVERTS THE CHEMICAL ENERGY FROM ATP INTO ELECTROCHEMICAL POTENTIAL ENERGY STORED IN SOLUTE GRADIENTS

The differences between passive diffusion, facilitated diffusion (or simple carrier-mediated transport), and coupled transport (cotransport and countertransport) were discussed in the preceding chapter. In our study of coupled transport we saw how energy from the Na^+ electrochemical gradient can be used to generate concentration (or electrochemical) gradients for other (coupled) solutes. This is sometimes called secondary active transport because a *pre-existing* electrochemical energy gradient is dissipated in one part of the transport process (e.g., the downhill movement of Na^+) to generate the chemical or electrochemical gradients of other solutes (e.g., glucose or Ca^{2+}). There is, however, no *net* expenditure of metabolic energy by these secondary active transport processes.

The question we need to address here is: How does the Na^+ concentration gradient (typically, $[Na^+]_o/[Na^+]_i \approx 10\text{-}15$) become established in the first place? This brings us to the direct role of ATP in powering some transport processes (i.e., **primary active transport**). During active ion transport, adenosine triphosphatases (ATPases) interconvert chemical (phosphate bond) energy

149

and electrochemical potential (ion gradient) energy. These straightforward chemical reactions can, depending on the concentrations of substrates and products, operate in either the forward or the reverse direction; that is, they can either utilize (hydrolyze) or synthesize ATP.

Three Broad Classes of ATPases Are Involved in Active Ion Transport

The three classes of ion transport ATPases are the F-, V-, and P-type ATPases. Mitochondria possess F-type (F_1F_0) ATPases that are used to synthesize ATP with energy from the proton electrochemical gradient across the inner mitochondrial membrane; the proton gradient is generated by oxidative metabolism. The vacuolar (V-type) H^+-ATPases lower intraorganellar pH by concentrating protons in a variety of vesicular organelles, including lysosomes and secretory and storage vesicles. Neither the F- nor the V-type ATPases form stable phosphorylated intermediates. The **P-type ATPases,** which do form stable **phosphorylated intermediates** that can be isolated chemically, transport a variety of ions and other solutes into and out of cells and organelles. Examples of P-type ATPases are the plasma membrane Na^+ pump (Na^+,K^+-ATPase), the plasma membrane and sarcoplasmic reticulum/endoplasmic reticulum Ca^{2+} pumps, and the gastric mucosa proton pump (H^+,K^+-ATPase). These P-type ATPases are the focus of much of this chapter.

■ THE PLASMA MEMBRANE Na^+ PUMP (Na,K-ATPase) MAINTAINS THE LOW Na^+ AND HIGH K^+ CONCENTRATIONS IN THE CYTOSOL

Nearly All Animal Cells Normally Maintain a High Intracellular K^+ Concentration ($[K^+]_i$) and a Low Intracellular Na^+ Concentration ($[Na^+]_i$)

In most cells in mammals, including man, $[K^+]_i \approx$ 120-130 mM and $[Na^+]_i \approx$ 5-10 mM (photoreceptors and, in a few species, red blood cells, which have a higher $[Na^+]_i$ and lower $[K^+]_i$, are notable exceptions). These cells are, however, bathed by an extracellular fluid that contains a high Na^+ concentration ($[Na^+]_o \approx$ 145 mM) and a low K^+ concentration ($[K^+]_o \approx$ 4-5 mM). Moreover, as we now know, cells are not impermeable to Na^+ and K^+. The Na^+ and K^+ channels and Na^+ gradient–dependent transport systems (see Chapters 7 and 10) permit Na^+ to enter cells and K^+ to exit as the ions move down their respective electrochemical gradients. Therefore all cells require a means to maintain these normal Na^+ and K^+ gradients by exporting Na^+ and importing K^+. Energy must be used to perform the work needed to generate these ion electrochemical gradients. The transport system that accomplishes this work is called the **sodium pump or Na^+-K^+ ATPase;** it uses energy in the form of ATP. In the nervous system and the kidneys, for example, the Na^+ pump accounts for a very large fraction (75%-85%) of total ATP hydrolysis. The transport of Na^+ and K^+ by the Na^+ pump thus compensates for the leak of these ions into and out of the cell, respectively. This is known as the **"pump-leak model"** of Na^+ and K^+ homeostasis. The *Na^+ pump not only maintains constant intracellular Na^+ and K^+ ion concentrations, but also influences cell volume.* The direct contribution of the Na^+ pump to cell volume maintenance is addressed below.

The Na^+ Pump Hydrolyzes ATP While Transporting Na^+ out of the Cell and K^+ into the Cell

The *Na^+ pump is an integral plasma membrane protein* whose major (α, or "catalytic") subunit, with a molecular weight of about 100,000 and 10 membrane-spanning helices (Figure 11-1), contains the ATP and ion binding sites. The α subunit is closely associated with a smaller (40,000-60,000 molecular weight),

Active Transport

highly glycosylated, β subunit that has a single membrane-spanning domain. Complexes of α and β subunits, in a 1:1 ratio, are required for Na⁺ pump activity, but the precise function of the β subunit is unknown. The Na⁺ pump is frequently called the "Na⁺,K⁺-ATPase" because the purified protein is an enzyme (specifically, an ATPase) that *requires both Na^+ and K^+ for its catalytic activity* (ATP hydrolysis).*

The Na⁺ pump hydrolyzes 1 ATP molecule to adenosine diphosphate (ADP) and inorganic phosphate (Pi) *while transporting 3 Na^+ ions out of the cell and 2 K^+ ions into the cell.* The transport cycle begins with the binding of ATP, in the form of MgATP (a magnesium ion complexed with ATP), at the hydrolytic site on the large cytoplasmic loop of the α subunit (Figure 11-1). When 3 Na⁺ ions bind to the pump on the cytoplasmic side, the ATP is cleaved and its terminal, high-energy phosphate is transferred to the α subunit. During this phosphorylation the protein undergoes a conformational change. The energy from the high-energy phosphate bond is transferred to the protein as the Na⁺ binding site conformation changes so that the bound Na⁺ becomes transiently inaccessible ("occluded") to both the intracellular and extracellular fluids. The Na⁺ binding site then opens to the extracellular fluid. Simultaneously, as a consequence of this conformational change, the affinity of the protein for Na⁺ is greatly reduced. Thus the 3 Na⁺ ions are able to dissociate even though $[Na^+]_o \approx 145$ mM. At the same time, a site that binds 2 K⁺ ions with high affinity is exposed at the external surface. When 2 K⁺ ions bind, the protein undergoes a second conformational change. As the low-energy α-subunit–phosphate bond is cleaved and inorganic phosphate (Pi) is released into the cytoplasm, the K⁺ binding site closes to the external surface (i.e., the 2 K⁺ ions are transiently occluded) and then opens to the internal surface. The 2 K⁺ ions are released into the cytoplasm because the affinity for K⁺ decreases markedly during this conformational change. This sequence of steps in the Na⁺ pump cycle is illustrated in Figure 11-2.

The net reaction for the Na⁺ pump (Box 11-1) can be written as Equation [1]:

$$3\ Na^+_{cyt} + 2\ K^+_{ECF} + 1\ ATP_{cyt} \rightleftharpoons 3\ Na^+_{ECF} + 2\ K^+_{cyt} + 1\ ADP_{cyt} + 1\ Pi_{cyt} \quad [1]$$

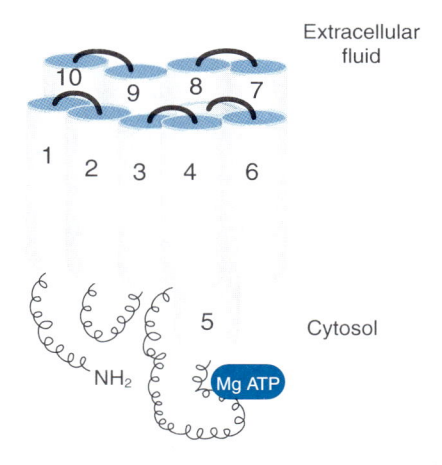

Figure 11-1 ■ Proposed three-dimensional structural model of the Na⁺ pump (ATPase) catalytic subunit (alpha). This subunit consists of 10 membrane-spanning domains (cylinders in the figure). The large cytoplasmic loop between transmembrane helices 4 and 5 contains the ATP binding domain (shown) and the aspartate phosphorylation site. The ion binding sites are probably located in transmembrane helices 4, 5, 6, and 8. Residues that bind ouabain are located on the external surfaces of helices 1, 2, 5, 6, and 7; thus bound ouabain may block access to the cation binding sites. (Modified from Lingrel JB, Croyle ML, Woo AL, Arguello JM: *Acta Physiol Scand Suppl* 643:69, 1998.)

---

*The Na⁺,K⁺-ATPase was first identified in 1957 by the Danish physiologist Jens Skou. He was awarded the Nobel Prize for this work in 1997.

BOX 11-1

The Na$^+$ Pump Is Reversible

The reaction diagram (Figure 11-3) appears to suggest that the reaction is unidirectional and only moves Na$^+$ out of, and K$^+$ into, cells. This is, however, a straightforward chemical reaction. By the law of mass action, if the concentrations of the products (right-hand side of Equation [1]) are high and the concentrations of the reactants (left-hand side of Equation [1]) are low, the net reaction could proceed from right to left. This is indeed the case. If little or no Na$^+$ or ATP is present in the cells and little K$^+$ is present in the extracellular fluid, while the intracellular concentrations of K$^+$, adenosine diphosphate, and inorganic phosphate and the extracellular concentration of Na$^+$ are all high, then the Na$^+$ pump can generate ATP. This is analogous to the mitochondrial F_1F_0 ATPase that synthesizes ATP by harnessing the energy derived from the transport of protons down their electrochemical gradient.

This net reaction can be diagrammed as shown in Figure 11-3. Note that this reaction is, in fact, reversible (Box 11-1).

As a result of the 3 Na$^+$:2 K$^+$ coupling ratio, *inhibition* of the Na$^+$ pump will lead to a net gain of solute (as Na$^+$ salts, to maintain electroneutrality) and a rise in osmotic pressure. The cells will therefore gain water and swell (see discussion of the Donnan effect in Chapter 4). Thus *the Na$^+$ pump participates directly in cell volume maintenance* (i.e., the "pump-leak model," mentioned previously).

The Na$^+$ Pump Is "Electrogenic"

The reaction sequence (Equation [1]) reveals that *during each Na$^+$ pump cycle one more positive charge leaves the cell than enters.* This *net* flow of charge (i.e., outward "pump current") across the membrane generates a small voltage (cytoplasm negative). The Na$^+$ pump is therefore said to be "electrogenic." Indeed, this voltage adds to the membrane potential, so that the actual resting membrane potential is slightly more negative than the potential calculated from the Goldman-Hodgkin-Katz equation (see Chapter 4). The maximum voltage that can be generated by the Na$^+$ pump with a coupling ratio of 3 Na$^+$:2 K$^+$, under *steady-state* conditions, is about 10 mV. In practice, however, the *contribution of the electrogenic Na$^+$ pump to the resting potential* (i.e., in the steady state) *in most cells is only a few millivolts* (1 to 4 mV) and is therefore often ignored. When cells are activated and the intracellular Na$^+$ concentration rises significantly (e.g., in nerve cells after a long burst of action potentials), the rate of Na$^+$ transport by the Na$^+$ pump can increase considerably. Under these *non*-steady-state conditions, the Na$^+$ pump may *transiently hyperpolarize* the cells by 10 to 20 mV or more. Such hyperpolarization can temporarily reduce the ability of stimuli to excite the cells.

The Na$^+$ Pump Is the Receptor for Cardiotonic Steroids Such as Ouabain and Digoxin

A special feature of the Na$^+$ pump α subunit is that it is uniquely sensitive to a class of drugs known as **cardiotonic steroids;** two examples are **digoxin** and **ouabain,** which are derived from plants (Box 11-2). The only known direct action of the cardiotonic steroids is inhibition of the Na$^+$ pump. As described below, this action on the Na$^+$ pump indirectly leads to the cardiotonic effect (increased force of contraction of the heart, or *positive inotropic effect*), which is the key feature of cardiotonic steroid therapeutic efficacy.

Four molecular **isoforms** of the **Na$^+$ pump α subunit** (α1, α2, α3, and α4) have been

Active Transport

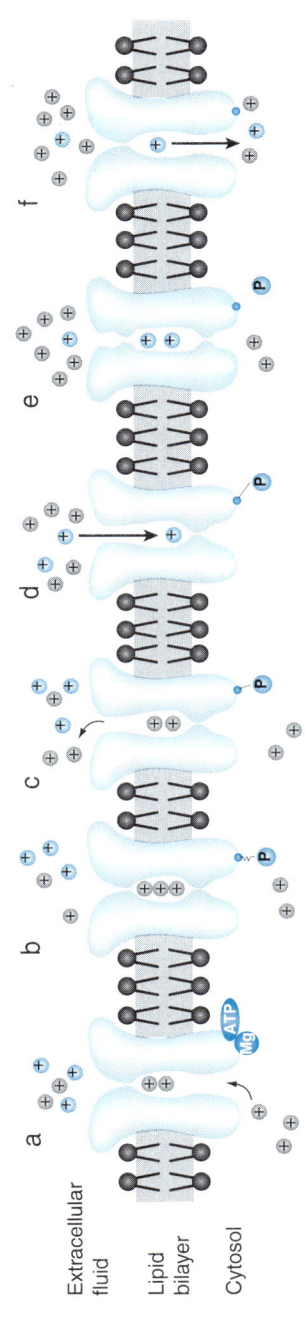

Figure 11-2 ■ Sequence of steps in the Na$^+$ pump cycle illustrates the mechanism of operation of the pump. The cycle begins with the binding of ATP to the large cytoplasmic loop (*a*), followed by the binding of three Na$^+$ ions (gray circles) from the cytosol (*a,b*). The three Na$^+$ are transiently occluded (*b*) and then released to the extracellular fluid (ECF; *c*). Two K$^+$ (blue circles) from the ECF bind (*d*) and, during the subsequent conformation change, are transiently occluded (*e*). The cycle ends with the hydrolysis of the low-energy covalent phosphate bond, dissociation of the phosphate (P$_i$, originally the terminal phosphate of the ATP), and release of the two K$^+$ into the cytosol (*f*). See text for further details.

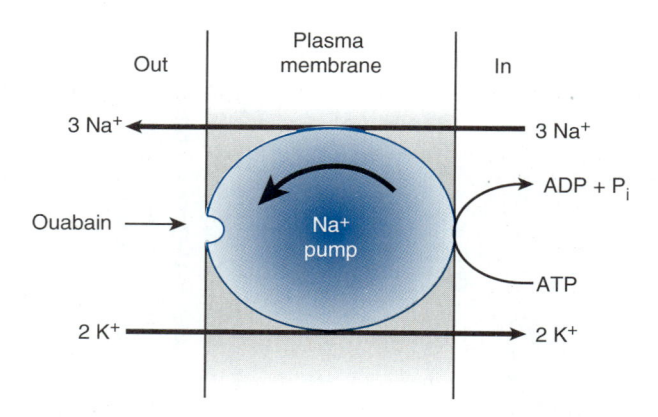

Figure 11-3 ■ Net reaction mediated by the Na⁺ pump. Note that the ouabain binding site faces the extracellular fluid.

identified. They differ in their affinities for Na⁺ and K⁺, and for ouabain (and digoxin). These isoforms, which have extensive sequence homology, resulted from gene duplication and have been conserved during vertebrate evolution. All cells express α1 and one other isoform; α1 is responsible for maintaining the low Na⁺ concentration in "bulk" cytoplasm.

The α-subunit isoforms are independently upregulated or downregulated under various physiological and pathophysiological conditions, and this may alter the sensitivity to ouabain. For example, thyroid hormone increases expression of α2, and heart failure decreases expression of the α2 isoform in the heart. In kidney distal tubules, aldosterone upregulates α1, which then promotes Na⁺ reabsorption and retention. Also, several hormones, such as dopamine, vasopressin, and serotonin (5-hydroxytryptamine, 5-HT), may modulate the activity of the Na⁺ pump in an isoform-specific manner. These hormones may activate the pump or may inactivate it by promoting phosphorylation of the pump at sites other than the site that is phosphorylated during ion transfer. The activity of some Na⁺ pumps, most notably those in the kidney, are up-regulated or downregulated by members of a family ("FXYD"*) of small integral membrane proteins with a single membrane-spanning region. Different members of the FXYD family are expressed in different portions of the kidney tubule and may exert different effects. New ideas about the significance of the isoforms and of these regulatory mechanisms are just beginning to emerge (Box 11-3 and Figure 11-4).

■ INTRACELLULAR Ca^{2+} SIGNALING IS UNIVERSAL AND IS CLOSELY TIED TO Ca^{2+} HOMEOSTASIS

Intracellular Ca^{2+} signaling (a change in the concentration of free Ca^{2+} ions in the cytoplasm) is directly or indirectly involved in most cell processes, from sexual reproduction and cell division to cell death. For example, Ca^{2+} ions

---

*The name of this protein family derives from the fact that they all have a core motif of 35 highly conserved amino acids, including the signature sequence: phenylalanine (F)-X-tyrosine (Y)-aspartate (D), where X can be any one of several amino acids.

BOX 11-2

Why Do Sodium Pumps Have a Cardiotonic Steroid Binding Site ("Receptor")?

The cardiotonic steroids derive their name from the fact that they improve the performance of the heart. Digoxin and ouabain come from the leaves of the foxglove plant, *Digitalis purpurea*, and the bark of the ouabaio tree, *Acokanthera ouabaio*, respectively. Some pharmacologically related cardiotonic steroids, the bufadienolides, are produced by poisonous toads of the genus *Bufo*. Digitalis steroids such as digoxin have been *used clinically to treat heart failure and certain cardiac arrhythmias* for more than 200 years, and they are still used frequently. Ouabain, a structurally similar molecule, is also effective, but it is poorly absorbed from the intestine and must be injected. In contrast, digoxin can be administered orally because it is lipid soluble and thus readily absorbed in the intestine.

All cells have Na^+ pumps with a binding site ("receptor") for cardiotonic steroids, but the physiological significance was unknown. Recently a molecule that is indistinguishable from ouabain (i.e., it is ouabain itself or a stereoisomer) was isolated from human plasma and shown to be a human hormone. This hormone is synthesized in, and secreted by, cells in the zona glomerulosa of the adrenal cortex. This "endogenous ouabain" has been postulated to play a role in the pathogenesis of some forms of hypertension (high blood pressure). About 50% of patients with "essential hypertension" (i.e., hypertension of unknown cause) have significantly higher blood plasma levels of this compound than the levels found in normotensive subjects (i.e., those with normal blood pressure).

BOX 11-3

Na⁺ Pump Isoform Localization and Function

A clue to the isoform-specific functions of the Na^+ pump is the fact that the high-affinity ouabain binding site has been conserved on the α2, α3, and α4 isoforms during vertebrate evolution, whereas the α1 ouabain binding affinity varies greatly. In addition, α1 is distributed relatively uniformly in the plasma membrane (PM) of many types of cells, whereas α2 and α3 (depending on cell type; α4 has not been studied) are confined to PM microdomains that overlie sub-PM ("junctional") components of the sarcoplasmic or endoplasmic reticulum (S/ER). Interestingly, the Na^+/Ca^{2+} exchanger colocalizes with the α2 and α3 Na^+ pumps, whereas the ATP-driven PM Ca^{2+} pump (PMCA) is, like α1, uniformly distributed but may be excluded from the junctional microdomains. It appears that diffusion of Na^+ and Ca^{2+} between the tiny sub-PM space separating the PM from junctional S/ER, and the "bulk" cytosol, may be markedly restricted. Thus the Na^+ and Ca^{2+} concentrations in these junctional cytosolic spaces and the adjacent S/ER may be governed exclusively by the α2 or α3 Na^+ pumps and the Na^+/Ca^{2+} exchanger. This organization of transporters, diagrammed in Figure 11-4, may help explain how low doses of ouabain and other cardiotonic steroids (including "endogenous ouabain") exert large effects on $[Ca^{2+}]_i$ and Ca^{2+} signaling. This is exemplified by increased cardiac contractility (the *cardiotonic* effect).

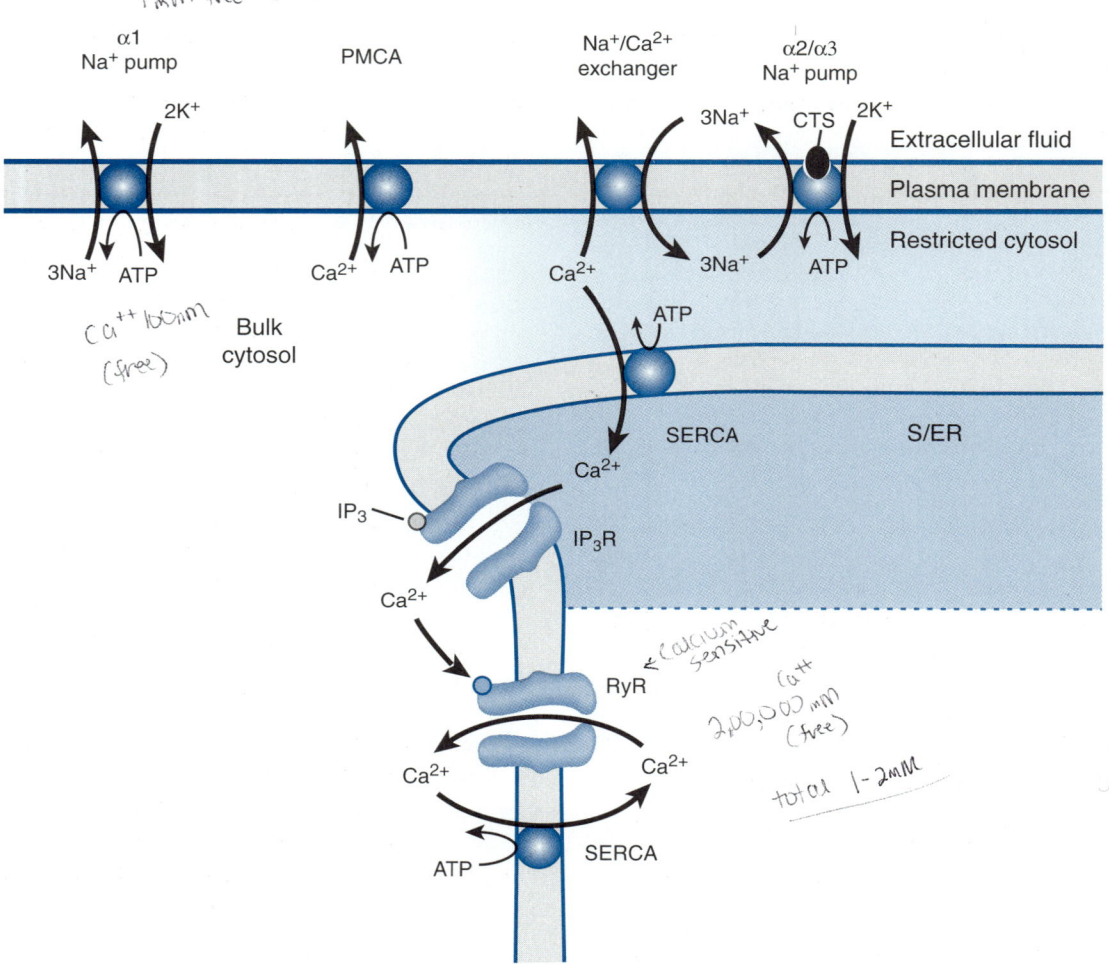

Figure 11-4 ■ Small portion of a cell showing the plasma membrane (PM)-junctional sarcoplasmic or endoplasmic reticulum (S/ER) region at the lower right. The PM that faces "bulk" cytosol contains α1 Na⁺ pumps and PM Ca²⁺ pumps (PMCA); the microdomain adjacent to junctional S/ER contains α2 or α3 Na⁺ pumps (depending on cell type) and Na⁺/Ca²⁺ exchangers. The S/ER membrane contains S/ER Ca²⁺ pumps (SERCA), inositol trisphosphate (IP₃) receptors, and ryanodine receptors (RyR, which are also activated by elevated [Ca²⁺]$_i$, as illustrated). Activation of these receptors (see Chapter 13) opens Ca²⁺ release channels in the S/ER membrane, and Ca²⁺ is released into the bulk cytosol. Diffusion of Na⁺ and Ca²⁺ between bulk cytosol and the tiny volume of cytosol located in the space between the PM and junctional S/ER is greatly restricted. Low-dose ouabain (or other cardiotonic steroids; CTS) acts on the α2/α3 Na⁺ pumps and raises the Na⁺ concentration primarily in the cytosol between the PM and junctional S/ER. The altered Na⁺ gradient across the PM in this region reduces the driving force that normally promotes Ca²⁺ extrusion by the Na⁺/Ca²⁺ exchangers. This raises the Ca²⁺ concentration in the restricted space. The SERCA then stores more Ca²⁺ in the junctional S/ER (shaded area of S/ER) so that more is released when the cells are activated. (Modified from Arnon A, Hamlyn JM, Blaustein MP: *Am J Physiol Heart Circ Physiol* 279:H679, 2000.)

play a role in the fertilization of the ovum and are directly involved in muscle contraction and in hormone and neurotransmitter secretion. Ca^{2+} ions are also involved in the control of electrical excitability (e.g., through Ca-activated K^+ channels; see Chapter 8) and in the regulation of many protein kinases, protein phosphatases, and other enzymes. Cell Ca^{2+} overload usually leads to cell death; protection from Ca^{2+} overload may rescue damaged cells. Thus an appreciation of cell Ca^{2+} homeostasis is essential for an understanding of many physiological and pathophysiological processes.

The Ca^{2+} involved in cell signaling comes from the extracellular fluid (it may enter through a variety of Ca^{2+}-permeable channels; see Chapter 8) or from **intracellular Ca^{2+} stores** in the **endoplasmic reticulum (ER)** or, in muscle, the **sarcoplasmic reticulum (SR)**. This "signal Ca^{2+}" must then either be extruded across the plasma membrane or be resequestered in the sarcoplasmic or endoplasmic reticulum (S/ER). A plasma membrane transport system that mediates the interrelationship between Na^+ homeostasis and Ca^{2+} (i.e., the Na^+/Ca^{2+} exchanger) was described in Chapter 10. Here we consider other mechanisms involved in Ca^{2+} transport and discuss their relative roles in Ca^{2+} homeostasis.

■ Ca^{2+} STORAGE IN THE SARCOPLASMIC/ ENDOPLASMIC RETICULUM IS MEDIATED BY A Ca^{2+}-ATPase

In Chapter 10 we noted that the *cytosolic free (ionized) Ca^{2+} concentration ($[Ca^{2+}]_i$) in most cells at rest is about 100 nM* (10^{-7} M or 0.0001 mM). The *total* intracellular Ca^{2+} concentration is generally about 1000 to 10,000 times higher than this, however, or about 0.1 to 1 millimoles per liter of cell water (i.e., 0.1 to 1 mM). Thus more than 98% of the intracellular Ca^{2+} is sequestered in intracellular organelles, although a small amount is buffered (i.e., bound to cytoplasmic proteins, such as calmodulin, and to other molecules). *The primary Ca^{2+} storage site is the ER or, in muscle, the SR,* although a small amount is also normally stored in mitochondria. The S/ER is an enclosed, interconnecting system of tubules and sacs within the cytoplasm that plays a central role in Ca^{2+} signaling. Some elements of the S/ER lie just beneath the plasma membrane and are specialized for Ca^{2+} signal initiation or amplification. When cells are activated (e.g., by hormones, neurotransmitters, or depolarization), Ca^{2+} is often released from the S/ER stores. This released (signal) Ca^{2+} can trigger such processes as contraction and secretion (depending, of course, on the type of cell). Subsequently, the Ca^{2+} is resequestered in the S/ER. How is this sequestration of Ca^{2+} accomplished?

The S/ER membrane has a Ca^{2+} pump, **SERCA (S/ER Ca^{2+}-dependent ATPase),** which, like the Na^+/K^+-ATPase, is a P-type ATPase. SERCA and the Na^+ pump (Figure 11-1) have extensive sequence and functional homology (Box 11-4), but *only* the Na^+ pump has a cardiotonic steroid binding site. SERCA uses 1 ATP to transport 2 Ca^{2+} ions from the cytosol (cyt) to the S/ER lumen and 2 protons (H^+ ions) from the lumen to the cytosol. The mechanism of transport is similar to that of the Na^+ pump.

$$2\ Ca^{2+}_{cyt} + 1\ ATP_{cyt} + 2\ H^+_{S/ER\ lumen} \rightleftharpoons$$
$$2\ Ca^{2+}_{S/ER\ lumen} + 1\ ADP_{cyt} + 1\ Pi_{cyt} + 2\ H^+_{cyt} \quad [2]$$

The 2 to 3 mM of ATP in the cytosol provides enough energy to enable SERCA to concentrate Ca^{2+} in the S/ER lumen more than 1000-fold relative to the cytosol. The intra-S/ER *free* Ca^{2+} concentration is about 0.15 to 0.5 mM, but in addition the lumen of the S/ER contains Ca^{2+} binding proteins (e.g., calsequestrin and calreticulin) that buffer the Ca^{2+}. Thus, if 80% to 90% of the intra-S/ER Ca^{2+} is bound, the *total* Ca^{2+} concentration in the lumen may be as high as several millimolar (Box 11-5).

> **BOX 11-4**
>
> ### Aspects of the Mechanism of Ca^{2+} Transport Revealed by the Crystal Structure of SERCA
>
> The structure of SERCA (sarcoplasmic or endoplasmic reticulum Ca^{2+}-dependent ATPase) from skeletal muscle (SERCA1) was recently determined by x-ray crystallography. This molecule, like the Na^+,K^+-ATPase α subunit (Figure 11-1), has a molecular weight of about 100,000, with 10 membrane-spanning helices and a large "regulatory" cytoplasmic loop between helices 4 and 5. The regulatory loop contains an ATP-binding domain and a phosphorylation domain with a critical aspartate that is phosphorylated. The Ca^{2+} binding pocket, with side-by-side sites for 2 Ca^{2+} ions, is surrounded by carbonyl oxygens from transmembrane helices 4, 5, 6, and 8; indeed, the intramembrane regions of helices 4 and 6 are disrupted to accommodate the 2 Ca^{2+}. When the aspartate is phosphorylated (Asp-P), the activator domain (the N-terminal tail and cytoplasmic loop between helices 2 and 3) moves toward the Asp-P. This movement transmits conformational changes to the Ca^{2+} binding site. How the energy from the high-energy phosphate bond induces the conformational changes to permit the Ca^{2+} to enter from the cytosol and then exit to the S/ER lumen is not yet known.

> **BOX 11-5**
>
> ### A Large Quantity of Ca^{2+} Is Stored in the Sarcoplasmic or Endoplasmic Reticulum
>
> A conservative estimate is that 80% to 90% of the Ca^{2+} in the sarcoplasmic or endoplasmic reticulum (S/ER) is bound to calsequestrin or calreticulin. The free (ionized) Ca^{2+} concentration in the S/ER is ~0.2 mM, and the total Ca^{2+} concentration (free + bound) in the S/ER is approximately 1 to 2 mM. If the S/ER encloses 2% to 5% of the cell volume, rapid release of *all* of the stored Ca^{2+} should increase the cytosolic free Ca^{2+} concentration ($[Ca^{2+}]_i$) by 0.02 to 0.10 mM. These values are about 10 to 50 times larger than the largest Ca^{2+} signals normally evoked by maximal concentrations of hormones or neurotransmitters (maximal cytosolic Ca^{2+} signals are typically on the order of several millimolar). Thus the S/ER stores contain more than sufficient Ca^{2+} to account for the cytosolic Ca^{2+} signals even in the absence of Ca^{2+} entry from the extracellular fluid. Indeed, as we will see in Chapter 13, *all* of the Ca^{2+} required to activate skeletal muscle contraction is derived from the SR.

SERCA Has Three Isoforms

The three isoforms of SERCA (SERCA1, SERCA2, and SERCA3) are the products of different genes. Expression of the different SERCA isoforms is cell type specific. For example, SERCA1 is expressed almost exclusively in skeletal muscle. Release of SR Ca^{2+} triggers contraction in skeletal muscle (see Chapter 13). Relaxation of contracted skeletal muscle requires resequestration of the released Ca^{2+} back into the SR; this is the job of SERCA1. Indeed, a mutation in the SERCA1 gene that impairs Ca^{2+} sequestration in the SR slows skeletal muscle relaxation in Brody disease (Box 11-6).

■ THE PLASMA MEMBRANE OF MOST CELLS ALSO HAS AN ATP-DRIVEN Ca^{2+} PUMP

The plasma membrane (PM) of most cells contains, in addition to the Na^+/Ca^{2+} exchanger, a P-type Ca-ATPase, **PMCA,** whose amino acid sequence differs from that of SERCA (i.e., the proteins are not homologous). The PMCA and Na^+/Ca^{2+} exchanger must function in parallel to regulate $[Ca^{2+}]_i$. The *PMCA has a 10-fold slower turnover (cycling) rate than the Na^+/Ca^{2+} exchanger* (see Table 10-1). Therefore the $Na^+/$

BOX 11-6

A Mutation in the SERCA1 Gene Impairs Skeletal Muscle Relaxation

Brody disease is a rare, nonlethal, inherited disorder of Ca^{2+} sequestration in the sarcoplasmic reticulum (SR) of skeletal muscle. It is the result of a mutation in the SERCA1 gene that markedly slows Ca^{2+} transport into the SR. The disease is manifested as defective skeletal muscle relaxation that worsens rapidly during exercise. This impairment of function can readily be explained by the markedly decreased rate of Ca^{2+} sequestration into the SR, which prolongs the contractile state (see Chapter 14).

Ca^{2+} exchanger, with its 10-fold higher rate (Table 10-1) of Ca^{2+} transport (per molecule), plays the dominant role in Ca^{2+} export during recovery from activation, especially in cells with a large entry of Ca^{2+} during activity (cardiac muscle is a good example). On the other hand, the PMCA has a 10-fold higher affinity for intracellular Ca^{2+} than the Na^+/Ca^{2+} exchanger, so the PMCA may be particularly important for keeping the $[Ca^{2+}]_i$ concentration very low under resting conditions.

The Relative Roles of the Several Na^+ and Ca^{2+} Transporters Differ in Different Cell Types

The functional interrelationships of the Na^+ pump, the Na^+/Ca^{2+} exchanger, and the PMCA and SERCA in Ca^{2+} homeostasis are complex and tissue specific. For example, in skeletal muscle almost all of the Ca^{2+} for contraction comes from the SR and is resequestered in the SR by SERCA during relaxation. In contrast, in cardiac muscle a much larger fraction of the Ca^{2+} for contraction comes from the extracellular fluid and enters through voltage-gated Ca^{2+} channels. This Ca^{2+} must be reextruded across the cardiac muscle plasma membrane (sarcolemma), and here the Na^+/Ca^{2+} exchanger plays a dominant role in removal of Ca^{2+} from the cytosol during the relaxation phase ("diastole") of each cardiac cycle.

The PMCA and SERCA, along with the Na^+/Ca^{2+} exchanger, govern Ca^{2+} homeostasis. In addition, several mitochondrial Ca^{2+} transport systems are involved in controlling intramitochondrial Ca^{2+}. Indeed, small increases in the intramitochondrial Ca^{2+} level result from rises in $[Ca^{2+}]_i$ during cell activity. The modestly elevated intramitochondrial Ca^{2+} stimulates the activity of Krebs (tricarboxylic acid) cycle enzymes and oxidative metabolism in the mitochondria and increases production of ATP.

Different Functions Account for the Different Distribution of the Na^+/Ca^{2+} Exchanger and PMCA in the Same Plasma Membrane

Why do cells express both the Na^+/Ca^{2+} exchanger and PMCA, both of which can be used to extrude Ca^{2+}? The specific localization of the Ca^{2+} transporters provides clues to transporter function (Box 11-3). In nerve terminals Ca^{2+} entry through voltage-gated Ca^{2+} channels (see Chapter 8) elevates the $[Ca^{2+}]_i$ concentration and triggers neurotransmitter release. The Na^+/Ca^{2+} exchanger, which is some distance from the release sites, plays an important role in extruding the Ca^{2+} that enters during neuronal activity. In contrast, the PMCA is concentrated in nerve terminal plasma membrane domains near the Ca^{2+} entry and transmitter release sites. This PMCA keeps the Ca^{2+} near these sites very low in the periods between depolarizations to maximize the sensitivity of the transmitter release sites to entering Ca^{2+}. The coordination of the several transport systems in the regulation of Ca^{2+} signaling is illustrated by the effects of low concentrations of cardiotonic steroid (Box 11-7 and Figure 11-4).

> **BOX 11-7**
>
> ### Cardiotonic Steroids Exert Their Cardiotonic Effect Without Elevating $[Na^+]_i$
>
> Cardiotonic steroids inhibit the Na^+ pump selectively and can be expected to elevate $[Na^+]_i$. Nanomolar concentrations of cardiotonic steroids such as digoxin or ouabain, however, exert their cardiotonic effects without measurably elevating $[Na^+]_i$ in the cell as a whole ("bulk" $[Na^+]_i$). How can this be explained? The high ouabain affinity of the α2 and α3 isoforms and the localization of the various Na^+ and Ca^{2+} transporters (see Box 11-3 and Figure 11-4) suggest the solution indicated by the sequence of events shown at the right.
>
> The main point is that negligible change in *total* cell Na^+ is needed to account for the augmented Ca^{2+} signaling induced by low-dose cardiotonic steroids. Increase in the Na^+ concentration in the tiny space between the PM and junctional S/ER is sufficient to explain the positive inotropic effect induced by cardiotonic steroids. Based on similar reasoning, a *reduction* of local $[Na^+]$ apparently underlies the relaxation of intestinal smooth muscle that is induced by β-adrenergic agonists such as isoproterenol, which stimulates the Na^+ pump (see study problems).
>
> Thus control of this local, sub-PM $[Na^+]$ apparently plays a critical role in regulating Ca^{2+} signaling in a large variety of cell types.
>
> Inhibition of Na^+ pump α2/α3 isoforms by nanomolar ouabain
> ⇓
> ↑$[Na^+]$ in the tiny space between the plasma membrane (PM) and junctional sarcoplasmic or endoplasmic reticulum (jS/ER)
> ⇓
> ↓Ca^{2+} exit and/or ↑Ca^{2+} entry via Na^+/Ca^{2+} exchangers in PM microdomains adjacent to jS/ER
> ⇓
> ↑$[Ca^{2+}]$ in the tiny space between the PM and jS/ER
> ⇓
> ↑Free and total $[Ca^{2+}]$ in the lumen of the jS/ER (mediated by SERCA; see Box 11-5)
> ⇓
> ↑Ca^{2+} release from the S/ER whenever the cells are activated

■ TRANSPORT SYSTEMS MAY BE FUNCTIONALLY COUPLED IN PARALLEL OR IN SERIES

As discussed earlier, the *Na^+ pump and Na^+/Ca^{2+} exchanger are arranged in parallel* in the plasma membrane so that the exchanger can use the energy from the Na^+ electrochemical gradient to transport Ca^{2+} out of cells. Moreover, as illustrated in Figure 11-4, these two transport systems are clustered within microdomains to facilitate their close functional coupling (Box 11-3). In contrast, the *Na^+/Ca^{2+} exchanger and SERCA operate in series* in adjacent membranes to help regulate the S/ER Ca^{2+} stores and control Ca^{2+} signaling (Figure 11-4).

■ SEVERAL OTHER PLASMA MEMBRANE TRANSPORT ATPases ALSO PLAY IMPORTANT PHYSIOLOGICAL ROLES

An H^+,K^+-ATPase Mediates Gastric Acid Secretion

The intracellular concentrations of many other solutes must also be carefully regulated, and a number of these are regulated by P-type ATPases. The **gastric H^+,K^+-ATPase**, however, is a P-type ATPase that mediates acid secretion into the *lumen* of the stomach. The gastric peptidase pepsin, which carries out the initial stages of proteolytic cleavage on the foods we eat, has optimum enzymatic activity at a pH of

~3. Consequently, the *gastric glands* must produce a secretion that is nearly isotonic HCl (145 mM, which would have a pH of 0.084). Dilution of this secretion in the gastric lumen produces a pH of ~3.

The gastric H^+,K^+-ATPase is a proton (H^+) pump that is located in the *apical* ("brush border") membrane of the *parietal cells* of the gastric epithelium. This pump, which moves H^+ out of the cells and into the gastric lumen in exchange for K^+, is structurally homologous and functionally similar to the Na^+ pump. The regulation of the H^+,K^+-ATPase is, however, markedly different. Few copies of this transporter are present in the parietal cell apical membrane between meals; the H^+ pump molecules are instead located in the membranes of *tubulovesicles* that lie just beneath the apical membrane. This prevents digestion of the gastric epithelium itself. Ingestion of a meal activates vagal neurons and promotes secretion of gastrin (a local hormone). Gastrin stimulates nearby enterochromaffin-like cells to release histamine. The histamine activates parietal cell histamine type-2 (H_2) receptors that, via a cyclic AMP–mediated mechanism, induce the tubulovesicles containing the H^+,K^+-ATPase to fuse temporarily with the apical membrane. The cells can then pump H^+ into the gastric lumen. At the same time, apical membrane Cl^- and K^+ permeabilities are both increased. The net effect is HCl secretion because Cl^- exits passively, through parallel apical membrane Cl^--selective channels, while K^+ is recycled across the apical membrane (Figure 11-5). The Cl^- comes from the plasma and enters the cells across the basolateral membrane in exchange for HCO_3^- (another role for Cl^-/HCO_3^- exchange). Carbonic acid (H_2CO_3) is formed by the hydration of CO_2, a reaction catalyzed by the enzyme carbonic anhydrase (CA). The H^+ and HCO_3^- are then formed by dissociation of the H_2CO_3. Knowledge of the mechanism of acid secretion has found widespread application in the treatment of gastric hyperacidity ("heartburn") and gastroesophageal reflux (Box 11-8).

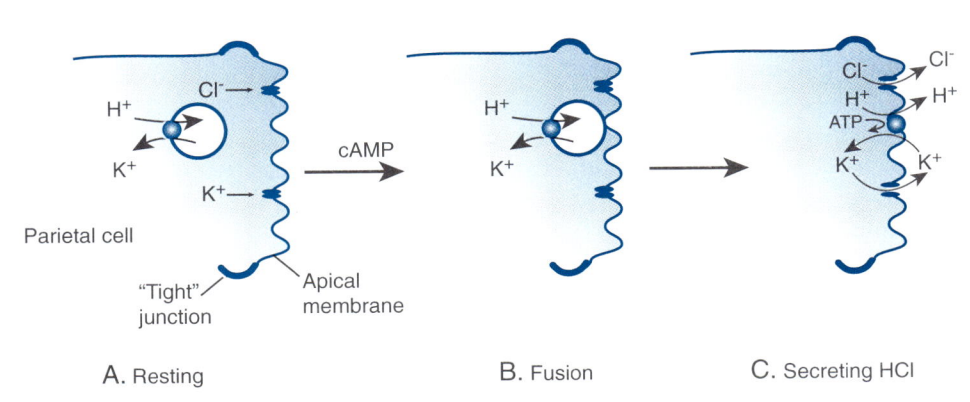

Figure 11-5 ■ Mechanism of acid (HCl) secretion by the gastric parietal cell. A, Before stimulation of the parietal cell by gastrin or histamine, most H^+,K^+-adenosine triphosphatase molecules are located in subapical vesicle membranes. Ingestion of a meal leads to stimulation of cyclic adenosine monophosphate (cAMP) production in the parietal cell. B, The elevated cAMP concentration promotes fusion of subapical vesicles with the apical membrane. C, At the same time, apical membrane Cl^- and K^+ channels are activated. The net effect is stimulation of HCl secretion and recycling of K^+ across the apical membrane.

> **BOX 11-8**
>
> ### Treatment of Gastric Hyperacidity ("Heartburn") with an H^+,K^+-ATPase Inhibitor
>
> Postprandial (i.e., after a meal) gastric hyperacidity is a very common clinical problem. The most common treatment is, of course, acid neutralization with a mild alkali such as Tums. A second, oft-used therapy involves block of parietal cell H_2-receptors with pharmacological agents such as cimetidine (Tagamet), ranitidine (Zantac), and famotidine (Pepcid). If these treatments are insufficient, the H^+,K^+-ATPase can be blocked directly with omeprazole (Prilosec) or lansoprazole (Prevacid). The latter two agents are irreversible inhibitors of the ATPase and are long acting because the cells must synthesize new H^+,K^+-ATPase molecules to compensate for the loss of the original molecules.

> **BOX 11-9**
>
> ### Some Essential Cu^{2+}-Requiring Metalloenzymes
>
> *Cytochrome c oxidase* is involved in mitochondrial electron transport. Impaired activity of this enzyme results in deficient energy production, leading to myopathies, ataxia, and seizures.
>
> *Dopamine β-hydroxylase* is involved in catecholamine synthesis. Reduced activity leads to severe defects in hypothalamic function, causing hypothermia, hypotension, and somnolence.
>
> *Lysyl oxidase* crosslinks collagen and elastin. Malfunction causes several connective tissue abnormalities, leading to tortuous blood vessels, bladder diverticula, and loose joints.
>
> *"Cross-linkase"* crosslinks keratin molecules. Malfunction causes "brittle hair."
>
> *Tyrosinase* is involved in melanin production. Malfunction results in a lack of pigmentation.

Two Copper-Transporting ATPases Play Essential Physiological Roles

Copper is an essential trace metal because a number of key metalloenzymes require Cu^{2+} (Box 11-9). Cu^{2+} is absorbed in the intestinal tract by a two-step process: it most likely enters the cells passively across the apical membrane and is then actively transported out across the basolateral membrane. The Cu^{2+} is bound to albumin in the plasma and is carried to the liver, the critical organ for Cu^{2+} homeostasis. The liver, which synthesizes *ceruloplasmin*, a Cu^{2+}-binding protein, secretes free Cu^{2+} into the bile and secretes Cu^{2+}-ceruloplasmin complexes into the plasma. The ceruloplasmin then ferries the Cu^{2+} to all cells that must use small amounts of this cation.

Deficiency of the Cu^{2+}-requiring metalloenzyme activities has serious medical consequences. Genetic analyses of two rare inherited diseases, *Menkes disease* and *Wilson disease* (Box 11-10), led to the discovery of two critical **Cu^{2+}-transporting** P-type **ATPases;** none had previously been identified in mammals. Serum Cu^{2+} and ceruloplasmin levels are low in both Wilson disease and Menkes disease. Menkes disease is manifested as an apparent copper deficiency because copper is accumulated in the intestinal mucosa, as well as in the spleen, lung, pancreas, and kidneys, but *not in the liver or brain* (where it is actually present in abnormally low amounts). The accumulation of Cu^{2+} in the intestine is due to a genetic defect in the ATPase that transports Cu^{2+} out of the intestinal mucosal cells across the basolateral membrane; thus, Cu^{2+} cannot be absorbed from the intestinal lumen.

In contrast, Wilson disease is manifested as a toxic accumulation of copper primarily in the

> **BOX 11-10**
>
> ### Menkes Disease and Wilson Disease Are Associated with Defects in Different Cu^{2+} Transport ATPases
>
> Menkes disease is characterized by mental retardation, convulsions, progressive neurodegeneration, and multiple connective tissue disorders. The classic feature is kinky, steely hair (like steel wool). The disease is lethal, usually by 3 years of age. The disorder is due to a defect in an X-linked recessive gene that encodes the copper-transporting ATPase that exports Cu^{2+} from intestinal mucosal cells or renal tubule cells, across the basolateral membrane to the interstitial space. Consequently, insufficient Cu^{2+} is absorbed from the intestinal lumen or reabsorbed by the kidneys. The manifestations of this disease indicate that Cu^{2+}-requiring metalloenzymes (see Box 11-9) cannot obtain the Cu^{2+} needed for their normal function.
>
> Wilson disease is characterized by hepatitis or cirrhosis, neurological manifestations (movement disorder, e.g., tremors), and psychotic symptoms. A diagnostic (*pathognomonic*) feature is greenish yellow Kayser-Fleischer rings in the cornea, caused by copper deposits. The disease results from a defect in an autosomal recessive gene that encodes for a copper-transporting ATPase that exports Cu^{2+} from hepatocytes (liver cells) to the bile canaliculi. The inability to export Cu^{2+} from the liver accounts for the toxic Cu^{2+} accumulation in the liver and the consequent liver disease.

liver and brain, as well as in the kidneys and cornea. The underlying problem is a genetic defect in another Cu^{2+}-transporting ATPase that normally plays a key role in the export of Cu^{2+} across the hepatocyte apical (canalicular) membrane and into the bile. These two Cu^{2+}-transporting ATPases are homologous.

ATP-Binding Cassette (ABC) Transporters Are a Superfamily of P-Type ATPases

Multidrug resistance transport ATPases transport many different types of agents The human genome codes for three classes of ATPases that actively transport drugs (often as conjugates) across plasma membranes. These classes are the P-glycoproteins, the breast cancer–resistant proteins, and the **multidrug resistance proteins (MRPs)**. To date, 12 such transporters have been identified. These proteins are all members of a superfamily of **ATP binding cassette (ABC) membrane transporters,** one of the largest superfamilies of proteins across all species. ABC proteins all use energy from ATP hydrolysis to transport, actively, a large variety of chemically unrelated substances, including *xenobiotics* (foreign biologically active substances). The various ABC transporters have different solute selectivities, but the precise mechanism of drug selectivity is not understood.

Two well-studied examples of the MRP class of transporters are MRP1 and MRP2. MRP1 is widely distributed, but its level of expression is normally low in the liver, where a homologous, functionally similar protein, MRP2, is highly expressed. Not only are these transporters physiologically important (e.g., MRP1 transports leukotriene C_4, and hepatic MRP2 plays a key role in bilirubin glucuronide secretion into the bile), but also they are involved in many medically important phenomena. These include cystic fibrosis, resistance to anticancer agents, and bacterial resistance to antibiotics.

Figure 11-6 illustrates the novel mechanism of transport used by some MRPs. Some neutral solutes are cotransported with glutathione (GSH, the tripeptide γ-glutamyl-cysteinyl-glycine); some solutes are conjugated to GSH and then

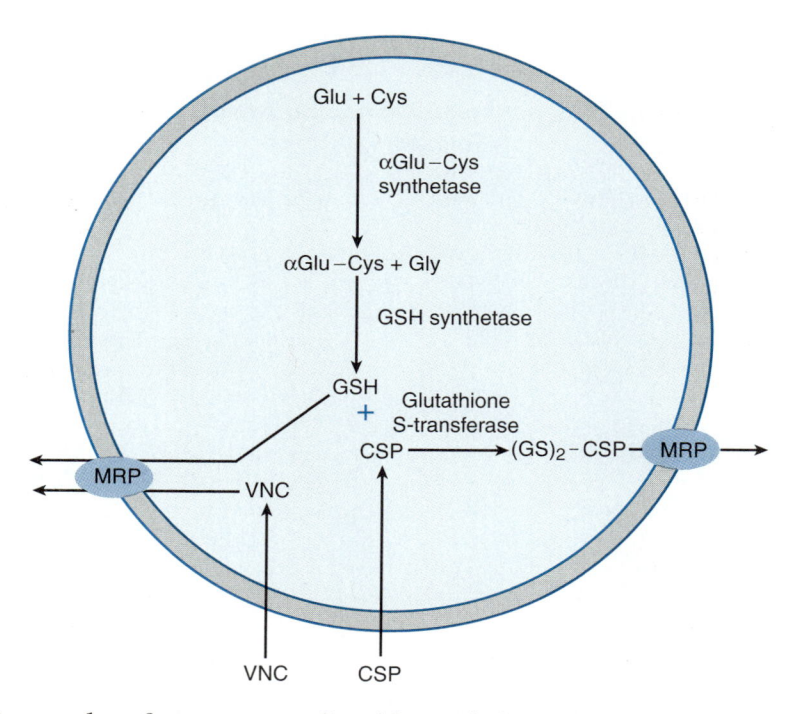

Figure 11-6 ■ Two modes of transport mediated by multidrug resistance proteins (MRPs) such as MRP1 and MRP2. The transport may involve cotransport of glutathione (GSH) with a neutral organic ligand (e.g., the vinca alkaloid, vincristine [VNC], an anticancer agent) or extrusion of a glutathione (GS)-coupled solute (e.g., cisplatin [CSP], another anticancer agent). Although not illustrated here, MRPs may also transport organic anions in an uncoupled manner or other solutes as glucuronate (e.g., bilirubin-glucuronide) or sulfate conjugates. Each MRP has its own, unique spectrum of substrates.

transported. In addition, MRPs transport some organic anions as free ions, and they also transport some solutes as glucuronate conjugates or sulfate conjugates.

In many instances administration of cytotoxic agents (including anticancer drugs) can cause upregulation of an MRP. Thus tumors that initially are sensitive to an agent such as adriamycin can become resistant (i.e., the MRPs are cytoprotective). Because many MRPs have broad selectivity, this upregulation may cause the tumor to become resistant to multiple drugs; hence the name "multidrug resistance proteins."

Interestingly, during upregulation, mutant MRP genes may be preferentially expressed, so the substrate selectivity of the gene product may change with time.

A number of agents, including the calcium channel blocker verapamil and the antiarrhythmic agent quinidine, block MRPs and thereby enhance the sensitivity to the antitumor agents. Use of these blockers has a serious drawback, however: normal cells are then also prevented from extruding these cytotoxic agents, which may lead to intolerable side effects. A goal in antitumor chemotherapy is to target the MRP in

> **BOX 11-11**
>
> ### Cystic Fibrosis Is Caused by Mutations in the Gene That Encodes the CFTR Cl⁻ Channel
>
> Cystic fibrosis is an inherited autosomal recessive disease characterized by thick, viscous secretions from the mucous gland and airway epithelium, pancreatic insufficiency (greatly reduced exocrine secretions), and unusually high concentrations of Na^+ and Cl^- in sweat. The cause of the disease is mutation of the gene that encodes an epithelial Cl^- channel and transport regulatory protein known as the cystic fibrosis transmembrane conductance regulator (CFTR). The disease is most prevalent in Caucasians, with a frequency of about 1 per 1600 births; the mutated gene frequency is about 1 in 20 in the Caucasian population.
>
> As a result of mutation, the Cl^- conductance through the CFTR Cl^- channel in a variety of epithelia is decreased in patients with cystic fibrosis. In addition, regulation of certain other epithelial Cl^- channels and Na^+ channels by CFTR may be altered in these patients. The consequent reduction in Cl^- (and Na^+) secretion greatly reduces secretory volume (because of the reduced osmotic driving force), so that the residual secretions are viscous. These thick secretions tend to plug small pancreatic ducts and pulmonary airways, leading to pancreatic insufficiency and a high rate of severe respiratory infections.

the cancer cells with these blocking agents or to prevent, selectively, cancer cell MRP from being upregulated after drug treatment.

The cystic fibrosis transmembrane conductance regulator is a Cl^- channel The **cystic fibrosis transmembrane conductance regulator** (**CFTR**) is another member of the ABC superfamily of transporters. CFTR is unusual in that it functions in part as a Cl^- channel and in part as a regulator of several other conductances. Mutations in CFTR play a central role in the pathogenesis of cystic fibrosis (Box 11-11).

■ NET TRANSPORT ACROSS EPITHELIAL CELLS DEPENDS ON THE COUPLING OF APICAL AND BASOLATERAL MEMBRANE TRANSPORT SYSTEMS

Epithelia Are Continuous Sheets of Cells

The cells in an epithelium are joined by special **"tight" junctions** with variable permeability. These cells form a continuous sheet, usually one cell layer thick (Figure 11-7). A good structural analogy is a six-pack of beer cans joined by a plastic sheet (the tight junctions) with holes for the six cans (the cells). As we shall see, the tightness of the junctions (measured as "leakiness" or electrical conductance) varies considerably among epithelia and is thereby responsible for markedly different functional properties.

The tight junctions separate the epithelial cell apical and basolateral membranes (Figures 11-7 and 11-8), which face solutions of different composition and have different sets of transport proteins. The apical and basolateral membranes can have different permeabilities to water. Solutes and water may move across the epithelium between cells, that is, through intercellular junctions (the **paracellular pathway**). Alternatively, these substances may move through the cells (the **transcellular pathway**). In the latter case the solutes are transported across the apical and basolateral membranes by different, selective transporters. This two-step process, in which the transporters are arranged in series, is exemplified by the net uptake of glucose in the proximal small intestine and proximal renal tubules, as described in Chapter 10. Another

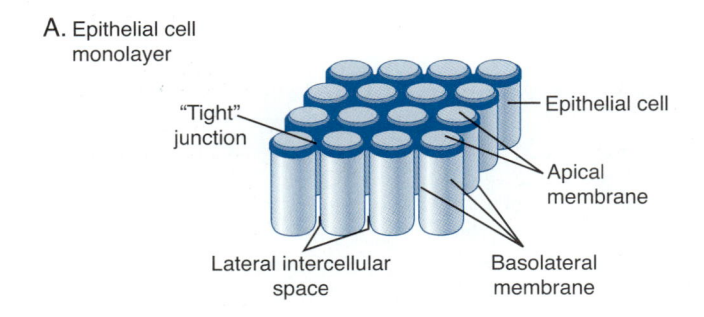

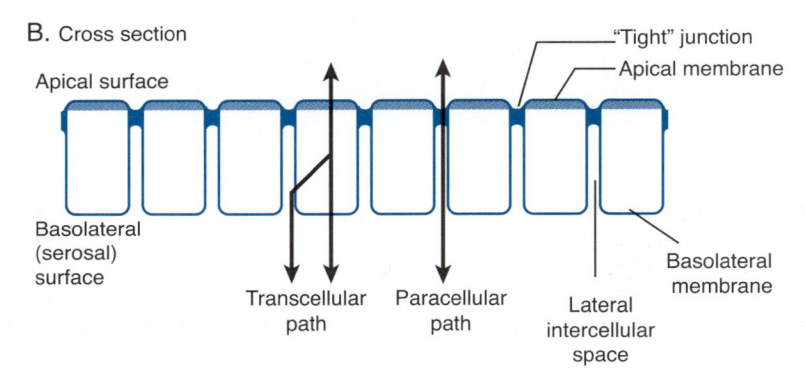

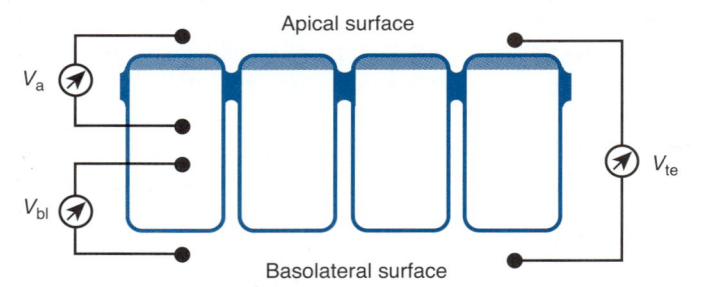

Figure 11-7 ■ **Epithelial cell monolayer. A,** Apical surface view. **B,** Cross section through the epithelial cells to illustrate the apical and basolateral surfaces, the lateral intercellular spaces, and the transcellular and paracellular pathways across the epithelium. **C,** Epithelial membrane potentials: V_a, potential across the apical membrane; V_{bl}, potential across the basolateral membrane; and V_{te}, the potential in the lumen relative to that in the interstitial space (i.e., the transepithelial potential = $V_a - V_{bl}$). (Redrawn and modified from Friedman MH: *Principles and models of biological transport,* Berlin, 1986, Springer-Verlag.)

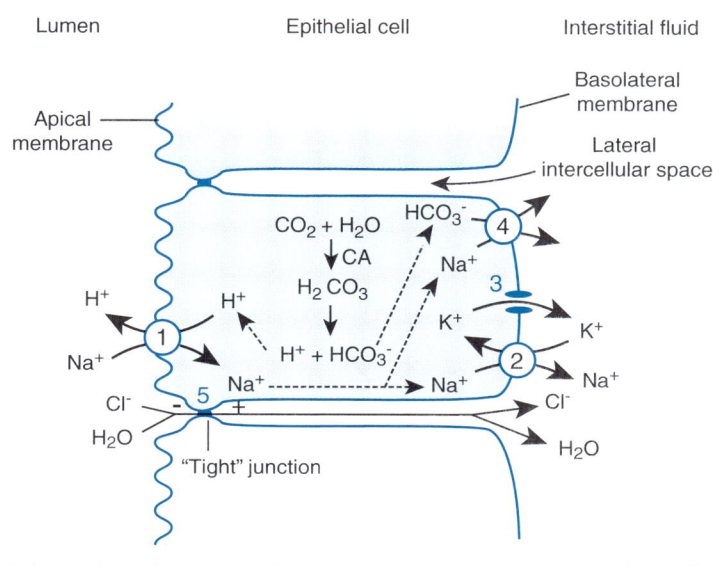

Active Transport

Figure 11-8 ■ Model epithelial cell such as a renal proximal tubule cell illustrates the net (re)absorption of NaCl and H_2O. The model shows the mechanism of Na^+ uptake via Na^+/H^+ exchange across the apical membrane (*1*), the extrusion of Na^+ via the basolateral membrane Na^+ pump (*2*), which exchanges 3 Na^+ for 2 K^+, the recycling of K^+ via basolateral K^+ channels (*3*), the cotransport of Na^+ and HCO_3^- (formed by the enzyme carbonic anhydrase, or CA) across the basolateral membrane (*4*), and the movement of Cl^- (down an electrochemical gradient) and H_2O (down an osmotic gradient) through the paracellular pathway (*5*). Although not shown in the diagram, Na^+ ions are also pumped into the narrow lateral intercellular spaces, so that a large buildup of unaccompanied Cl^- ions does not occur in these spaces. In addition, some Cl^- is transported through the transcellular pathway (not shown). Note that the ATP needed to drive the Na^+ pump is not shown.

---

example is the renal secretion of organic cations and anions, also described in Chapter 10.

Epithelia Exhibit Great Functional Diversity

In this section we discuss the general principles of transepithelial transport and the integration and coordination of multiple transport processes that contribute to the overall function of the intestinal, renal, and other epithelia. We explore first the source of the Na^+ that is required for the numerous Na^+-coupled apical transport systems. Anion transport is then considered, followed by water transport. Although epithelia are functionally diverse, one common feature is the presence of Na^+ pumps in the basolateral membranes. The identities of other transport proteins in apical and basolateral membranes of the epithelial cell, as well as the leakiness of the paracellular pathway (regulated by small molecules called *claudins*), determine the specific transport properties of the various epithelia. These other transport proteins then determine whether net transport of the various solutes is from lumen to interstitial fluid (absorption) or from interstitial fluid to lumen (secretion).

In Chapter 10 we learned how expression of different glucose transporters (SGLT-2 and SGLT-1) along the nephron maximizes the reabsorption of glucose from the luminal fluid in kidney proximal tubules. Similarly, other specific transport systems are expressed in the various epithelial cell types along the gastrointestinal tract and the renal tubules. In the more proximal segments this maximizes salt and water absorption, and in the more distal segments it fine-tunes the absorption of solutes and water and the secretion of solutes.

Ion gradients across the apical and basolateral membranes are established by the Na^+ pump and various secondary active transport processes. The membrane potentials across the apical and basolateral membranes, V_a and V_{bl}, are determined by these ion concentration gradients and by the relative ion permeabilities across the two membranes. The transepithelial potential, V_{te}, is thus defined as the electrical potential in the lumen relative to that in the interstitial space surrounding the basolateral surface of the epithelial cells (see Figure 11-7). V_{te} is equal to the difference, $V_a - V_{bl}$, where V_{te} may be either negative or positive. As we shall see, these electrical potentials are important for solute transport because the passive movement of an ion is driven not only by its concentration gradient, but also by the electrical potential gradient (see Chapter 9).

What Are the Sources of Na^+ for Apical Membrane Na^+-Solute Cotransport?

Humans normally ingest a modest amount of Na^+ (on average about 100 to 150 mmol/day), and dietary Na^+ may be exceedingly low (<15 mmol/day) in some nonindustrialized societies, such as the Yanomamo Indians of Northern Brazil. Nevertheless, extracellular Na^+ salts play an important role in maintaining extracellular fluid volume. This implies that the body's Na^+ must be carefully conserved and that the Na^+ required for Na^+-solute cotransport must be recycled in the body. This principle is illustrated by transport processes in the gastrointestinal tract.

As noted earlier in the chapter, HCl is secreted into the lumen of the stomach. This acid must be neutralized in the small intestine because most digestion in the intestine occurs at a neutral or alkaline pH. Consequently, the exocrine pancreas secretes an alkaline solution that contains primarily sodium bicarbonate ($NaHCO_3$). Some of the HCO_3^- is used to neutralize the HCl from the stomach, leaving NaCl in the intestinal lumen. This Na^+ then drives Na^+-solute cotransport across the apical membrane of the small intestine columnar epithelial cells (Figure 11-8). Thus the Na^+ secreted by the pancreas is recycled into the plasma as a result of the sequential transport across the apical and basolateral membranes of the intestinal epithelial cells (Figure 11-8). Na^+/H^+ exchange across the apical membrane not only mediates Na^+ uptake across the apical membrane, but also provides additional protons to neutralize the remainder of the luminal HCO_3^- (Figure 11-8). The protons are produced in the epithelial cell cytoplasm—for example, by the action of the enzyme carbonic anhydrase on CO_2, a product of oxidative metabolism ($CO_2 + H_2O \rightarrow H_2CO_3 \rightarrow H^+ + HCO_3^-$). The resulting cytosolic HCO_3^- can then be transported across the basolateral membrane into the plasma (Figure 11-8), or it can be exchanged for Cl^- across the apical membrane (Figure 11-9).

A different but comparable situation regarding the origin and transport of the Na^+ prevails in the kidneys. Here, the glomeruli filter the blood and produce a nearly protein-free **ultrafiltrate** of plasma that, in normal adults, amounts to about 180 liters per day of a solution isoosmotic to plasma ($\approx$290 mosmoles/kg), in which the predominant ions are Na^+ and Cl^-. This fluid then enters the proximal tubules, but 99% of the Na^+, Cl^-, and H_2O is reabsorbed before the final urine (about 1.5 liters/day) is formed. About 67% of the Na^+ is reabsorbed in the proximal tubules. Some of this Na^+ is

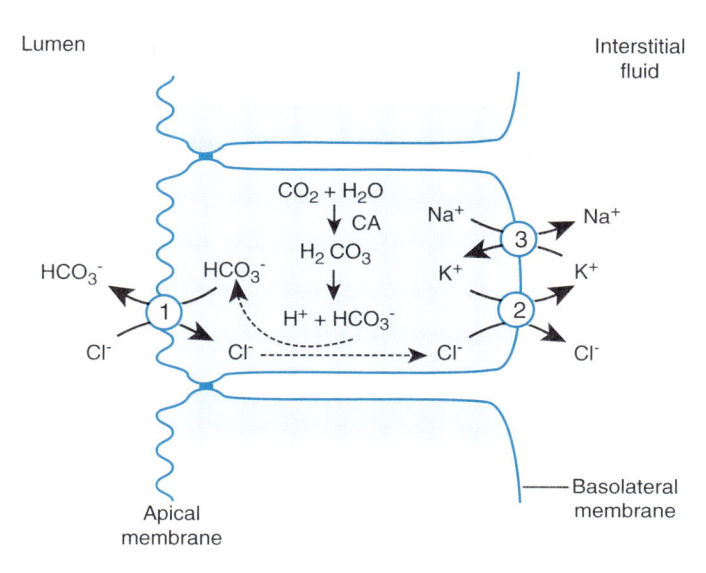

Active Transport

Figure 11-9 ■ Model epithelial cell showing the mechanism of Cl^- absorption by the transcellular route. Cl^- is taken up across the apical membrane by a Cl^-/HCO_3^- exchanger (*1*). The Cl^- is then extruded across the basolateral membrane by a K^+-Cl^- cotransporter (*2*), using energy from the K^+ electrochemical gradient that is maintained by the Na^+ pump (*3*). Note that the ATP needed to drive the Na^+ pump is not shown.

cotransported with sugars and amino acids, but much of it is reabsorbed by Na^+/H^+ exchange (Figure 11-8). Some of the H^+ transported into the lumen is recycled through the organic cation/H^+ exchanger (see Chapter 10), and some of the H^+ reacts with HCO_3^- in the tubular fluid to form H_2O and CO_2. The CO_2 can then reenter the cells to start another hydration cycle (i.e., to form more H^+). We know that the primary active transport of Na^+ (i.e., the ATP-driven exchange of 3 Na^+ for 2 K^+) across the basolateral membrane of epithelial cells maintains the Na^+ and K^+ electrochemical gradients. The examples given above demonstrate that these gradients, directly or indirectly, drive *all* of the aforementioned transport processes. Thus it is not surprising that the *Na^+ pump accounts for 75% to 85% of all the ATP hydrolysis in the kidneys.*

Another important aspect of the Na^+ pump activity in epithelia is the very large amount of K^+ transported into the cells. Most of this K^+, *in most epithelia, is normally recycled across the basolateral membranes and into the plasma* by efflux through K^+-selective channels (Figure 11-8) or K^+-Cl^- cotransport (Figure 11-9).

Absorption of Cl^- Occurs by Several Different Mechanisms

Na^+ cannot be (re)absorbed without an accompanying anion. The main anion in the intestinal lumen and renal tubular lumen is Cl^-, which also must be recycled, and a variety of mechanisms are involved. The cytoplasm of the intestinal and renal cells is electrically negative relative to the intestinal or kidney tubule lumen. Thus the Cl^- electrochemical gradient across the apical membrane may favor Cl^- movement from cell to lumen. Nevertheless, the lumen-negative transepithelial potential (V_{te} ~ -3 to -5 mV) in the small intestine and kidney proximal tubule provides an electrical driving force that favors the net movement of Cl⁻ across the epithelium from lumen to interstitial space. Then, because *the small intestine and renal proximal tubule tight junctions are in reality somewhat "leaky"* (i.e., they have relatively low electrical resistances), *Cl⁻ moves through the junctions between cells (the paracellular pathway) from lumen to plasma* (Figure 11-8).

In some epithelial cells, specific Cl⁻ transport mechanisms are involved in Cl⁻ movement. Two important Cl⁻ transporters in some intestinal and renal epithelial cell apical membranes are a Cl⁻/HCO_3^- exchanger (Figure 11-9) and a 1 Na⁺-1 K⁺-2 Cl⁻ cotransporter (Figure 11-10). The basolateral membranes of the intestinal epithelial cells contain a K⁺-Cl⁻ cotransporter (Figure 11-9) or Cl⁻-selective channels (Figure 11-10). The Cl⁻ taken up at the apical membrane is transported across the basolateral membrane by one of these mechanisms, thereby averting a rise in the cytosolic Cl⁻ concentration. In the case of the basolateral Cl⁻ channels, Cl⁻ moves down its electrochemical gradient across the basolateral membranes when the intracellular Cl⁻ concentration rises sufficiently that E_{Cl}, the Cl⁻ equilibrium potential, becomes more positive than V_{bl} (see Chapter 4).

Substances Can Also Be Secreted by Epithelia

Epithelia not only transport solutes (and fluid) from the lumen to the plasma (absorption), but also may move some substances in the opposite

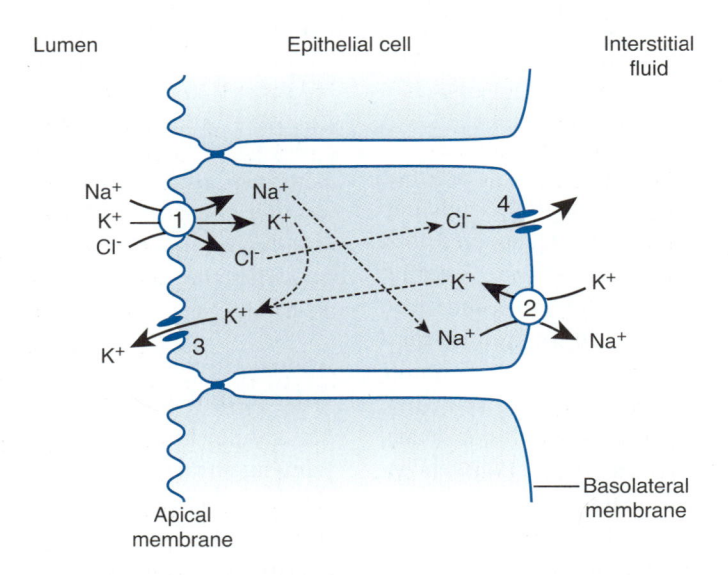

Figure 11-10 ■ Mechanism of net K⁺ secretion across an epithelium (the thick ascending limb of Henle's loop). In this case, Na⁺, K⁺, and Cl⁻ enter the cell via an *apical* Na⁺-K⁺-2 Cl⁻ cotransporter (*1*), driven by the Na⁺ electrochemical gradient. K⁺ also is pumped into the cell across the basolateral membrane in exchange for Na⁺, via the Na⁺ pump (*2*). K⁺ leaves the cell, down its electrochemical gradient, via K⁺-selective channels in the apical membrane (*3*). Cl⁻ moves down its electrochemical gradient, from cell to interstitial space, via Cl⁻-selective channels in the basolateral membrane (*4*). Note that these cells also have K⁺ channels and a K⁺-Cl⁻ cotransporter in their basolateral membranes (not shown). Note also that the ATP needed to drive the Na⁺ pump is not shown.

BOX 11-12

Salt Wasting, Salt Retention, and Blood Pressure

About 30% of the Na^+ filtered in the kidney glomerulus is reabsorbed in the thick ascending limb of Henle's loop. The mechanisms involved are illustrated in Figure 11-10. Genetic loss-of-function defects in the Na^+-K^+-2 Cl^- cotransporter, the apical K^+ channels (which enable K^+ recycling), or the basolateral Cl^- channels (which permit Cl^- to accompany Na^+ to maintain electroneutrality) result in severe salt (NaCl) wasting. All of these defects cause low blood pressure (hypotension), which may be life threatening in newborns. The syndrome of salt wasting, excessive urinary Ca^{2+} loss, and hypotension is known as Bartter's syndrome.

In contrast, salt retention and hypertension result from excessively high levels of aldosterone secretion, as may occur with certain tumors or hyperplasia (increased cell number) of the adrenal cortical glomerulosa cells (Conn's syndrome, or primary aldosteronism). The aldosterone increases apical Na^+ permeability and the number of Na^+ pumps in the basolateral membrane of kidney cortical collecting tubule cells.

As these examples imply, salt transport and net salt balance play a key role in the regulation of plasma volume and blood pressure. Pathological conditions that cause salt retention without a large decrease in plasma protein invariably lead to hypertension. Conversely, pathological conditions that cause salt wasting invariably lead to hypotension.

---

direction (i.e., secretion). We have already discussed two examples of net secretion: organic cations and organic anions (see Chapter 10).

Another example of secretion is that of K^+ in some epithelia. In this case the K^+ is transported into the cells by the basolateral Na^+ pump. The secretion is then mediated by K^+-selective channels in the apical membrane (Figure 11-10). A genetic defect in these channels in the thick ascending limb of Henle's loop (TALH) in the kidney results in reduced K^+ permeability and reduced K^+ secretion. The inability of K^+ to recycle back into the kidney tubule lumen limits Na^+ absorption via Na^+-K^+-2 Cl^- cotransport and thus causes salt (NaCl) wasting and low blood pressure, or hypotension (Bartter's syndrome; Box 11-12).

Now, consider an epithelium (such as the intestinal mucosa) in which the epithelial cells possess a Cl^- entry mechanism (1 Na^+-1 K^+-2 Cl^- cotransport), as well as Na^+ pumps and K^+ channels in their basolateral membranes and Cl^--selective channels in their apical membranes (Figure 11-11). Under these circumstances, Na^+ drives Cl^- (and K^+) into the cells, across the basolateral membranes, by secondary active transport. Then, while the Na^+ is pumped out (recycled) across these membranes, the Cl^- is driven into the lumen, across the apical membrane, by its electrochemical gradient. At the same time, Na^+ moves from intestinal fluid to lumen through the paracellular pathway, driven by the transepithelial electrical potential gradient (V_{te}, lumen negative) that is set up by the secretion of Cl^- (Figure 11-11).

The apical Cl^- channels and thus Cl^- secretion in intestinal epithelial cells are regulated by cyclic nucleotide–dependent protein phosphorylation. When cyclic AMP or cyclic guanosine monophosphate (GMP) is pathologically increased by enterotoxins, however, the result may be a massive loss of Cl^-, Na^+, and water in the stool. This is a *secretory diarrhea* (Box 11-13) and may be contrasted with the *osmotic diarrhea* described in Chapter 10 (Box 10-8).

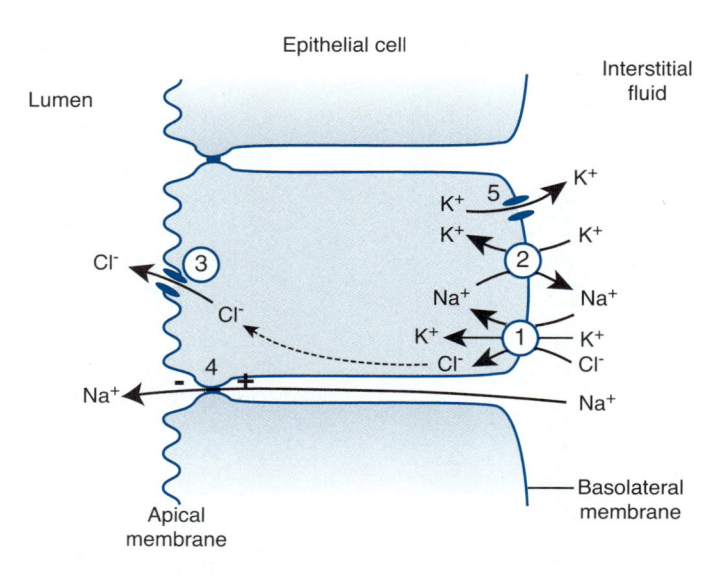

Figure 11-11 ■ Mechanism of net NaCl secretion across an epithelium. In this case Cl^- enters the cell via a *basolateral* membrane Na^+–K^+–2 Cl^- cotransporter (*1*), driven by the Na^+ electrochemical gradient that is maintained by the Na^+ pump (*2*). As the Cl^- concentration rises within the epithelial cell, the Cl^- electrochemical gradient across the apical membrane drives Cl^- out through Cl^--selective channels in this membrane (*3*) that are regulated by cyclic nucleotides. The resulting transepithelial electrical gradient, V_{te} (lumen negative), drives Na^+ from the interstitial space to the lumen through the paracellular pathway (*4*). The K^+ that enters the cell across the basolateral membrane is recycled across this membrane through K^+-selective channels (*5*). Secretion of NaCl provides the osmotic driving force for concomitant H_2O movement into the lumen. Note that the ATP needed to drive the Na^+ pump is not shown.

Net Water Flow Is Coupled to Net Solute Flow Across Epithelia

The preceding discussion provides some examples of how solutes can be either absorbed or secreted across epithelia. We now need to consider the movement of water across epithelia. No active transport of water occurs across epithelia; water must move passively, driven by the (vanishingly small) osmotic gradients that are set up by the net solute transport. *Water may move through the cells* (i.e., *the transcellular pathway*) *or*, if the "tight junctions" are sufficiently leaky, *through the paracellular pathway*

Water transport across leaky epithelia is osmotic and obligatory The small intestine and the renal proximal tubule are examples of "leaky" epithelia. In these tissues, which have a high rate of net solute transfer, the apical membrane permeability to water is high, in part because the membranes contain constitutive water channels (aquaporin-1). Thus most of the net (osmotic) water flow occurs through the transcellular pathway. In addition, however, the net solute transport, from lumen to interstitial space, establishes a very small osmotic gradient across the epithelium. This drives water flow through the paracellular pathway tight junctions and into the lateral intercellular spaces (Figure 11-8), which are actually quite narrow. Local hydrostatic pressure then propels the fluid

BOX 11-13

Enterotoxins That Activate Cl⁻ Channels Induce Secretory Diarrhea

Heat-stable enterotoxins from *Escherichia coli* activate guanylate cyclase and increase the production of cyclic guanosine monophosphate (cGMP), whereas enterotoxins from *Vibrio cholerae* augment the production of cyclic adenosine monophosphate (cAMP). These cyclic nucleotides activate cGMP- or cAMP-dependent protein kinases, which in turn activate the cystic fibrosis transmembrane conductance regulator (CFTR) Cl⁻ channels in the apical membrane of small intestinal epithelial cells. The consequent increase in Cl⁻ conductance enhances secretion of Cl⁻ and Na⁺ (Figure 11-11) and thereby provides an osmotic driving force so that water flows from interstitial space to the intestinal lumen. The result is the excretion of large volumes of watery stool, called a *secretory diarrhea*. The loss of NaCl and water often causes severe dehydration and may be fatal if not treated rapidly and aggressively. This is an especially critical problem in underdeveloped regions of the world where unsanitary conditions prevail and where the enterotoxin-producing bacteria are endemic. As discussed in Chapter 10, these diarrheas can often be treated with oral rehydration using a solution containing NaCl and glucose. The cotransport of glucose and Na⁺ and, consequently, Cl⁻ into the body provides a source of nutrient and replenishes the salt and water lost through the secretory diarrhea.

The action of the enterotoxins is blunted in individuals with a loss-of-function mutation in the CFTR gene, as might be expected from the aforementioned role of the CFTR Cl⁻ channels (see Box 11-11). This has fostered the hypothesis that the high frequency of cystic fibrosis may have been the result of its protective effect against secretory diarrheas.

(solvent and solutes) out of these lateral intercellular spaces and into the blood. Despite the large amount of solute transfer, there is never a very large osmotic gradient because the constant osmotic water flow prevents the buildup of a large osmotic pressure difference between the lumen and the interstitial space.

Another feature of water flow through "leaky epithelia" is that some solutes may move with the water through the paracellular pathway. This phenomenon, known as **solvent drag**, may be an important mechanism for the reabsorption of K^+ and Ca^{2+} in renal proximal tubules. The explanation is that the complete separation of water from solute takes a lot of energy. Therefore, if tight junctions are sufficiently leaky (i.e., they have large "pores"), dissolved solute will flow through these junctions along with the water (also called **"bulk flow"**).

Water transport across tight epithelia is regulated The colon and renal late distal tubule and cortical and medullary collecting ducts are examples of **tight epithelia.** In these epithelia the transepithelial conductance is very low, and very little water normally flows across the tight junctions (i.e., through the paracellular pathway). Moreover, the apical membranes of these cells normally have very low water permeability unless water channels (aquaporins) are inserted into the membranes. When an increase in plasma osmolality signals a need to increase water reabsorption in the distal segments of the renal tubules, the posterior pituitary gland secretes antidiuretic hormone (ADH, or vasopressin). ADH acts on the cells in the distal nephron segments to promote the synthesis of cyclic AMP. The cyclic AMP, in turn, stimulates the temporary fusion of sub–plasma membrane vesicles containing aquaporins with the apical membrane. In tight epithelia in the renal cortex the solute uptake systems generate a very small osmotic gradient across the apical membranes of the epithelial cells. Solute extrusion across the basolateral membrane then sets up a small osmotic gradient that drives water into the interstitial space. As a result, net water reabsorption is increased.

In contrast, if more water excretion is required to maintain water balance, the ADH level will remain low. In this case very little water is reabsorbed in the distal nephron and a dilute urine (i.e., with a low osmotic pressure) is excreted. Defects either in the ADH secretory mechanism or in the hormone receptors on the renal tubule cells, or mutations of the aquaporin-2 gene, result in pathological excretion of large amounts of dilute urine (diabetes insipidus; see Chapter 10).

The ultimate example of a "tight" epithelium is the mammalian urinary bladder. Once the urine is formed in the renal tubules, it is temporarily stored in the bladder. Virtually no transport of solute or water occurs either across the apical membranes of the bladder epithelial cells or through the tight junctions in this epithelium because of the impermeability of these barriers. The urinary bladder is therefore simply a "storage organ."

■ SUMMARY

1. Some integral membrane proteins, known as "pumps" or ATPases, harness the energy from the hydrolysis of ATP to transport specific solutes such as Na^+, H^+, and Ca^{2+} against their electrochemical gradients. These transporters are said to mediate "primary active transport."
2. The PM Na^+ pump mediates the export of 3 Na^+ ions and import of 2 K^+ ions, while hydrolyzing 1 ATP to ADP and inorganic phosphate. By exporting one positive charge per cycle, this pump generates a small voltage and is therefore called an electrogenic pump. The Na^+ pump is uniquely sensitive to cardiotonic steroids such as ouabain and digoxin.
3. The Na^+ pump maintains the large Na^+ and K^+ electrochemical gradients across the PM of most cells. These gradients are critical for the electrical activity of excitable cells (Chapters 7 and 8) and for powering secondary active transport (see Chapter 10). By maintaining a low intracellular Na^+ concentration, the Na^+ pump also plays a critical role in cell volume regulation: it enables cells to behave as if they are impermeable to Na^+ (see discussion of the Donnan effect in Chapter 4).
4. The Ca^{2+} pump in the sarcoplasmic/endoplasmic reticulum (SERCA) has striking sequence homology to the Na^+ pump. SERCA plays a key role in storing the Ca^{2+} in the S/ER that is required for Ca^{2+} signaling.
5. The structures of two conformations of SERCA, including one in which two Ca^{2+} ions are bound, have been determined by X-ray crystallography. These structures reveal how SERCA binds the Ca^{2+} ions when the pump ion access channel is open to the cytosolic fluid, and how, when ATP is hydrolyzed, the conformation changes so that the Ca^{2+} can be transferred to the lumen of the S/ER.
6. Certain Na^+ pump catalytic subunit isoforms and the Na^+/Ca^{2+} exchanger act cooperatively to help regulate the Na^+ and Ca^{2+} concentrations in the small volume of cytosol between the PM and sub-PM ("junctional") S/ER in many cell types. This influences the storage of Ca^{2+} in the junctional S/ER and thus the Ca^{2+} signaling that depends on Ca^{2+} release from the S/ER.
7. Other transport ATPases such as the PM Ca^{2+} pump and two Cu^{2+} pumps help to regulate

ions in cells or their environment. For example, the gastric H^+,K^+-ATPase secretes protons into the lumen of the stomach to optimize the action of pepsin.
8. ABC proteins are involved in the ATP-dependent extrusion of some endogenous compounds and xenobiotics (foreign substances such as anticancer drugs) from cells. The cystic fibrosis transmembrane conductance regulator protein, which behaves in part as a Cl^- channel, is also an ABC protein.
9. Transepithelial transport occurs in part through the paracellular pathway and in part through the transcellular pathway.
10. The Na^+ electrochemical gradient generated by the Na^+ pump provides the energy for absorption and reabsorption of water and for net transport (either absorption or secretion) of most solute species across epithelia.
11. Net transport of solutes across epithelia through the transcellular pathway requires two different transport mechanisms for each transported solute species, one in the apical membrane and one in the basolateral membrane.
12. Net solute transport through the paracellular pathway depends on the permeability of the "tight junctions" between cells and on the osmotic and electrical driving forces across the epithelium.

■ KEY WORDS AND CONCEPTS

- Primary active transport
- P-type ATPases
- Sodium pump (Na^+,K^+-ATPase)
- Pump-leak model
- Cardiotonic steroids (e.g., digoxin and ouabain)
- Sodium pump catalytic (α) subunit isoforms
- Intracellular Ca^{2+} stores
- Endoplasmic reticulum (ER)
- Sarcoplasmic reticulum (SR)
- SERCA (S/ER Ca^{2+}-dependent ATPase)
- PMCA (plasma membrane Ca^{2+}-dependent ATPase)
- Gastric H^+,K^+-ATPase
- Cu^{2+}-transporting ATPases
- ATP binding cassette (ABC) membrane transporters
- Multidrug resistance protein (MRP)
- Cystic fibrosis transmembrane conductance regulator (CFTR)
- Tight junction
- Transcellular pathway
- Paracellular pathway
- Ultrafiltrate
- Leaky epithelium
- Solvent drag
- Bulk flow
- Tight epithelium

STUDY PROBLEMS

1. Some intestinal smooth muscles relax when they are exposed to β-adrenergic agonists such as isoproterenol, which stimulate the Na^+ pump through a cyclic AMP-mediated mechanism. The Na^+ pump stimulation is required for this relaxation. What is a likely mechanism for the relaxation?
2. Explain why so many secondary active transport systems are all coupled (indirectly) to the Na^+ pump.
3. Most transport systems, including the Na^+ pump, SERCA, PMCA, the Na^+/H^+ exchanger (NHE), the Na^+-glucose cotransporter (SGLT), and the simple glucose carrier (GLUT) are expressed in several different isoforms or splice variants. What are some possible reasons for this multiplicity of these transport systems?

■ BIBLIOGRAPHY

Anderson JM: Molecular structure of tight junctions and their role in epithelial transport, *News Physiol Sci* 16:126, 2001.
Arnon A, Hamlyn JM, Blaustein MP: Ouabain augments Ca^{2+} transients in arterial smooth muscle without raising cytosolic Na^+, *Am J Physiol Heart Circ Physiol* 279:H679, 2000.
Blanco G, Mercer RW: Isozymes of the Na-K-ATPase: heterogeneity in structure, diversity in function, *Am J Physiol* 275:F633, 1998.
Borst P, Evers R, Kool M, Wijnholds J: A family of drug

transporters: the multidrug resistance-associated proteins, *J Natl Cancer Inst* 92:1295, 2000.

Deen PM, Croes H, van Aubel RA, et al: Water channels encoded by mutant aquaporin-2 genes in nephrogenic diabetes insipidus are impaired in their cellular routing, *J Clin Invest* 95:2291, 1995.

Green NM, MacLennan DH: Structural biology: calcium calisthenics, *Nature* 418:598, 2002.

Harris ED: Cellular copper transport and metabolism, *Annu Rev Nutr* 20:291, 2000.

James PF, Grupp IL, Grupp G, et al: Identification of a specific role for the Na,K-ATPase $\alpha 2$ isoform as a regulator of calcium in the heart, *Molec Cell* 3:555, 1999.

Koeppen BM, Stanton BA: *Renal physiology*, ed 3, St Louis, 2001, Mosby.

Kutchai HC: The gastrointestinal system. In Berne RM, Levy MN, editors: *Physiology*, ed 4, St Louis, 1998, Mosby.

Lifton RP, Gharavi AG, Geller DS: Molecular mechanisms of human hypertension, *Cell* 104:545, 2001.

Lingrel JB, Croyle ML, Woo AL, Arguello JM: Ligand binding sites of Na,K-ATPase, *Acta Physiol Scand Suppl* 643:69, 1998.

MacLennan DH, Green NM: Structural biology: pumping ions, *Nature* 405:633, 2000.

Sachs G, Wallmark B: Biological basis of omeprazole therapy, *J Gastroenterol Hepatol* 4(suppl 2):S7, 1989.

Schwiebert EM, Benos DJ, Egan ME, et al: CFTR is a conductance regulator as well as a chloride channel, *Physiol Rev* 79(suppl 1):S145, 1999.

Sweadner KJ, Rael E: The FXYD gene family of small ion transport regulators or channels: cDNA sequence, protein signature sequence, and expression, *Genomics* 68:41, 2000.

CHAPTER 12

SECTION IV Molecular Motors and Muscle Contraction

Molecular Motors and the Mechanisms of Muscle Contraction

Objectives:

1. Understand the common principles that apply to all molecular motors: myosin, kinesin, and dynein.
2. Describe the structure of a skeletal muscle cell and the organization of its contractile elements, and compare and contrast this with the structure of cardiac and smooth muscle.
3. Understand the sliding filament theory of muscle contraction.
4. Understand the coupling between the mechanical motions of the myosin motor and the steps involved in ATP hydrolysis during cross-bridge cycling.
5. Describe how Ca^{2+} interacts with the regulatory proteins troponin and tropomyosin to activate contraction in skeletal and cardiac muscle.
6. Describe how Ca^{2+} activates contraction in smooth muscle by promoting the phosphorylation of myosin light chain kinase.

■ MOLECULAR MOTORS PRODUCE MOTILITY BY CONVERTING CHEMICAL ENERGY INTO KINETIC ENERGY

Movement is one of the defining characteristics of all living things. Cell motility is an essential feature of many biological activities, such as the beating of cilia and flagella, cell movement, cell division, development and maintenance of cell architecture, and muscle contraction, the main topic of this and the next two chapters. Moreover, the normal functioning of all cells requires the directional transport, *within* the cell, of numerous substances and organelles, such as vesicles, mitochondria, chromosomes, and macromolecules (e.g., mRNA and protein).

The Three Types of Molecular Motors Are Myosin, Kinesin, and Dynein

All types of cellular motility are driven by **molecular motors** that produce unidirectional movement along structural elements in the cell. The structural elements are two types of protein polymer structures: filaments, composed of **actin** monomers arranged in strands, and **microtubules**, which are polymers of the protein tubulin. Three distinct types of molecular motors that move along these structures have been described: **myosin, kinesin,** and **dynein**. Myosin is an "actin-based" motor that moves along actin filaments. Myosin motors produce muscle contraction. Kinesin and dynein transport organelles along microtubules. Kinesins are involved in mitotic and meiotic spindle formation and in chromosome separation, as well as in mRNA and protein transport. Dyneins are involved in the beating of cilia, movement of flagella, and vesicular trafficking.

Several principles apply to the operation of all molecular motors. *Molecular motors convert chemical energy into kinetic energy (movement).* The chemical energy is stored in the high-energy phosphate bond of ATP. The motors (myosin, kinesin, and dynein) all have adenosine triphosphatase (ATPase) activity. The binding of ATP, its hydrolysis, and the subsequent release of products are important steps in the generation of movement. In all cases movement is produced through repetitive cycles of interaction between the motor and a structural element in the cell (either an actin filament or a microtubule). In recent years a combination of biochemical, biophysical, and structural studies of muscle contraction and kinesin-based vesicle transport has demonstrated how the enzymatic steps involving ATP hydrolysis are coupled to the conformational and structural changes that produce movement. Based on these studies, animated models for the motility cycles of muscle myosin and kinesin have been developed. These models present a particularly clear picture of how movement is produced by these motors. The kinesin motor is described in Box 12-1, and the myosin motor is described in this chapter. (QuickTime movies of these animated models can be seen at www.sciencemag.org/feature/data/1049155.shl.)

■ SINGLE SKELETAL MUSCLE FIBERS ARE COMPOSED OF MANY MYOFIBRILS

Muscle cell types are classified primarily according to their structural and functional properties. An understanding of the detailed ultrastructure of single muscle cells provides insight into their functional properties. **Skeletal muscle cells** (skeletal myocytes) are attached to the skeleton by tendons and are under voluntary control. Their primary function is to shorten and generate force in order to produce movement of skeletal levers. The other two types of muscle, cardiac and smooth, are described later in this chapter.

Skeletal muscle is composed of many individual *muscle fibers*, each of which is an elongated cell. Each cell is 10 to 100 μm in diameter and may reach several centimeters in length. Electron micrographs reveal that a single skeletal muscle fiber is composed of bundles of filaments, called **myofibrils**. The myofibrils lie parallel to one another and run along the long axis of the cell (Figure 12-1). Surrounding each myofibril is an extensive membrane-enclosed intracellular compartment called the **sarcoplasmic reticulum (SR)**, which plays a key role in activating muscle contraction. Enlarged portions of the SR, the terminal cisterns, come in close contact with invaginations of the surface membrane (plasma membrane or *sarcolemma*) called **transverse tubules (T-tubules)** (Figure 12-1). Although the T-tubule membrane is continuous with the surface membrane, the SR membrane is not. The SR membrane is an intracellular membrane that is electrically isolated from the surface membrane. The relevance of this point will become clear when we consider the role of the T-tubule and the SR in excitation-contraction coupling in Chapter 13. Viewed parallel to its long axis, a skeletal muscle cell has a striped appearance, with alternating light and dark bands (Figure 12-2), which has led to its classification as *striated muscle*. The banding pattern is due to the alignment of thin (actin) and thick (myosin) filaments.

■ THE SARCOMERE IS THE BASIC UNIT OF CONTRACTION IN SKELETAL MUSCLE

The Sarcomere Consists of Interdigitating Thin and Thick Filaments

The banding pattern in striated muscle is produced by the regular arrangement of **thick**

BOX 12-1

Kinesin Motors Exemplify the Mechanism by Which Molecular Motors Produce Movement

More than 50 genes in the human genome code for a family of kinesin-related proteins. The first microtubule-based kinesin motor to be discovered is now called "conventional" kinesin. This molecular motor transports vesicular cargo along microtubule "tracks." Multiple functional domains have been identified in the structure of conventional kinesin. The protein is a heterotetramer, with two heavy peptide chains and two light chains (Figure B-1). At the N-terminus of the heavy chain is the motor domain, which contains the sites for microtubule binding and ATP hydrolysis. The neck linker and neck domains play a critical role in the directional movement of the two motor domains along the microtubule, as described below. One important role of the heavy chain tail domain is to inhibit its own ATPase activity by interacting with the motor domain in a folded configuration of the molecule. This self-inhibition keeps the molecule in an inactive state when it is not transporting cargo. The light chains are involved in cargo binding.

Conventional kinesin walks along a microtubule, with the two motor domains (one on each of the heavy chains in the tetramer) alternately stepping from one tubulin subunit to another. Some of the events in this process are illustrated in Figure B-2. When kinesin is bound to a microtubule with the leading head free of nucleotide and the trailing head bound to adenosine diphosphate (ADP), both of the neck linkers are mobile (Figure B-2, *A*). When ATP binds to the leading head, the neck linker becomes docked on, or bound to, the leading head (Figure B-2, *B*), which throws the trailing head forward toward the next tubulin binding site (Figure B-2, *C*). At about the same time, events occur independently in the two motor domains (Figure B-2, *D*). The new leading head binds to the microtubule and releases ADP. The trailing head hydrolyzes ATP to ADP and phosphate (P_i), which becomes covalently bound to the head. When this P_i is cleaved from the trailing head, its neck linker undocks and a new cycle can begin with ATP binding to the leading head (Figure B-2, *E*). An animation of this model can be viewed at the website www.sciencemag.org/feature/data/1049155.shl.

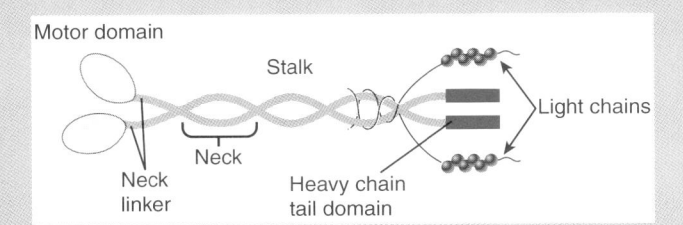

Figure B-1 ■ Conventional kinesin is a heterotetramer consisting of two heavy chains (*color*) and two light chains (*black*). The heavy chain contains the following functional domains: At the N-terminus is the catalytic motor domain, with sites for ATP hydrolysis and microtubule binding. The neck linker connects the motor domain to the neck and stalk and plays a critical role in directional movement along the microtubule. The tail region contributes to the regulation of kinesin activity. The light chains are believed to be involved in the binding of vesicular cargos to the kinesin molecule. (Modified from Verhey KJ, Rapoport TA: *Trends Biochem Sci* 26:545, 2001.)

BOX 12-1

Kinesin Motors Exemplify the Mechanism by Which Molecular Motors Produce Movement—Cont'd

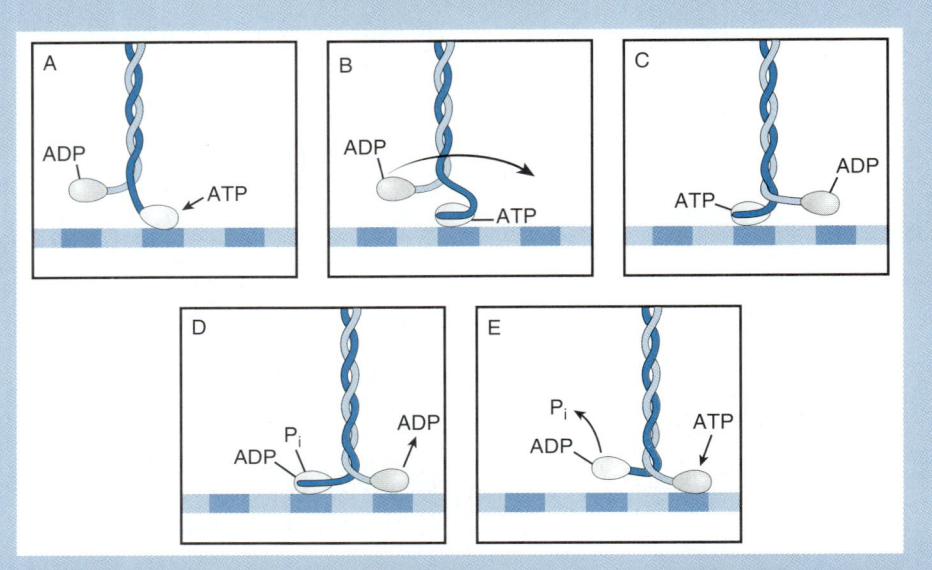

Figure B-2 ■ This model of the motility cycle for conventional kinesin is derived from a variety of biochemical, biophysical, and structural studies. The two motor domains in conventional kinesin produce directional movement through a sequence of coordinated steps. A, The nucleotide-free leading head *(to the right)* is tightly bound to tubulin. The ADP-bound trailing head is not bound to tubulin, and its neck linker is mobile. B, ATP binding to the leading head causes the neck linker to dock. C, The docking of the neck linker on the leading head throws the loosely bound trailing head forward toward the next tubulin binding site. D, The new leading head binds to the microtubule and then releases ADP. At the same time the trailing head hydrolyzes ATP to ADP and phosphate (P_i). E, After the trailing head releases P_i and undocks its neck linker, the cycle can be repeated. (From Vale RD, Milligan RA: *Science* 288:88, 2000.)

---

and **thin filaments** in the myofibrils. The light bands are I bands, which contain thin filaments that extend in both directions from a thin dense line, called the Z line (Figure 12-3). The region of myofibril between two adjacent Z lines is called a **sarcomere**. The dark bands, called A bands, contain thick (myosin) filaments arranged in parallel (Figure 12-3). At the center of the A band is a dense line called the M line. The thin (actin) filaments extend into the A bands but are not present in the central H zone,* which therefore appears lighter. The regular arrangement of thick and thin filaments is clearly shown in a cross section of a myofibril taken in the

---

*The darker bands are called A bands because they are anisotropic; the I bands are isotropic. Anisotropic material has different refractive indices for different planes of polarized light; isotropic material has a single refractive index. The Z line takes its name from the first letter of *Zwischenscheibe* (intervening disk, in German). The H in H zone stands for *heller* (lighter, in German).

Molecular Motors and the Mechanisms of Muscle Contraction

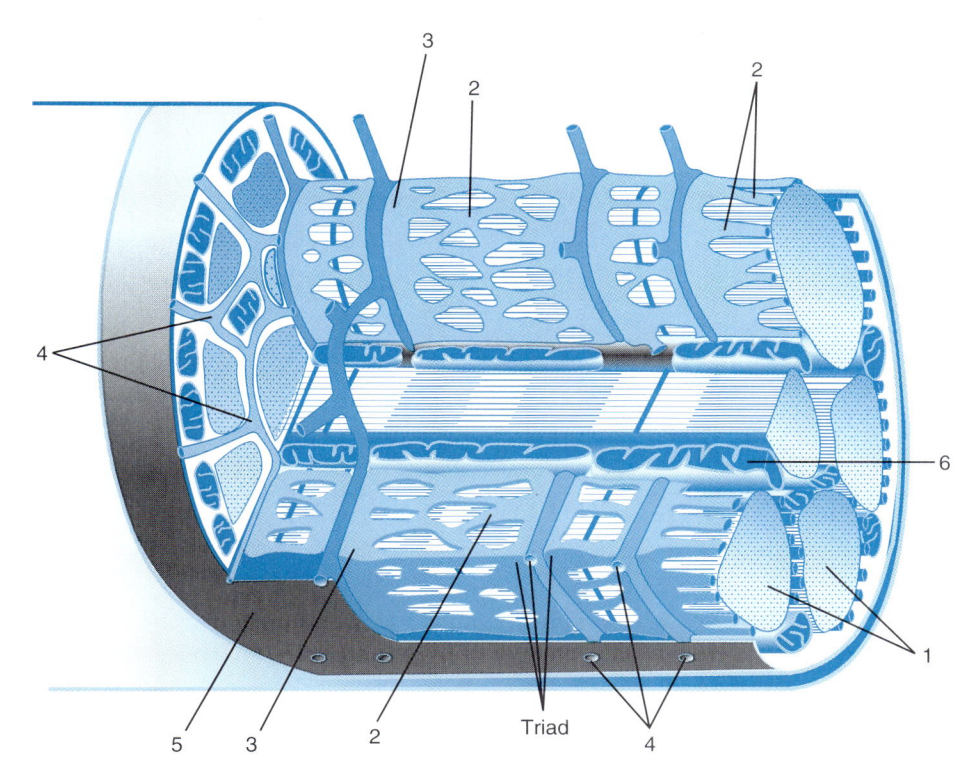

Figure 12-1 ■ Ultrastructure of a mammalian skeletal muscle cell. In this drawing a portion of the surface membrane (*5*) has been removed to reveal the parallel arrangement of myofibrils (*1*). The cut ends of the myofibrils reveal that they are composed of arrays of thick and thin filaments. Each myofibril is surrounded by elements of the sarcoplasmic reticulum (*2*) with their terminal cisterns (*3*). The transverse tubules (*4*) are invaginations of the surface membrane that form a network of tubules extending into the center of the cell. Note that the lumen of the T-tubule is continuous with the extracellular space (see Figure 13-3); the *triad* is the conjunction of a T-tubule with a pair of SR terminal cisterns (see Figure 13-5). Numerous mitochondria (*6*) lie between myofibrils. (Modified from Krstic RV: *Ultrastructure of the mammalian cell,* New York, 1979, Springer-Verlag.)

region of the A band where the filaments overlap (Figure 12-3). The thick filaments interdigitate with thin filaments so that each thick filament is surrounded by a hexagonal array of thin filaments. This precise filament geometry is maintained by various cytoskeletal proteins that link filaments within a sarcomere and also link the sarcomeres of adjacent myofibrils. One of these important cytoskeletal proteins, **α-actinin,** is a major component of the Z line structure to which the thin filaments attach. **Titin** is a giant (2.5 to 4 megaDaltons = 2.5 to 4×10^6 Daltons) muscle protein that has an important role in muscle elasticity (see Chapter 14). One end of the titin molecule is inserted into the Z line; the other end forms a portion of the thick filament. The titin molecule constitutes most of the passive parallel elastic element in muscle (see Chapter 14).

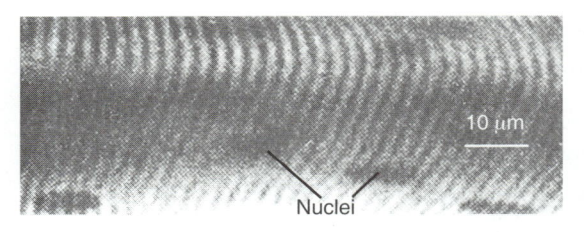

Figure 12-2 ■ Skeletal muscle cells have striations. A short segment of a single muscle fiber from human gastrocnemius (calf) muscle clearly shows the alternating light and dark bands that characterize striated muscle. Several nuclei are also visible. (From Berne RM, Levy MN, Koeppen BM, Stanton BA, editors: *Physiology*, ed 4, New York, 1998, Mosby.)

Thick Filaments Are Composed Mostly of Myosin

Myosin is a large protein, with a molecular weight of about 470,000 Daltons, consisting of two heavy chains and two pairs of different light chains. The myosin molecule has a long, rodlike tail with two globular heads (Figure 12-4). The rodlike portion of the molecule contains an "arm" adjacent to the globular heads. At each end of the arm is a flexible region that acts as a hinge, allowing rotation at that point. Many myosin molecules aggregate to form a thick filament (Figure 12-5). The tail regions of the molecules are bundled to form the body of the thick filament. The globular heads and arm regions project out from the bundle. The heads of the myosin molecules can bind to the thin filaments to form **cross-bridges** between the two filaments. The myosin heads in each half of the thick filament are oriented in opposite directions; the heads are not present in the central region (Figure 12-5).

Thin Filaments in Skeletal Muscle Are Composed of Four Major Proteins: Actin, Tropomyosin, Troponin, and Nebulin

Actin is a globular protein (G-actin) with a molecular weight of 41,700 Daltons. G-actin monomers aggregate to form strands resembling a string of pearls. The thin filament consists primarily of two helical strands of G-actin wound around each other (Figure 12-6). The 600-kDa protein molecule **nebulin** runs along the thin filament and forms a template that limits the length of the actin filaments. The thin filament also contains the regulatory proteins **tropomyosin** and troponin. Tropomyosin is a long, rod-shaped dimeric protein with a molecular weight of about 66,000 Daltons. This molecule lies along both sides of the thin filament in grooves formed by the two strands of actin molecules (Figure 12-6). Each tropomyosin molecule binds to seven actin monomers in one of the strands. Troponin, which is bound to tropomyosin, is a complex of three proteins: **troponin T, troponin C,** and **troponin I.** The role of tropomyosin and troponin in the Ca^{2+}-dependent regulation of skeletal muscle contraction is discussed later in this chapter.

■ ACCORDING TO THE "SLIDING FILAMENT" MECHANISM, MUSCLE CONTRACTION RESULTS FROM THIN AND THICK FILAMENTS SLIDING PAST EACH OTHER

Current understanding of the mechanism of muscle contraction can be traced back to the **sliding filament** theory proposed in 1954, independently, by A.F. Huxley and H.E. Huxley. This theory was based primarily on the observed changes in striation pattern that occur in skeletal muscle during contraction. The studies demonstrated that the sarcomere length decreased as the muscle shortened (Figure 12-7). Before the contraction a relatively wide I band and lighter H zone are visible (Figure 12-7, *A*). When stimulated to contract, muscle shortening is accompanied by sarcomere shortening (Figure 12-7, *B*). After the muscle shortens, the width of the A band is unchanged but the widths of the I band and H zone decrease. The sliding

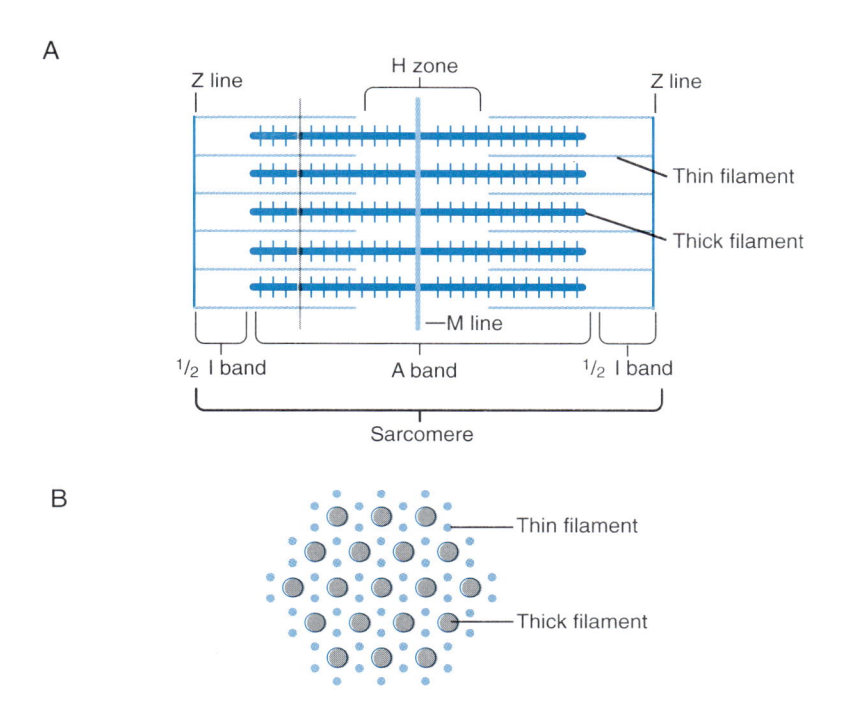

Figure 12-3 ■ Thick and thin filaments are arranged in regular arrays in the myofibril. A, Schematic drawing of a longitudinal section of a single sarcomere, which is the region of myofibril between two adjacent Z lines. For a detailed description, see text. B, Diagram of a cross section of the myofibril through the A band at the position indicated by the thin gray line in A. In this region, thick and thin filaments overlap, and each thick filament is surrounded by a hexagonal array of thin filaments. (Modified from Huxley HE, Hanson J: The molecular basis of contraction in cross-striated muscles. In Bourne GH, editor: *The structure and function of muscle,* vol 1, New York, 1960, Academic Press.)

---

filament theory proposed that the change in sarcomere length was caused by a change in the degree of overlap between thick and thin filaments, as if they were sliding past one another.

Electron micrographs of skeletal muscle at different degrees of shortening demonstrate that changes in muscle length are accompanied by changes in the overlap between thick and thin filaments. In a resting muscle there is only partial overlap between thick and thin filaments (Figure 12-8, *A*). The region of the thin filament that does *not* overlap the thick filaments corresponds to the I band; the H zone (of the A band) is the region of the thick filaments that does *not* overlap the thin filaments. When the muscle shortens during a contraction, the region of overlap between thin and thick filaments increases (Figure 12-8, *B*). In this contracted state the I bands and H zones are narrower because the nonoverlapped portions of both thick and thin filaments are shorter. The A band corresponds to the entire length of the thick filament. Since the filament length is constant,

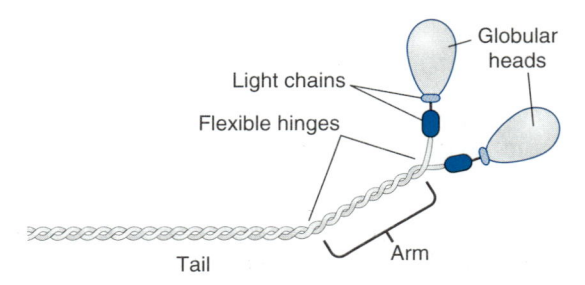

Figure 12-4 ■ **Structure of myosin.** Myosin is composed of two identical heavy chains and two different pairs of light chains. Each heavy chain has a globular head attached to an elongated, rodlike tail. The two tails are twisted together; most of each tail is buried in the thick filament. The arm projects out from the thick filament and has flexible hinges at both ends. The arm and the globular head can form a cross-bridge to the thin filament. One of each type of light chain is associated with each heavy chain near the globular head. The light chains play a role in the regulation of contraction. (Modified from Berne RM, Levy MN, Koeppen BM, Stanton BA, editors: *Physiology,* ed 4, New York, 1998, Mosby.)

the length of the A band remains constant during changes in muscle length.

In the region of filament overlap, short connections, or cross-bridges, project from the thick filaments toward the thin filaments (Figure 12-8). H.E. Huxley proposed that the molecular basis for filament sliding involved cross-bridge movement. He suggested that the cross-bridges first attach to the thin filaments and then pull on them. This causes the thick and thin filaments to slide past each other, leading to increased overlap between the filaments and shortening of the sarcomere. Subsequent biochemical, biophysical, and structural studies confirmed that cross-bridge movement is the molecular basis for muscle contraction, as described in the next section.

■ THE CROSS-BRIDGE CYCLE POWERS MUSCLE CONTRACTION

Cross-bridge movement produces filament sliding in the following way (Figure 12-9). The

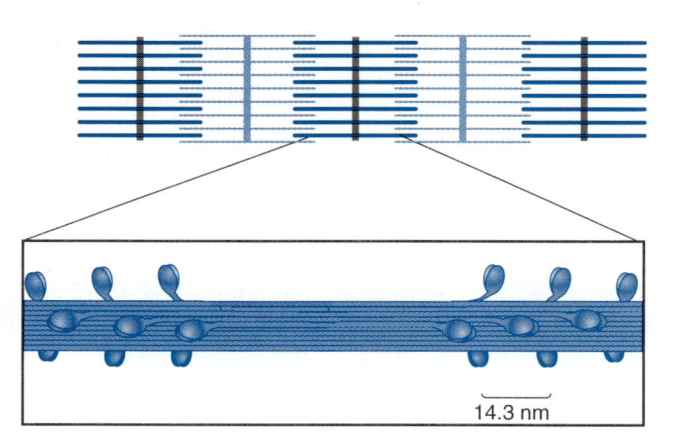

Figure 12-5 ■ **Structure of the thick filament. A,** Schematic drawing of the structure of the sarcomere. **B,** The proposed structure of the thick filament. The body of the thick filament is formed from the tail regions of a large number of myosin molecules. The arms and heads of the myosin molecules project out from the thick filament at regular intervals. Successive projections are rotated 120 degrees around the thick filament. Three pairs of myosin heads project out at intervals of 14.3 nm along the thick filament.

Molecular Motors and the Mechanisms of Muscle Contraction

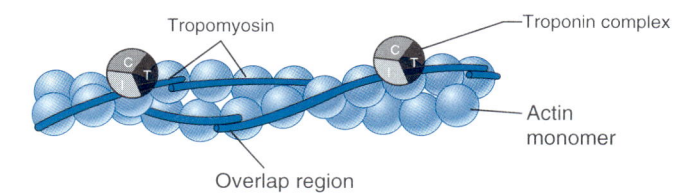

Figure 12-6 ■ The thin filament consists of two helical strands of actin monomers. Double-stranded tropomyosin molecules (drawn as a single strand) lie in each of the two grooves formed by the actin strands. Each tropomyosin molecule binds to seven actin monomers in one strand. The ends of two adjacent tropomyosin molecules overlap slightly, and near this overlap region a troponin complex is bound to tropomyosin. The troponin (Tn) complex consists of three proteins, TnC (C), TnI (I), and TnT (T).

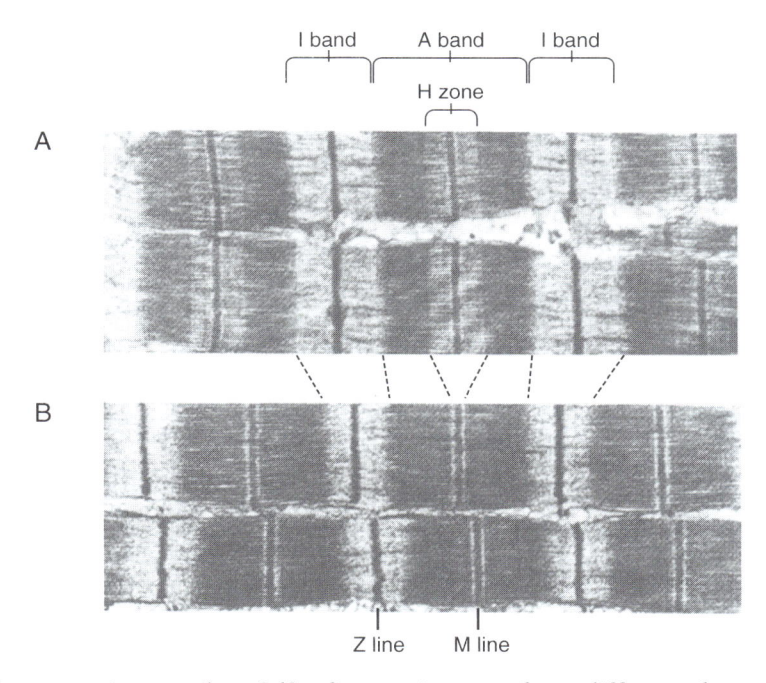

Figure 12-7 ■ Electron micrographs of (frog) sartorius muscle at different degrees of shortening. Muscle shortening in B is greater than in A. Sarcomere shortening accompanied muscle shortening: the sarcomere length in B (the shorter muscle) is shorter than in A. The shorter sarcomere length is due to a shorter I band and H zone. The length of the A band (i.e., the length of the thick filament) is constant. (From Huxley HE: Structural evidence concerning the mechanism of contraction in striated muscle. In Paul WM, Daniel EE, Kay CM, Monckton G, editors: *Muscle: proceedings of a symposium held at the Faculty of Medicine, University of Alberta,* Oxford, Eng, 1964, Pergamon.)

Cellular Physiology

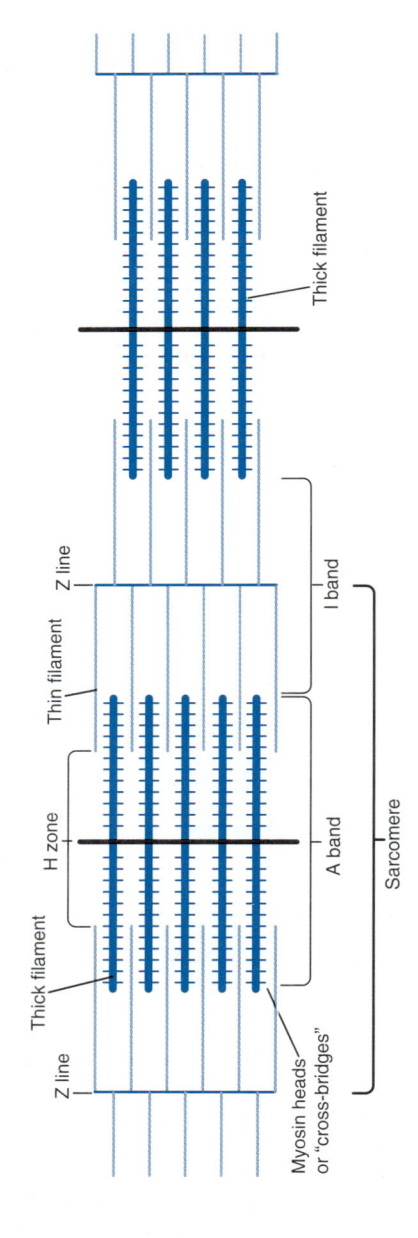

A. Relaxed muscle

B. Contracted muscle

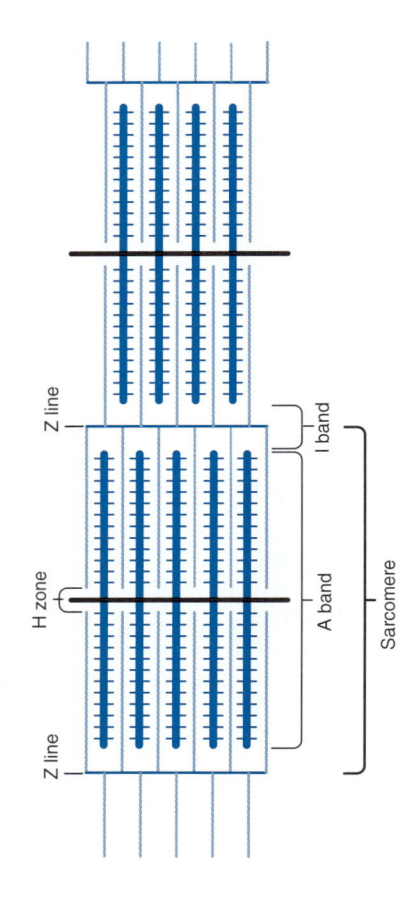

Figure 12-8 ■ The sliding filament mechanism. A, Schematic drawing based on an electron micrograph of a muscle in a relaxed state. There is little overlap between thin and thick filaments. The projections from the thick filaments are the arm and globular head regions of the myosin molecules that form cross-bridges to the thin filaments. B, Schematic drawing of the same muscle during a contraction. The thin filament has slid along the thick filament so that they overlap each other to a greater extent. Note that in the contracted state, both the H zone and the I band are narrower but the A band is unchanged.

Molecular Motors and the Mechanisms of Muscle Contraction

myosin head attaches to an actin filament, forming a cross-bridge. The head then rotates toward the myosin tail, thus pulling on the thin filament and causing it to move relative to the thick filament. The head detaches and rotates back to its original orientation, and the cycle can repeat. This mechanism is analogous to the rowing of a boat. The oar is dipped into and pulled through the water (myosin binding and rotation; the "power stroke"), the oar is pulled out of the water and pushed back to its original position (myosin detachment and "recocking" of the head), and a new stroke can begin. These mechanical steps are coupled to the hydrolysis of ATP, which is catalyzed by the myosin head during its interaction with actin (i.e., myosin is an ATPase). The cyclical sequence of steps (Figure 12-9), called the **cross-bridge cycle,** illustrates the mechanism by which the muscle cell converts chemical energy, in the form of the high-energy phosphate bond in ATP, into mechanical energy in the form of force generation.

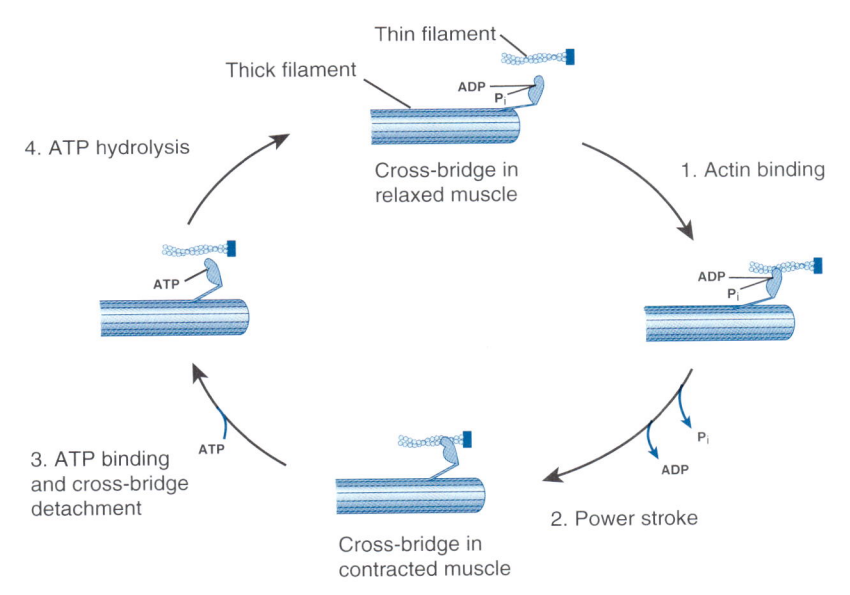

Figure 12-9 ■ The cross-bridge cycle illustrates the coupling between ATP hydrolysis and movement. The top of the figure shows the state of the contractile proteins in a relaxed muscle cell. With the products of ATP hydrolysis (adenosine diphosphate [ADP] and phosphate [P_i]) bound to the myosin, it has high affinity for actin. Thus, if [Ca^{2+}]$_i$ is elevated, the regulatory proteins enable myosin to bind to actin (step 1). In step 2 the myosin head rotates by 45 degrees when ADP and P_i are released, causing filament sliding. This is the "power stroke," or the force-generating step in the cross-bridge cycle. In the absence of ATP, cross-bridges are locked in this state of "rigor" (rigor mortis). In step 3 ATP binds to the myosin head. In this state, myosin has a low affinity for actin and the cross-bridge detaches. In step 4, the final step, ATP is hydrolyzed, rephosphorylating the myosin head and restoring it to an angle of 90 degrees.

In resting muscle, cross-bridges are not attached and the myosin heads are oriented at an angle of 90 degrees to the thin filaments. In this state, the myosin head is phosphorylated and adenosine diphosphate (ADP) is bound to the head. Actin-myosin interactions are prevented because the myosin binding sites on the thin filament are covered by tropomyosin. When the muscle is activated and $[Ca^{2+}]_i$ increases (see below), the tropomyosin molecules move to expose the myosin binding sites on actin molecules. The myosin head then binds to the thin filament with low affinity, forming a weakly attached cross-bridge. In the next step, ADP and phosphate (P_i) are released to allow a high-affinity (strong) attachment to form between actin and myosin. This is accompanied by a conformational change whereby the myosin head rotates by 45 degrees. This bending of the cross-bridge generates a force on the thin filament that causes it to slide relative to the thick filament, and the sarcomere therefore shortens. When bound to actin, myosin has high affinity for ATP. The binding of ATP causes the cross-bridge to detach. Hydrolysis of ATP results in a return to the myosin-ADP-P_i complex, with the myosin head again poised at an angle of 90 degrees with respect to the thin filament. As long as $[Ca^{2+}]_i$ remains elevated, the cycle can repeat itself.

■ IN SKELETAL AND CARDIAC MUSCLES, Ca^{2+} ACTIVATES CONTRACTION BY BINDING TO THE REGULATORY PROTEIN TROPONIN C

A necessary step in the activation of contraction in all types of muscle cells is an increase in $[Ca^{2+}]_i$. The process by which muscle cell activation leads to an increase in $[Ca^{2+}]_i$ (excitation-contraction coupling) is described in Chapter 13. Here we describe the mechanism by which an increase in $[Ca^{2+}]_i$ initiates contraction. In both skeletal and cardiac muscle, Ca^{2+} activation of contraction involves the regulatory proteins troponin and tropomyosin.

The ends of consecutive tropomyosin molecules overlap each other, and one troponin complex binds to each tropomyosin molecule near the overlap region (Figure 12-6). Troponin consists of three subunits: troponin I (TnI), troponin C (TnC), and troponin T (TnT). TnT binds to TnI, TnC, and tropomyosin and is responsible for linking the troponin complex to tropomyosin. TnI binds to actin, TnC, and tropomyosin and plays an inhibitory role in actin-myosin interactions. In skeletal and cardiac muscle, Ca^{2+} initiates contraction by binding to TnC.

In a resting (relaxed) skeletal muscle cell $[Ca^{2+}]_i$ is ~100 nM. At this low $[Ca^{2+}]_i$, TnI is tightly bound to actin and tropomyosin covers the myosin binding sites on actin and prevents cross-bridges from forming. When an action potential causes $[Ca^{2+}]_i$ to rise transiently into the micromolar range (see Chapter 13), Ca^{2+} binds to TnC. This weakens the bond between TnI and actin so that tropomyosin can move laterally on the thin filament to expose the myosin binding sites on actin. This permits attachment of myosin heads to the actin filament to form cross-bridges and generate force.

■ THE STRUCTURE AND FUNCTION OF CARDIAC MUSCLE AND SMOOTH MUSCLE ARE DISTINCTLY DIFFERENT FROM THOSE OF SKELETAL MUSCLE

Cardiac Muscle Is Striated

The heart functions as a pump and is designed for continuous, rhythmic activity over the life of an individual. Several structural and functional differences between cardiac and skeletal muscle cells play important roles in this continuous pumping activity. However, the contractile mechanism in an individual **cardiac muscle cell** (cardiac myocyte) is very similar to that in skeletal muscle. Like skeletal muscle, cardiac muscle is striated (Figure 12-10). The contractile elements are arranged in sarcomeres, with myosin-containing thick filaments interdigitated

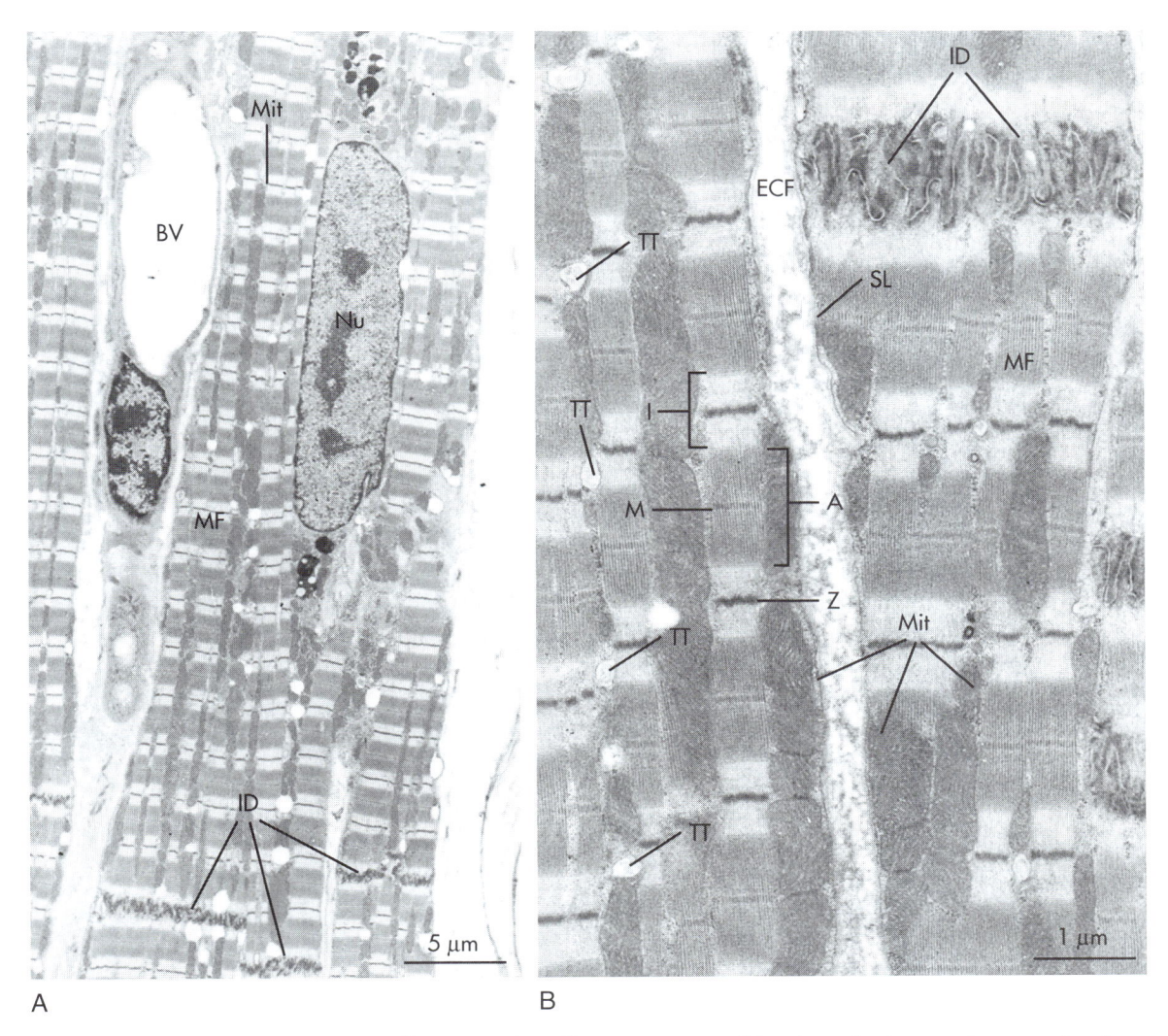

Figure 12-10 ■ Structure of a cardiac muscle cell. A, Low-magnification electron micrograph of a ventricular myocyte. Typical features of cardiac myocytes include myofibrils (*MF*) with clear striations, numerous mitochondria (*Mit*) arranged in columns between the myofibrils, intercalated disks (*ID*), and an elongated nucleus (*Nu*). A blood vessel (*BV*) lies between two cells. B, Details of the structure are shown in a higher magnification electron micrograph. The figure shows portions of two cells separated by extracellular fluid (*ECF*) between the cells. The surface membrane, or sarcolemma (*SL*), is folded many times at the intercalated disk (*ID*). Mitochondria (*Mit*) are located in columns between myofibrils and are clustered next to the sarcolemma. The structure of the sarcomere is similar to that of skeletal muscle and includes the A band (*A*), I band (*I*), Z line, and M line. T-tubules (*TT*) are larger in diameter than in skeletal muscle. (From Berne RM, Levy MN, Koeppen BM, Stanton BA, editors: *Physiology*, ed 4, New York, 1998, Mosby.)

with thin filaments containing actin. As in skeletal muscle, Ca^{2+} initiates contraction by binding to TnC, which causes tropomyosin to expose myosin binding sites on actin. Shortening is then produced by cross-bridge cycling, which causes the filaments to slide.

Cardiac Muscle Cells Require a Continuous Supply of Energy

Cardiac muscle requires an uninterrupted supply of ATP to support the continuous, repetitive contraction-relaxation cycles. The main source of this ATP is oxidative phosphorylation in mitochondria, which are present in cardiac muscle cells at very high density (compared with skeletal muscle) (Figure 12-10). A large number of mitochondria are needed to keep ATP production in pace with its continuous utilization by the contractile machinery and other metabolic activities. The high rate of oxidative phosphorylation requires an uninterrupted supply of oxygen; this is provided by the extensive capillary network throughout the heart. Every cardiac muscle cell is in contact with a capillary. This ensures continuous and efficient delivery of oxygen and nutrients to, and removal of metabolic waste from, each cardiac muscle cell.

To Act as a Pump, the Muscle Cells That Make Up Each Chamber of the Heart Must Contract Synchronously

The heart consists of four chambers: right and left atria and right and left ventricles. The cardiac muscle cells that make up the wall of each chamber must contract synchronously so that the chamber can eject its contents efficiently. In a cardiac muscle cell, as in skeletal muscle, an action potential in the surface membrane initiates a contraction (see Chapter 13). Heart muscle contracts synchronously because the action potential spreads rapidly from cell to cell through electrical connections, called **gap junctions**, between the cells. Gap junctions are high-conductance ion channels that allow the action potential in one cell to bring an adjacent cell rapidly to the action potential threshold. This is important in the heart, in which the muscle cells must contract synchronously to reduce the lumen volume. The gap junctions are located in the **intercalated disks**, which are dense segments of the sarcolemma that separate the ends of cells (Figure 12-10). Thus the heart behaves as an electrical syncytium* in which the cardiac muscle cells are electrically coupled longitudinally (i.e., end to end). This is in contrast to skeletal muscle cells, which do not contain gap junctions and are electrically isolated from one another. In addition, in the heart the intercalated disks transmit force from cell to cell. This connection of individual cardiac myocytes functionally mimics a single, long skeletal muscle fiber.

Smooth Muscles Do Not Exhibit the Striations Observed in Other Muscle Types

Smooth (nonstriated) muscles are the types of muscle cells contained within the walls of hollow organs such as the gastrointestinal tract, arteries and veins, urinary bladder, bronchi, and ureters. These muscles are diverse in their regulation. They are under involuntary control and are regulated by the **autonomic nervous system** (*sympathetic* and *parasympathetic* nerves) and by hormones. Not only must smooth muscle cells perform work by shortening, as other types of muscle do, but many smooth muscles must remain tonically contracted to *maintain* organ volume.

The name "smooth muscle" derives from the fact that these muscles do not exhibit the

---

*In general, a syncytium is a large multinucleated cell formed by fusion of smaller cells. An electrical syncytium refers to a group of cells interconnected by numerous gap junctions, so that ionic currents can flow freely from cell to cell.

striation or banding pattern observed in skeletal and cardiac muscles. Smooth muscles do contain actin and myosin filaments, however, and these filaments are organized in sarcomere-like units between **dense bodies** that are the equivalent of skeletal and cardiac muscle Z lines. Moreover, smooth muscles do contract by a sliding filament mechanism that causes increased overlap of these two types of filaments.

The special feature of smooth muscle is the organization of the contractile elements (actin and myosin filaments) into small bundles that run obliquely across the long axis of the cells. The two ends of these bundles are inserted into *plasma membrane–associated dense bodies* on opposite sides of the cell, as illustrated in Figure 12-11. Within the contractile unit bundles the actin and myosin filaments are organized into sarcomeres and exhibit partial overlap, just as in skeletal and cardiac muscle (see magnified diagram at the upper right of Figure 12-11). Because of the different orientation of the individual bundles of contractile filaments, the filaments in adjacent bundles are not in register; hence the lack of striation.

The actin filaments are attached to dense bodies (Figure 12-11). The dense bodies are composed primarily of α-actinin, which is also a major component of skeletal and cardiac muscle Z line structures. The dense bodies are thus both structurally and functionally equivalent to the Z line structures of skeletal muscle. These dense bodies are held in position by attachment to cytoskeletal elements, the **"intermediate filaments."** Intermediate filaments are thicker than actin filaments but thinner than myosin filaments. Two major components of the intermediate filaments are the cytoskeletal proteins **desmin** and **vimentin**.

The plasma membrane (PM) attachment sites of the bundles of contractile units (i.e., the PM-associated dense bodies) may be arranged in either a helical pattern around the cell or a criss-cross pattern, as shown in the figure. The PM attachment sites in neighboring cells often abut one another to maximize the transmission of force from cell to cell (Figure 12-11). Because the contractile fiber bundles are oriented obliquely to the long axis of the smooth muscle cells (Figure 12-11), some contractile force is transmitted laterally. Most of the force is, however, transmitted longitudinally. Thus in a cylindrical organ such as an artery or the intestine, smooth muscle cells that are oriented nearly end to end (with some overlap) around the lumen constrict the lumen when they contract. In contrast, contraction of longitudinally oriented smooth muscle cells, as in the longitudinal muscle layer of the intestine, causes the organ to shorten. In saccular organs such as the urinary bladder, both lateral and longitudinal forces cause the wall of the organ to contract relatively uniformly, leading to a reduction in organ volume.

In Smooth Muscle, Elevation of the Cytosolic Ca^{2+} Concentration Activates Contraction by Promoting the Phosphorylation of the Myosin Regulatory Light Chain

Elevation of $[Ca^{2+}]_i$ activates contraction in smooth muscle as in skeletal and cardiac muscle, but the mechanism of activation of the contractile apparatus by the Ca^{2+} is entirely different. Smooth muscles lack troponin. Instead, in smooth muscle the Ca^{2+} binds to the Ca^{2+}-binding protein **calmodulin,** and the Ca^{2+}-calmodulin complex binds to and activates **myosin light chain kinase (MLCK).** The activated enzyme catalyzes the *phosphorylation of the myosin regulatory light chain* (Figure 12-12). Phosphorylation induces a conformational change in the myosin. This is the "switch" that enables the cross-bridges to form between actin and myosin (Figure 12-13), thereby generating force and shortening the muscle cells. Thus in smooth

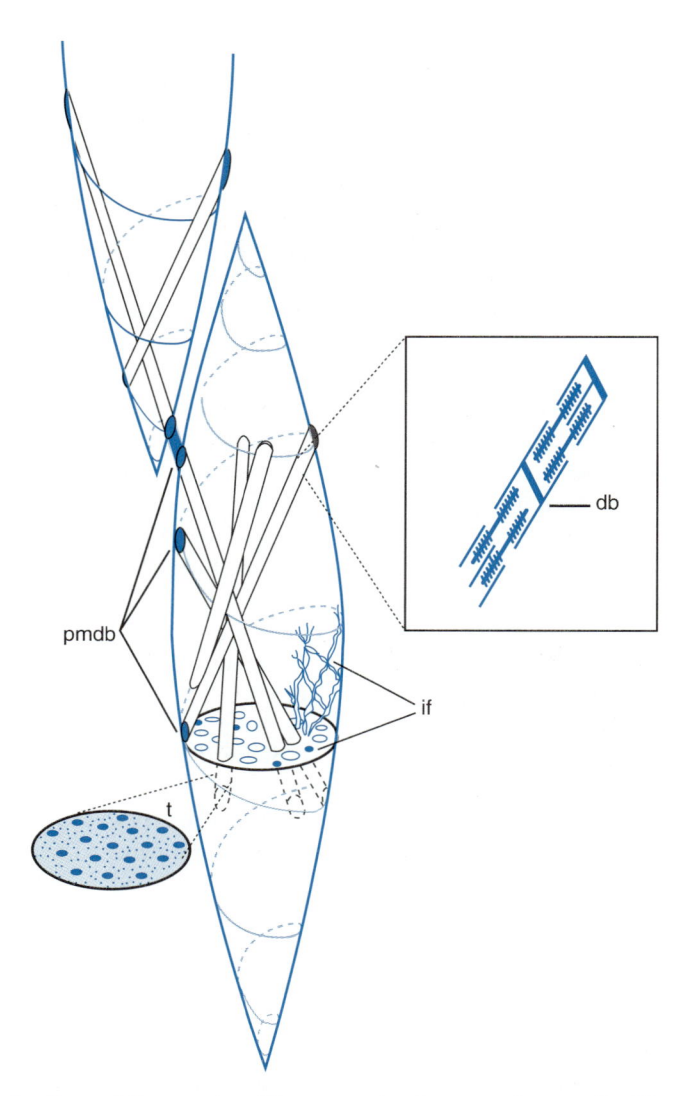

Figure 12-11 ■ **Organization of the contractile apparatus in smooth muscle.** The contractile units are arranged in columns containing thick (myosin) and thin (actin) filaments *(t* shows a cross section of a column); as shown in the box, the interdigitation of the thick and thin filaments is similar to that in skeletal muscle. The columns are shown in a helical arrangement. The actin filaments are anchored to dense bodies (*db*), and the dense bodies are held in place by a cytoskeletal scaffold composed of intermediate filaments (*if*). Some dense bodies are inserted into the plasma membrane (*pmdb*). The insertion points in adjacent cells may abut one another, as depicted in the upper left portion of the figure. (Modified from Small JV, Sobieszek A: *Int Rev Cytol* 64:241, 1980.)

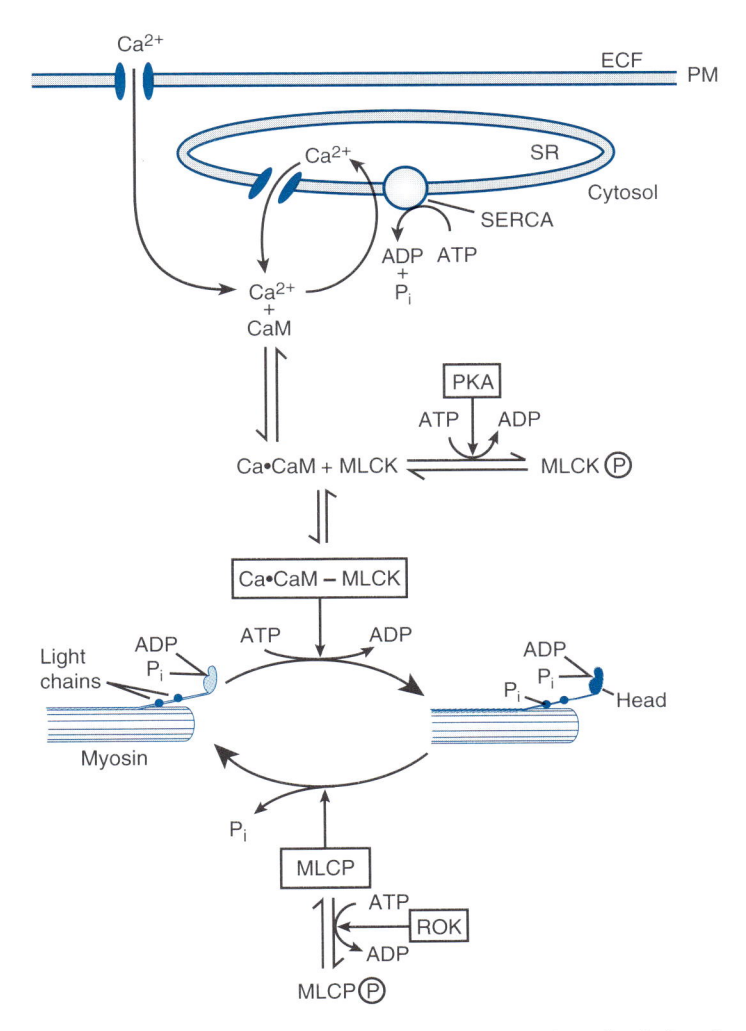

Figure 12-12 ■ Schematic diagram of the chemical processes involved in the phosphorylation and dephosphorylation of smooth muscle myosin regulatory light chain. The Ca^{2+} that triggers contraction comes from either the extracellular fluid (*ECF*) or the sarcoplasmic reticulum (*SR*). The Ca^{2+} combines with calmodulin (*CaM*) to form a complex with myosin light chain kinase (*Ca·CaM+MLCK*). Ca·CaM+MLCK catalyzes the phosphorylation of the myosin regulatory light chain (the "essential" light chain is not phosphorylated). This light chain phosphorylation is the switch that initiates the smooth muscle myosin-actin interaction (see Figure 12-13) that generates force and promotes shortening. Relaxation is promoted by the dephosphorylation of myosin that is catalyzed by myosin light chain phosphatase (*MLCP*). The sensitivity of the contractile apparatus to Ca^{2+} (Box 12-2) is regulated, in part, by cyclic AMP–dependent protein kinase (*PKA*) and by Rho-associated protein kinase (*ROK*). *ECF*, Extracellular fluid; *SERCA*, sarcoplasmic or endoplasmic reticulum Ca^{2+} pump; *PM*, plasma membrane.

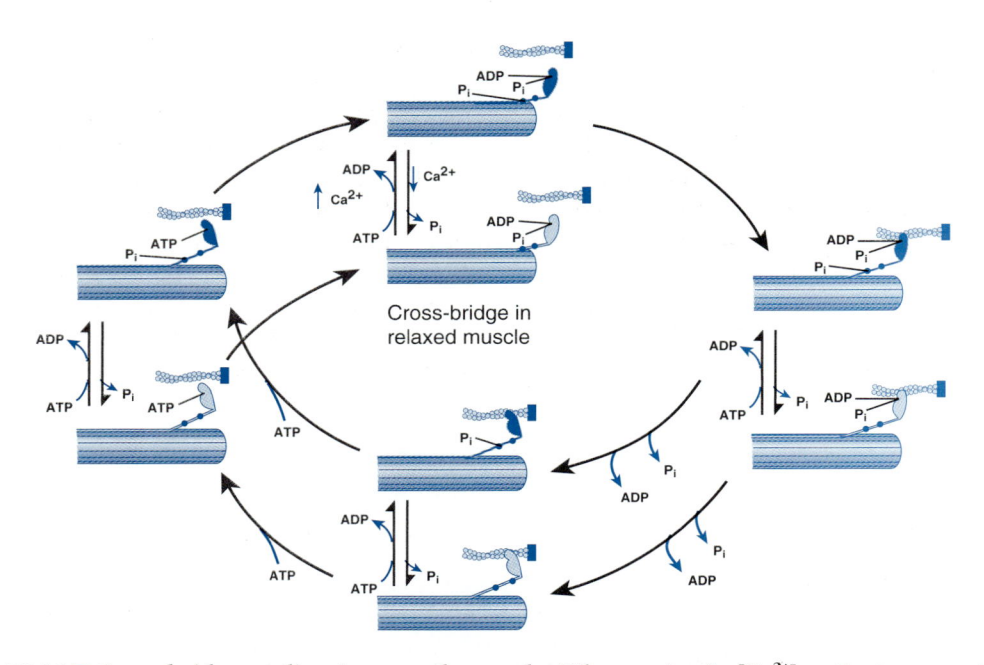

Figure 12-13 ■ Cross-bridge cycling in smooth muscle. When a rise in [Ca^{2+}]$_i$ activates myosin light chain kinase (MLCK), the cycle begins with the phosphorylation of the myosin regulatory light chain (*at the top*) catalyzed by MLCK. This enables myosin to attach to actin to form the actin-myosin cross-bridge (*at the right*). ADP and phosphate (P$_i$) then dissociate from the myosin head, which then rotates to produce force (*at the bottom*). ATP binds (*circling clockwise to the left*) and promotes cross-bridge detachment. The ATP bound to the myosin head is hydrolyzed to ADP and P$_i$ (*at the top*) so that a new cycle can begin. The myosin light chain can be dephosphorylated by myosin light chain phosphatase (MLCP) at any time during the cycle. If this occurs (as indicated by the lighter-colored myosin heads), once the myosin head becomes detached, it cannot reattach to actin (as indicated by the break in the cycle) until the light chain is rephosphorylated. (Modified from Murphy RA: Smooth muscle. In Berne RM, Levy MN, Koeppen BM, Stanton BA, editors: *Physiology,* ed 4, New York, 1998, Mosby.)

---

muscle the "switch" that turns on cross-bridge cycling is located on the thick filament (myosin), whereas in skeletal and cardiac muscle the switch (TnC) is located on the thin filament (actin).

Another enzyme, **myosin light chain phosphatase (MLCP),** promotes the dephosphorylation of myosin regulatory light chains (Figure 12-12). This halts actin-myosin cross-bridge cycling (Figure 12-13). This dephosphorylation may occur either when the actin is attached to the myosin head or when it is detached (Figure 12-13).

As long as the regulatory light chain is phosphorylated, the cross-bridge cycling will continue. As in skeletal muscle, the cross-bridge cycle is associated with the hydrolysis of ATP (Figure 12-13). This ATP is needed *in addition to* the ATP involved in the phosphorylation of the myosin regulatory light chain. If the cross-bridges are still attached when the myosin regulatory light chain is dephosphorylated, detachment of the cross-bridges is slowed (see Chapter 14). This slow detachment is believed to contribute to the maintenance of **tonic contraction** and force in smooth muscle. This tonic force (**"tone"**) and shortening are maintained with little expenditure of energy because the cross-bridges cycle very slowly, so that these processes consume little ATP. Ca^{2+} is required not only to initiate the contraction, but also to maintain tone. If after an initial transient increase, $[Ca^{2+}]_i$ declines and remains below the contraction threshold, no new cross-bridges will form and previously formed cross-bridges will detach. The several chemical reactions directly involved in the contractile activation and relaxation of smooth muscle contraction are diagrammed in Figures 12-12 and 12-13.

The sensitivity of smooth muscles to Ca^{2+} can be modulated so that a given $[Ca^{2+}]_i$ level can produce more or less contractile force. Some

BOX 12-2

Smooth Muscle Contraction Can Be Regulated by Modulating Ca^{2+} Sensitivity

The contraction of smooth muscle clearly depends on Ca^{2+} (see text and Figures 12-12 and 12-13). The contraction is also regulated by modulation of the sensitivity of the Ca^{2+}-dependent reactions to Ca^{2+} as a result of a change in the balance between the activity of myosin light chain kinase (MLCK) and myosin light chain phosphatase (MLCP). For example, stimulation by a hormone such as norepinephrine, acting on β-adrenergic receptors (α receptors activate smooth muscle contraction; see Chapter 13), stimulates adenylyl cyclase. This promotes the synthesis of the second messenger, cyclic adenosine-3′,5′-monophosphate (cAMP). The cAMP then activates a cAMP-dependent protein kinase (A-kinase or PKA) that catalyzes the phosphorylation of MLCK (Figure 12-12). In its phosphorylated form (MLCK-P), this enzyme is unable to bind the Ca^{2+}-calmodulin complex. Thus, in effect, cAMP reduces the sensitivity of the contractile apparatus to Ca^{2+}. Stimulation of cAMP synthesis can thereby decrease force production and relax tonic smooth muscle without altering $[Ca^{2+}]_i$.

Smooth muscles are also regulated by the Rho/Rho-kinase pathway. A variety of smooth muscle agonists (contractile activators), such as norepinephrine, serotonin (5-HT), and histamine, increase the concentration of the guanosine triphosphate (GTP)-bound (active) form of the small GTPase, RhoA. RhoA-GTP then activates the Rho-associated protein kinase, ROK. In turn, ROK phosphorylates MLCP, and this inhibits the phosphatase activity of the enzyme (Figure 12-12). The net effect is "sensitization" of the smooth muscle to Ca^{2+}. That is, the activating effect of Ca^{2+}-dependent phosphorylation is prolonged because dephosphorylation is delayed. In this way the Rho/Rho-kinase pathway apparently contributes to the tonic contraction of smooth muscles. In contrast, stimulation of cyclic guanosine-3′,5′-monophosphate (cGMP)-dependent protein kinase (G-kinase or PKG), for example, by endothelium-derived nitric oxide, promotes the phosphorylation of RhoA. Phosphorylated RhoA (RhoA-P) cannot bind GTP and is therefore unable to activate ROK. Thus MLCP can remain active and continue to dephosphorylate the myosin regulatory light chain. For example, this promotes desensitization of arterial smooth muscle to Ca^{2+} and results in blood vessel dilation. Again, these effects on smooth muscle contraction and relaxation, mediated by RhoA/ROK, can occur without changes in $[Ca^{2+}]_i$; therefore they are frequently referred to as "Ca^{2+}-independent regulatory mechanisms." Note, however, that all of these mechanisms actually exert their effect by tuning the sensitivity of the contractile apparatus to Ca^{2+}.

important mechanisms that regulate contraction without a change in $[Ca^{2+}]_i$ (so-called **Ca^{2+}-independent regulatory mechanisms**) are described in Box 12-2. These mechanisms hint at the complex regulation of contraction and relaxation in smooth muscles. Moreover, these regulatory mechanisms are important targets for pharmacological intervention.

■ SUMMARY

1. The three types of muscle are skeletal, cardiac, and smooth. In all three types of muscle, contraction is produced by a myosin motor that converts chemical energy into kinetic energy through the hydrolysis of ATP.
2. A single skeletal muscle fiber contains many myofibrils, which lie parallel to one another and run along the long axis of the cell. The sarcoplasmic reticulum surrounds each myofibril.
3. The region of myofibril between two Z lines is called a sarcomere.
4. There is an ordered arrangement of thick and thin filaments within the myofibril. Thick filaments, composed mostly of myosin, interdigitate with thin filaments. Thin filaments are composed of actin, tropomyosin, and troponin.
5. Each myosin molecule has a long tail and two globular heads. The heads of myosin molecules bind to actin in the thin filaments, forming cross-bridges between the two filaments.
6. Sarcomere length shortens during muscle contraction. The shortening is caused by thick and thin filaments sliding past one another. Cross-bridge movement is the molecular basis for filament sliding.
7. The cross-bridge cycle is the mechanism by which the chemical energy stored in the high-energy phosphate bond in ATP is converted into force generation.
8. When skeletal muscle is activated, myosin heads bind to actin in the thin filaments, forming cross-bridges. In the force-generating step of the cross-bridge cycle, the myosin head rotates 45 degrees as ADP and P_i are released. Subsequent binding of ATP causes the cross-bridge to detach.
9. In skeletal and cardiac muscle, Ca^{2+} initiates contraction by binding to troponin C. This causes a movement of tropomyosin that exposes myosin binding sites on actin, permitting cross-bridges to form.
10. Smooth muscles do not exhibit the regular striations observed in skeletal and cardiac muscles. The bundles of contractile elements run obliquely with respect to the longitudinal axis of the muscle cell and are not parallel to one another.
11. The diameters and volumes of many hollow organs are controlled by smooth muscles. Thus many smooth muscles must contract tonically to maintain these diameters and volumes.
12. The contraction of smooth muscles is regulated in part by the autonomic nervous system.
13. Smooth muscles are activated by elevation of the $[Ca^{2+}]_i$. This promotes the phosphorylation of myosin light chain kinase. The phosphorylation of myosin light chain enables the actin-myosin cross-bridges to form.
14. Smooth muscle contraction is also regulated by mechanisms that alter the sensitivity of the contractile apparatus to Ca^{2+}.

■ KEY WORDS AND CONCEPTS

- Molecular motor
- Actin
- Microtubule
- Myosin
- Kinesin
- Dynein

Molecular Motors and the Mechanisms of Muscle Contraction

- Skeletal muscle cell
- Myofibril
- Sarcoplasmic reticulum (SR)
- Transverse tubule (T-tubule)
- Thick and thin filaments
- Sarcomere
- α-Actinin
- Titin
- Cross-bridge
- Nebulin
- Tropomyosin
- Troponin T (TnT), troponin C (TnC), and troponin I (TnI)
- Sliding filament
- Cross-bridge cycle
- Cardiac muscle cell
- Gap junctions
- Intercalated disks
- Smooth (nonstriated) muscle
- Autonomic nervous system
- Dense bodies
- Intermediate filaments
- Desmin and vimentin
- Calmodulin
- Myosin light chain kinase (MLCK)
- Myosin regulatory light chain
- Myosin light chain phosphatase (MLCP)
- Tonic contraction (tone)
- Ca^{2+}-independent regulatory mechanisms

STUDY PROBLEMS

1. Compare and contrast the mechanisms by which elevation of the intracellular Ca^{2+} concentration activates the contractile proteins in skeletal, cardiac, and smooth muscles.
2. Contrast the function of skeletal, cardiac, and smooth muscle, and discuss how muscle cell structure and organization are related to these functions.
3. Why do you think that mechanisms that regulate the Ca^{2+}-sensitivity of the contractile machinery are especially important in smooth muscle?

■ BIBLIOGRAPHY

Alberts B, Johnson A, Lewis J, et al: *The molecular biology of the cell,* ed 4, New York, 2002, Garland Science.

Bagby RM: Organization of contractile/cytoskeletal elements. In Stephens NL, editor: *Biochemistry of smooth muscle*, vol 1, Boca Raton, Fla, 1983, CRC Press.

Berne RM, Levy MN, Koeppen BM, Stanton BA, editors: *Physiology*, ed 4, New York, 1998, Mosby.

Gordon AM, Huxley AF, Julian FJ: The variation in isometric tension with sarcomere length in vertebrate muscle fibres, *J Physiol* 184:170, 1966.

Huxley HE: Structural evidence concerning the mechanism of contraction in striated muscle. In Paul WM, Daniel EE, Kay CM, Monckton G, editors: *Muscle: proceedings of a symposium held at the Faculty of Medicine, University of Alberta*, Oxford, Eng, 1964, Pergamon.

Huxley HE, Hanson J: The molecular basis of contraction in cross-striated muscles. In Bourne GH, editor: *The structure and function of muscle*, vol 1, New York, 1960, Academic Press.

Krstic RV: *Ultrastructure of the mammalian cell*, New York, 1979, Springer-Verlag.

Leeson CR, Leeson TS: *Histology*, ed 3, Philadelphia, 1976, WB Saunders.

Murphy RA: Smooth muscle. In Berne RM, Levy MN, Koeppen BM, Stanton BA, editors: *Physiology*, ed 4, St Louis, 1998, Mosby.

Ruegg JC: Vertebrate smooth muscle. In *Calcium in muscle contraction,* Berlin, 1992, Springer-Verlag.

Small JV, Sobieszek A: The contractile apparatus of smooth muscle, *Int Rev Cytol* 64:241, 1980.

Vale RD, Milligan RA: The way things move: looking under the hood of molecular motor proteins, *Science* 288:88, 2000.

Verhey KJ, Rapoport TA: Kinesin carries the signal, *Trends Biochem Sci* 26:545, 2001.

CHAPTER 13

Excitation-Contraction Coupling in Muscle

Objectives:

1. Compare and contrast the mechanisms of excitation-contraction coupling in skeletal, cardiac, and smooth muscle cells.
2. Understand that in skeletal muscle:
   a. All of the Ca^{2+} required for contraction is released from the sarcoplasmic reticulum (SR) through Ca^{2+} release channels.
   b. Movement of a voltage sensor couples sarcolemmal depolarization to the opening of SR Ca^{2+} release channels.
   c. Almost all of the released Ca^{2+} is pumped back into the SR by the SR Ca^{2+} pump (SERCA).
3. Understand that in cardiac muscle, intracellular Ca^{2+} release channels are opened by Ca^{2+} ions in a process known as Ca^{2+}-induced Ca^{2+} release (CICR).
4. Describe the role of SERCA, Na^+/Ca^{2+} exchange, and the plasma membrane Ca^{2+} pump in the relaxation of cardiac muscle.
5. Understand that smooth muscles are highly diversified and that:
   a. Some smooth muscles are activated by depolarization.
   b. Some smooth muscles are activated by agonists through a process known as pharmacomechanical coupling.
6. Understand the different roles of the inositol trisphosphate receptors (IP_3R) and ryanodine receptors (RyR) in smooth muscle.

■ SKELETAL MUSCLE CONTRACTION IS INITIATED BY A DEPOLARIZATION OF THE SURFACE MEMBRANE

Skeletal muscle fibers (cells) are innervated by α motor neurons, which are large (with cell bodies up to 70 μm in diameter) multipolar neurons that originate in the ventral horn of the spinal cord. Terminal branches of α motor neuron axons form specialized connections with skeletal muscle cells called **neuromuscular junctions**. As discussed in Chapter 8, a single action potential in an α motor neuron causes the release of enough acetylcholine at a single neuromuscular junction to produce an action potential that is propagated along the entire muscle fiber.

In Skeletal Muscle, Depolarization Initiates Contraction

The muscle action potential is the initial event in a sequence of steps that leads to contraction. It is the *depolarization* of the muscle fiber membrane beyond a critical level, known as the mechanical threshold, that triggers contraction. Under normal physiological conditions an action potential causes this depolarization. However, the depolarization can also be produced experimentally with a voltage clamp or by an increase in the K^+ concentration in the extracellular solution. The relationship between the membrane potential and the amount of force generated by skeletal muscle is shown in Figure 13-1. The mechanical responses illustrated in Figure 13-1, which are produced by depolarizations that last several seconds, are called **contractures**. As the membrane potential becomes more positive than about –55 mV (the mechanical threshold), force increases very steeply with further depolarization. The process by which depolarization of the surface membrane causes contraction of the muscle cell is termed **excitation-contraction coupling** (E-C coupling). The fact that force increases with membrane potential indicates that the process of E-C coupling, which is the main topic of this chapter, involves a **voltage sensor** in the sarcolemma that couples depolarization to contraction.

Skeletal Muscle Has a High Resting Cl⁻ Permeability

In skeletal muscle the resting membrane potential (about –90 mV) is much more negative than in neurons (about –70 mV) because of the relatively high permeability of the sarcolemma to both K^+ and Cl^-. Because of the high resting Cl^- permeability, a relatively large stimulus is necessary to bring the membrane potential to

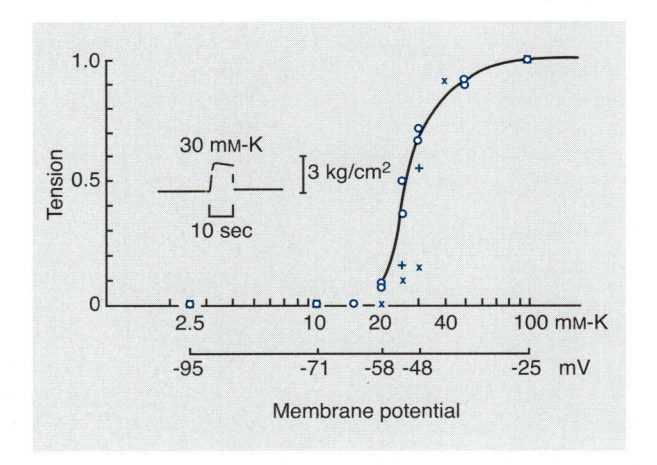

Figure 13-1 ■ Relationship between force and membrane potential. The membrane potential of single muscle fibers was depolarized to different levels by increasing the extracellular K^+ concentration ($[K^+]_o$). The membrane potential was measured with an intracellular electrode and is plotted on the lower scale. The force developed by the muscle cell was measured with a force transducer. The inset shows the force resulting from a 10-second depolarization in 30 mM $[K^+]_o$. The graph is a plot of the normalized tension (i.e., the tension at that membrane potential, divided by the maximum tension) as a function of $[K^+]_o$ or membrane potential. Depolarizations to voltages more positive than about –55 mV result in force production (in the form of contractures). The force increases steeply over a very narrow range of membrane potentials. (Modified from Hodgkin AL, Horowicz P: *J Physiol* 153:386, 1960.)

Excitation-Contraction Coupling in Muscle

> **BOX 13-1**
>
> ### Becker's Myotonia and Thomsen's Disease Are Caused by Mutations in a Cl⁻ Channel
>
> Two inherited forms of nondystrophic myotonia congenita* involve the Cl⁻ conductance (g_{Cl}) of the skeletal muscle sarcolemma. One form is Thomsen's disease, with an autosomal dominant inheritance. The other is the more severe Becker's myotonia, which has an autosomal recessive inheritance. Both forms are characterized by attacks of muscle stiffness that are caused by a delay in muscle relaxation after stimulation. Under conditions in which normal muscle responds with a single action potential, myotonic muscle cells respond to a single stimulation with repetitive action potentials. Thus a single α motor neuron action potential evokes a twitch in normal skeletal muscle, but a *tetanus* in myotonic muscle. A tetanus is a sustained contraction that is evoked in normal skeletal muscle only when it is stimulated by a train, or burst, of closely spaced action potentials (see Chapter 14). The rigidity and delayed relaxation of myotonic muscle are caused by the tetanic response to a *single* stimulus.
>
> The hyperexcitability of myotonic muscle is caused by a mutation in the gene encoding the predominant skeletal muscle Cl⁻ channel, CLCN1. This mutation reduces the Cl⁻ conductance of the skeletal muscle sarcolemma. Because of the reduction in g_{Cl} and thus an increase in membrane resistance, a stimulus will produce a larger change in V_m in myotonic muscle than in normal muscle (see Ohm's Law in Chapter 6). As a result, the current required to reach action potential threshold is less and the muscle becomes hyperexcitable.
>
> *Myotonia is muscle rigidity characterized by delayed muscle relaxation. It is a characteristic of several distinct diseases, including myotonic dystrophy, which is a relatively common neuromuscular disorder characterized by abnormal expression of CTG-trinucleotide repeats. The diseases discussed in this box are nondystrophic myotonias.

mechanical threshold. In some skeletal muscle diseases the membrane Cl⁻ permeability is reduced because of loss-of-function mutations in skeletal muscle Cl⁻ channels. As a result, the skeletal muscle action potential threshold can be reached more easily and the muscle becomes hyperexcitable (Box 13-1).

A Twitch Is a Brief Contraction That Results from a Single Action Potential

The temporal relationship between the skeletal muscle action potential and the force generated by the muscle is illustrated in Figure 13-2. The skeletal muscle action potential is similar to the nerve axon action potential (see Chapter 7) in that it is generated by the activity of voltage-gated Na⁺ and K⁺ channels. The development of force by the muscle cell begins several milliseconds after the action potential. The transient contraction produced by a muscle cell

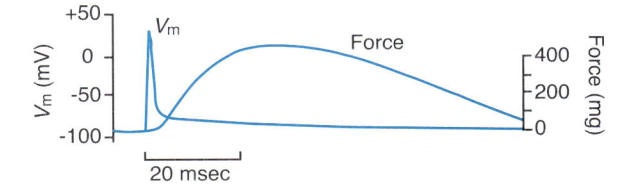

Figure 13-2 ■ The temporal relationship between the sarcolemmal action potential and a twitch contraction. The trace labeled V_m shows the time course of the skeletal muscle action potential. The twitch contraction (trace labeled force) begins a few milliseconds after the action potential. Peak twitch force is reached in about 30 msec, and the muscle then relaxes over the next 50 msec. After the peak of the action potential, a period of rapid repolarization occurs and is followed by a prolonged period of much slower repolarization (which is called an afterdepolarization). The afterdepolarization in skeletal muscle is caused by accumulation of K⁺ in the lumen of the T-tubule during fast repolarization. This transiently increases E_K.

in response to a single action potential is called a **twitch**. During the twitch the contractile force rises to a peak in 30 to 50 msec and then declines over the next 50 to 100 msec. The duration of the twitch is about two orders of magnitude longer than the duration of the action potential.

How Does Depolarization Increase $[Ca^{2+}]_i$ in Skeletal Muscle?

In Chapter 12 we learned that the activation of contraction in all types of muscle cells requires an increase in $[Ca^{2+}]_i$. Thus the central question in E-C coupling is, "How does a depolarization of the surface membrane bring about an increase in $[Ca^{2+}]_i$?" A related question is, "How does the $[Ca^{2+}]_i$ surrounding the myofibrils deep down, at the center of the muscle cell, increase fast enough for these myofibrils to contract synchronously with those close to the cell surface?" These questions are addressed in the following section.

■ DIRECT MECHANICAL INTERACTION BETWEEN SARCOLEMMAL AND SARCOPLASMIC RETICULUM MEMBRANE PROTEINS MAY MEDIATE EXCITATION-CONTRACTION COUPLING IN SKELETAL MUSCLE

In Skeletal Muscle, Depolarization of the T-Tubule Membrane Is Required for Excitation-Contraction Coupling

Can diffusion of a soluble factor from the surface membrane (such as Ca^{2+} ions entering the cell through voltage-gated Ca^{2+} channels) to the interior of the cell occur fast enough to explain the rapid activation of skeletal muscle? A molecule would take about a second to diffuse to the center of a 100-μm diameter skeletal muscle cell (see Chapter 2). This is much too slow to account for the development of force during a twitch contraction, which begins just a few milliseconds after the action potential (Figure 13-2).

How then does the action potential in the surface membrane rapidly activate the myofibrils in the center of the cell? A.F. Huxley and R. Taylor offered the first clue: they demonstrated that "hot spots" distributed over the surface membrane provided a pathway for the surface depolarization to spread into the interior of the cell. These hot spots were later shown to be openings of T-tubules. T-tubules are invaginations (inward extensions) of the plasma membrane that form an intricate network extending throughout the skeletal muscle cell (Figure 13-3). Thus the T-tubule lumen is a narrow extension of the extracellular space into the interior of the muscle cell. The T-tubule membrane contains voltage-gated Na^+ and K^+ channels, and action potentials from the surface of the cell are propagated along the T-tubule membrane into the interior of the cell.

In Skeletal Muscle, Extracellular Ca^{2+} Is *Not* Required to Activate Contraction

The T-tubule membrane of skeletal muscle contains receptors for the dihydropyridine derivatives that block L-type voltage-gated Ca^{2+} channels (see Chapter 8). Voltage clamp studies in skeletal muscle demonstrate that inward Ca^{2+} currents are generated by depolarization (Figure 13-4) and that these currents are blocked by dihydropyridines. Thus the **dihydropyridine receptors (DHPRs)** in the T-tubule membrane are also L-type Ca^{2+} channels. Therefore we might reasonably expect that it is the Ca^{2+} entry through these channels that raises $[Ca^{2+}]_i$ and activates contraction, but this is *not* the case. Skeletal muscle continues to contract normally when bathed in a solution containing *no* Ca^{2+} ions. This indicates that Ca^{2+} entry is not essential for skeletal muscle contraction and that *all* of the Ca^{2+} required for activating the contractile machinery is derived from intracellular sources. This is in marked contrast to the mechanism of E-C coupling in cardiac muscle, where Ca^{2+}

Excitation-Contraction Coupling in Muscle

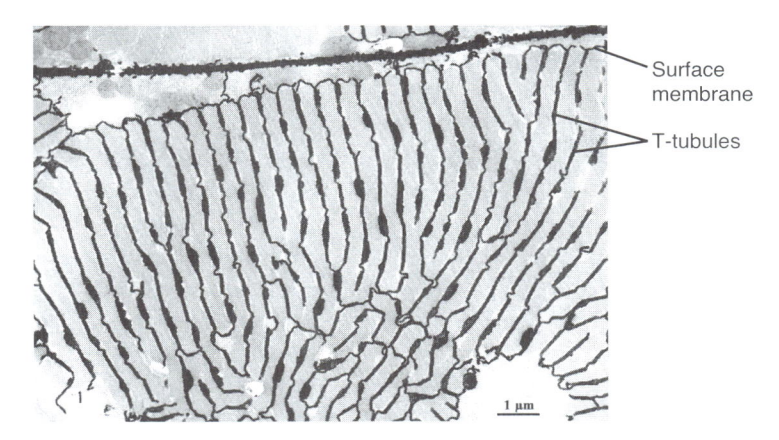

Figure 13-3 ■ The extensive network of T-tubules in skeletal muscle. A Golgi stain was used to infiltrate the T-tubule system from the extracellular space. The resulting black areas in this electron micrograph of skeletal muscle clearly delineate the extensive network of tubules. Longitudinal elements of the T-tubules interconnect transverse elements. The enlarged areas of the tubules are regions of functional couplings between the T-tubule membrane and sarcoplasmic reticulum membrane. (Courtesy D. Appelt and C. Franzini-Armstrong.)

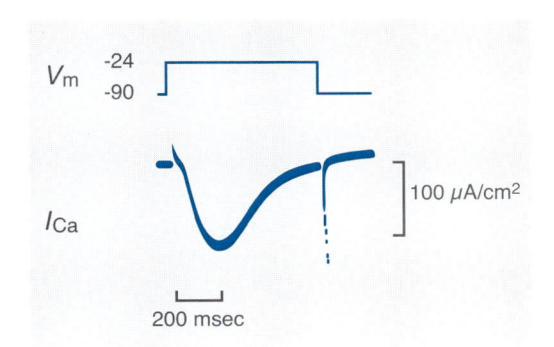

Figure 13-4 ■ Depolarization activates a slow inward Ca^{2+} current (I_{Ca}) in skeletal muscle cells. A voltage clamp was used to record I_{Ca} in skeletal muscle after current flow through other channels was eliminated. The I_{Ca} that develops in response to a voltage clamp step from -90 mV to -24 mV is a slowly developing inward current that reaches a peak in about 200 msec at this membrane potential. Surprisingly, although L-type Ca^{2+} channels generate I_{Ca} in skeletal muscle, their activation is nearly two orders of magnitude slower than in other cell types (see Figure 8-2). (From Sanchez JA, Stefani E: *J Physiol* 37:1, 1983.)

entry through voltage-gated Ca^{2+} channels is required (see below). We shall see, however, that even though Ca^{2+} entry through DHPRs is not required for E-C coupling in skeletal muscle, the DHPRs *do* play a crucial role in this mechanism.

In Skeletal Muscle, the Sarcoplasmic Reticulum Stores All of the Ca^{2+} Needed for Contraction

The SR is an extensive intracellular membrane-enclosed system of sacs and tubules that surrounds the myofibrils in skeletal muscle cells (see Figure 12-1). The consistent placement of the SR around all myofibrils has long suggested that it plays an important role in skeletal muscle contraction. The SR is a specialized development of the endoplasmic reticulum that has enhanced expression of three specific proteins: the **sarcoplasmic or endoplasmic reticulum Ca^{2+} pump (SERCA)** (see Chapter 11); the **ryanodine receptor (RyR)** that is the Ca^{2+} **release channel** in the SR membrane; and **calsequestrin**. The location of these proteins in various regions of the SR and the spatial relationship between the SR membrane and the T-tubule membrane have important functional consequences for E-C coupling. SERCA pumps are extremely abundant in the SR membrane. Consequently, virtually all of the Ca^{2+} released during a contraction is rapidly and efficiently transported back into the SR by the SERCA pumps. This rapid removal of Ca^{2+} from the cytoplasm causes relaxation. Because nearly all of the Ca^{2+} is recycled through the SR in this way, extracellular Ca^{2+} is not required in the short term and skeletal muscle contraction can proceed even in the absence of extracellular Ca^{2+}. The capacity of the SR to store all of this Ca^{2+} is greatly enhanced by the Ca^{2+}-binding protein calsequestrin, which is abundant in the lumen of the SR and acts as a Ca^{2+} buffer.

The Ca^{2+} release channels in the SR membrane are called ryanodine receptors because they bind ryanodine, a paralyzing plant alkaloid, with high affinity. Molecular cloning has identified three RyR isoforms: RyR1 in adult skeletal muscle, RyR2 in cardiac muscle, and RyR3 in embryonic skeletal muscle, brain, and other tissues. Each Ca^{2+} release channel is a homotetramer of four identical RyR protein subunits. These channels open when $[Ca^{2+}]_i$ reaches micromolar levels. Malignant hyper-

---

BOX 13-2

Malignant Hyperthermia Is Caused by a Sustained Increase of $[Ca^{2+}]_i$ in Skeletal Muscle

Malignant hyperthermia (MH) is a disorder of skeletal muscle characterized by hypermetabolism. MH is triggered by exposure to volatile, halogenated anesthetics, such as halothane. In children undergoing anesthesia, the incidence is about 1 in 3000 to 15,000. Thus about one case will occur in a busy metropolitan hospital every other year. Although relatively rare, MH is life threatening.

An episode of MH is characterized by an uncontrolled, sustained increase in $[Ca^{2+}]_i$ in skeletal muscle. This results in hypermetabolism: as cross-bridges continuously cycle and sarcoplasmic reticulum (SR) Ca^{2+} pumps attempt to restore normal $[Ca^{2+}]_i$, ATP is rapidly consumed in both processes. The maintained high $[Ca^{2+}]_i$ produces muscle rigidity. The rapid ATP consumption leads to a dramatic increase in aerobic and anaerobic metabolism, an increase in CO_2 production, and a sustained rise in body temperature. If untreated, this clinical syndrome is usually fatal. The skeletal muscle relaxant dantrolene is a lifesaving therapy for MH. This drug inhibits SR Ca^{2+} release through the ryanodine receptor (RyR) Ca^{2+} release channels. It rapidly reduces the uncontrolled increase in $[Ca^{2+}]_i$ in skeletal muscle and suppresses the hypermetabolism that threatens the patient with MH.

MH is a genetically heterogeneous disease. Most cases are associated with a point mutation in the gene encoding the skeletal muscle SR Ca^{2+} release channel (RyR1). To date, 24 different gain-of-function mutations have been identified. The altered channels exhibit several abnormalities that cause enhanced Ca^{2+} release from the SR. For example, MH muscle is more sensitive than normal muscle to depolarization and to caffeine, both of which open RyR Ca^{2+} release channels. The standard test for MH susceptibility involves exposing a muscle sample from the patient to halothane and caffeine and measuring the contracture response. Muscle from patients with MH produces larger caffeine contractures than does normal muscle, and the contractures occur at a lower caffeine concentration.

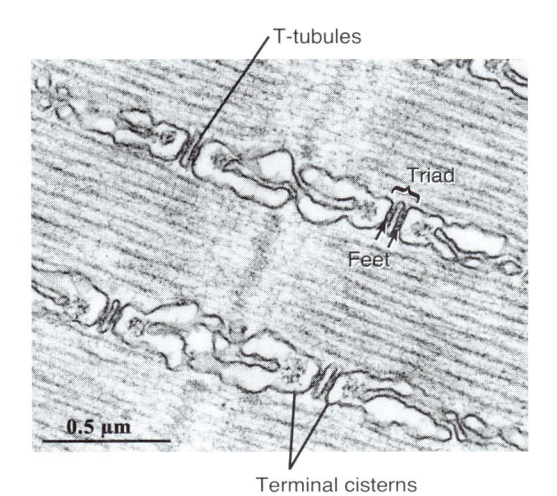

Figure 13-5 ■ **A triad in skeletal muscle consists of a T-tubule sandwiched between two terminal cisterns of the sarcoplasmic reticulum (SR). This longitudinal section shows the three elements of the triad. The flattened, oval elements are cross-sectional views of T-tubules. On either side of each T-tubule is a terminal cistern of the SR. Junctional feet *(arrows)* span the space between the T-tubule and SR membranes.** (Courtesy C. Franzini-Armstrong.)

thermia is a genetic disease of skeletal muscle caused by mutations in the skeletal muscle RyR (Box 13-2).

The Triad Is the Structure That Mediates Excitation-Contraction Coupling in Skeletal Muscle

The SR and T-tubule membranes in skeletal muscle are associated with each other at specialized junctions called **triads** (Figure 13-5). The triad consists of a T-tubule that is flanked on either side by enlarged terminal sacs of the SR, called **terminal cisterns**. The Ca^{2+} release channels (RyRs) are located in the terminal cisterns of the SR at the triads. A large cytoplasmic domain of the RyR spans the narrow gap between the T-tubule and SR membranes (Figure 13-5). At the skeletal muscle triads the T-tubule membrane contains clusters of DHPRs that are located in precise register with the RyR subunits on the underlying SR membrane (Figure 13-6). The DHPRs are grouped into tetrads, or groups of four DHPRs, and each DHPR molecule in the T-tubule membrane is aligned with and opposed to a subunit of the RyR in the SR. However, alternate RyR tetrads are unopposed by DHPRs (Figure 13-6). This arrangement, which is not present in cardiac muscle, apparently is the structural basis of the E-C coupling mechanism in skeletal muscle.

In Skeletal Muscle, Excitation-Contraction Coupling Is Believed to Be Mechanical

The SR Ca^{2+} release channels open in response to a depolarization of the T-tubule membrane. This enables Ca^{2+} to flow out of the SR, down its concentration gradient, into the cytoplasm, where it binds to troponin C (TnC) and activates contraction. How does depolarization of the T-tubule membrane open the SR Ca^{2+} release channel? This has been a central question in E-C coupling. The fact that the SR membrane is electrically isolated from the T-tubule membrane rules out the idea that depolarization spreads directly from the T-tubule to the SR. Two classes of indirect coupling models have been proposed. First, T-tubule membrane depolarization could generate a *chemical* messenger that diffuses to the RyR and activates the Ca^{2+} release channel. The second type of coupling mechanism involves a *mechanical* link between a *voltage sensor* in the T-tubule membrane and the gating mechanism of the Ca^{2+} release channel in the SR membrane. The available evidence supports the mechanical coupling model in skeletal muscle.

The L-type Ca^{2+} channel (DHPR) is homologous to the voltage-gated Na^+ channel. Like the Na^+ channel (Chapter 5), the DHPR has a positively charged, membrane-spanning segment

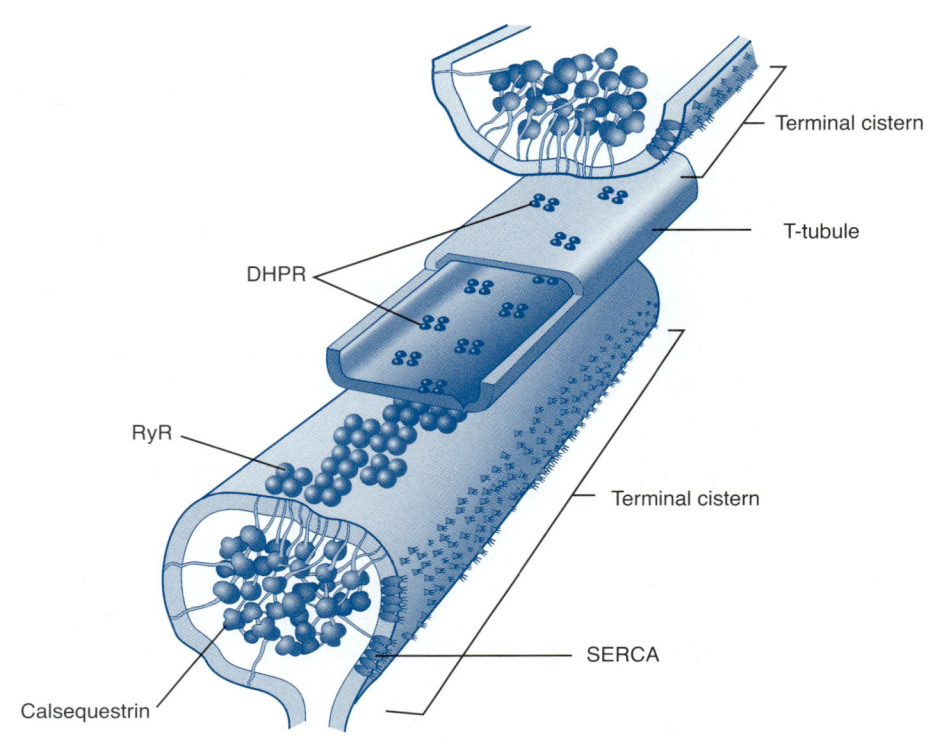

Figure 13-6 ■ The three dimensional structure of a triad. Each ball represents a ryanodine receptor (RyR) subunit, and four of these subunits form the Ca^{2+} release channel. The four subunits of the Ca^{2+} release channel form the foot protein that connects the sarcoplasmic reticulum (terminal cistern) membrane to the cytoplasmic face of the T-tubule membrane. In the T-tubule membrane, dihydropyridine receptors (DHPRs) are grouped into tetrads and each member of the tetrad is opposite a subunit of the Ca^{2+} release channel. However, every other Ca^{2+} release channel lacks the opposing tetrad of DHPRs. Calsequestrin and SERCA are also shown (see text). (Modified from Block BA, Imagawa T, Campbell KP, Franzini-Armstrong C: *J Cell Biol* 107:2587, 1988.)

(S4 region) that acts as the voltage sensor for the voltage-gated Ca^{2+} channel. In the T-tubules of skeletal muscle the DHPR also acts as the voltage sensor for E-C coupling: its ability to act as a voltage sensor is *independent* of its ability to conduct Ca^{2+} ions. The movement of the positive charges in the S4 segment of the DHPR (the voltage sensor) in response to depolarization generates a current that can be measured with a voltage clamp (Box 13-3). Studies of this charge movement in skeletal muscle reveal that it is an essential first step in E-C coupling. The relationship between voltage-dependent activation of DHPRs, charge movement, and E-C coupling has been demonstrated in elegant experiments with animals having mutated DHPRs (Box 13-4). These studies have led to models in which the movement of the voltage sensor in the DHPR is mechanically linked to the opening of the Ca^{2+} release channel in the SR (Figure 13-7). The main elements of E-C coupling in skeletal muscle are illustrated in Figure 13-8.

> **BOX 13-3**
>
> ### Nonlinear Charge Movement Reflects Movement of the Voltage Sensor In Skeletal Muscle
>
> In skeletal muscle the voltage clamp can be used to measure a nonlinear component of the capacitive current that is qualitatively similar to Na^+ channel gating current (see Box 7-3). With ionic and linear capacitive currents eliminated, a depolarizing voltage clamp step generates an outward current. This current reflects the movement of intramembrane charged amino acid residues in the S4 segment of the dihydropyridine receptor that act as the voltage sensor for excitation-contraction (E-C) coupling in skeletal muscle. Several lines of evidence indicate that this nonlinear intramembrane charge movement is related to E-C coupling. For example, the magnitude of the charge movement increases with the size of the depolarization and this occurs over the same range of potentials where muscle force increases (see Figure 13-1). Furthermore, Ca^{2+} release from the sarcoplasmic reticulum (SR) and charge movement are tightly correlated in several ways. Finally, no experimental or physiological conditions have been found that eliminate charge movement while maintaining depolarization-induced SR Ca^{2+} release in skeletal muscle.

> **BOX 13-4**
>
> ### A Dysgenic Muscle Model Reveals That Dihydropyridine Receptors Are the Voltage Sensors for Excitation-Contraction Coupling in Skeletal Muscle
>
> An animal model has provided some of the evidence that dihydropyridine receptors (DHPRs) act as the voltage sensors for excitation-contraction (E-C) coupling in skeletal muscle. A lethal autosomal recessive mutation in mice, termed muscular dysgenesis *(mdg)*, is functionally expressed as a failure of E-C coupling in skeletal muscle. The mutation alters the gene encoding the DHPR of skeletal muscle, producing a loss-of-function mutation. The α subunit of the L-type Ca^{2+} channel, which contains the dihydropyridine binding site, is missing in *mdg* mice. As a result, the inward Ca^{2+} current is absent. All other proteins are expressed at normal levels, and the skeletal muscle cells are normal in all other respects. The nonlinear intramembrane charge movement (Box 13-3) is also absent in *mdg* skeletal muscle, demonstrating that the DHPRs are the source of the charge movement. When *mdg* skeletal muscle cells are injected with cDNA encoding the normal skeletal muscle DHPR, normal E-C coupling, inward Ca^{2+} current, *and* the nonlinear charge movement are all restored. These findings support the idea that the DHPR is the voltage sensor that generates the charge movement, which is then coupled to the opening of the ryanodine receptor Ca^{2+} release channel in the sarcoplasmic reticulum of skeletal muscle.

Skeletal Muscle Relaxes When Ca^{2+} Is Returned to the Sarcoplasmic Reticulum by the Sarcoplasmic Reticulum Ca^{2+} Pump

As $[Ca^{2+}]_i$ increases during contraction, Ca^{2+} ions bind not only to TnC, but also to SERCA pumps. The SERCA pumps immediately begin to pump Ca^{2+} back into the SR. SERCA has higher affinity for Ca^{2+} than does TnC. Thus, after the Ca^{2+} release channels have closed, SERCA pump activity restores $[Ca^{2+}]_i$ to its resting level and brings about relaxation. Nearly all of the Ca^{2+} that is released from the SR during a contraction is pumped back into the SR by SERCA.

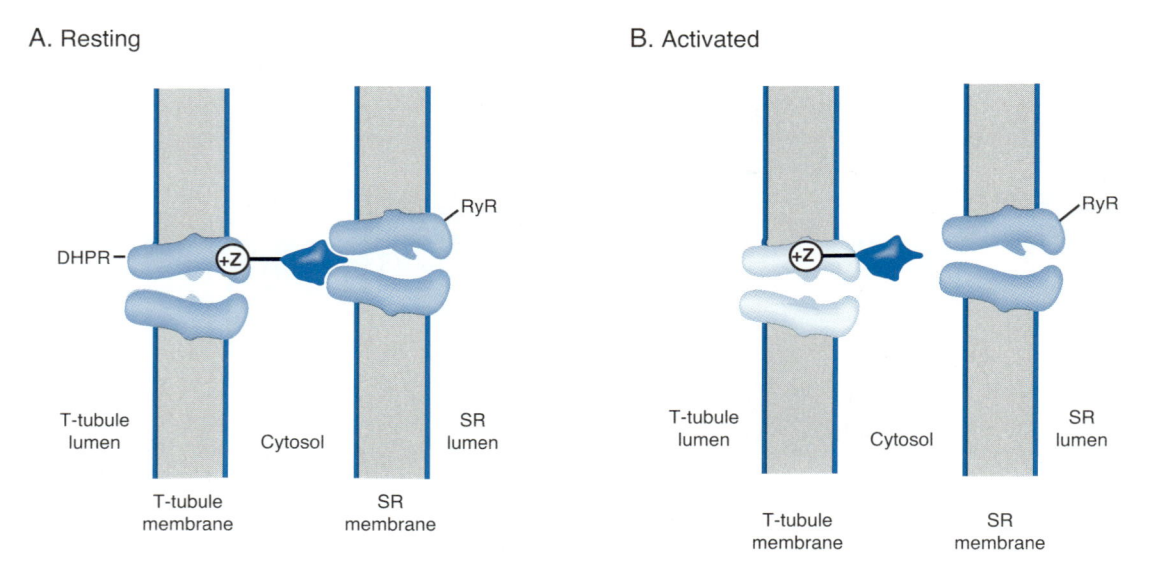

Figure 13-7 ■ Coupling of charge movement to the opening of a Ca^{2+} release channel in skeletal muscle. The T-tubule and sarcoplasmic reticulum (SR) membranes are shown separating the T-tubule lumen, the cytosol, and the SR lumen. A, The voltage sensor is shown as a charge of +Z in the dihydropyridine receptor (DHPR), which is mechanically linked to a plug that moves to open and close the ryanodine receptor (RyR) Ca^{2+} release channel. At rest, the voltage sensor is electrostatically attracted to the inner surface of the T-tubule membrane by the negative membrane potential, and the plug blocks the Ca^{2+} release channel. B, On depolarization, the voltage sensor moves outward, driven by the positive-going membrane potential, pulling the plug that opens the Ca^{2+} release channel. (Modified from Chandler WK, Rakowski RF, Schneider MF: *J Physiol* 254:285, 1976.)

■ Ca^{2+}-INDUCED Ca^{2+} RELEASE IS CENTRAL TO EXCITATION-CONTRACTION COUPLING IN CARDIAC MUSCLE

There are several important differences between cardiac and skeletal muscle E-C coupling mechanisms. Nevertheless, the general process of E-C coupling is similar. Contraction of a cardiac cell is initiated by an action potential that rapidly propagates over the surface of the cell and into the T-tubules. The cardiac T-tubule and sarcolemmal action potential leads to the opening of the Ca^{2+} release channels in the SR, allowing Ca^{2+} to flow out of the SR, bind to TnC, and activate contraction, as in skeletal muscle.

The mechanism by which the action potential is coupled to the opening of Ca^{2+} release channels in cardiac myocytes is, however, entirely different from the charge-coupled (electromechanical) mechanism just described for skeletal muscle. In addition, initiation of the cardiac sarcolemmal action potential does not occur through neuromuscular transmission, as it does in skeletal muscle. The sinoatrial node of the heart contains special pacemaker cells that spontaneously generate action potentials. Each action potential is conducted from myocyte to myocyte throughout the heart because the cells are electrically coupled to one another through *gap junctions* (see Chapter 12).

Excitation-Contraction Coupling in Muscle

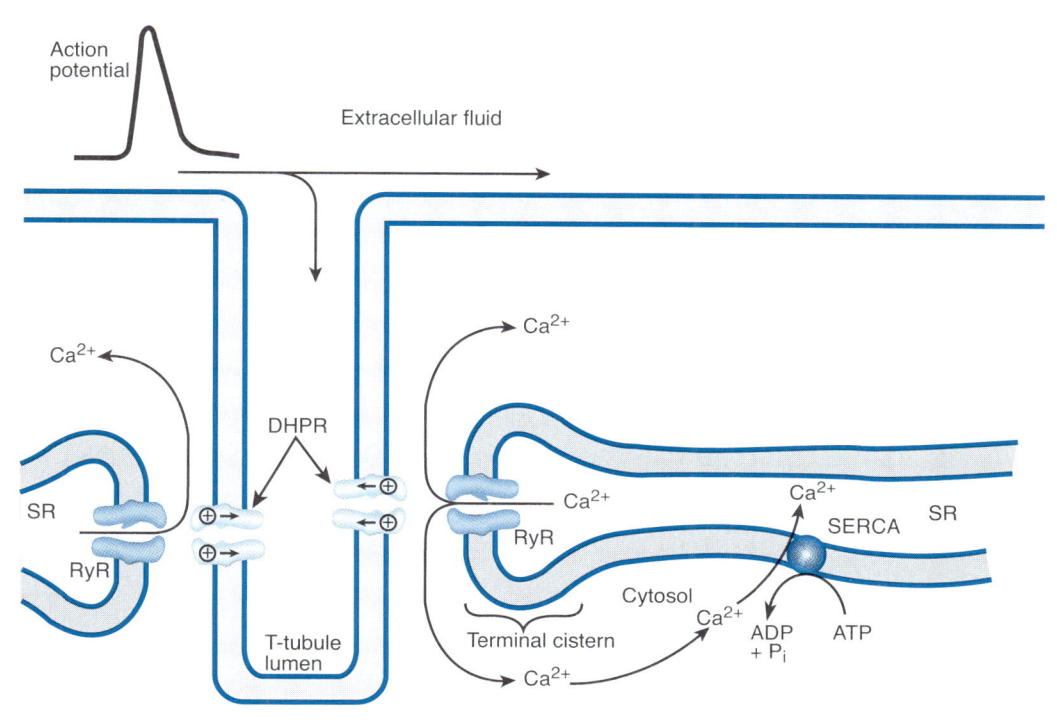

Figure 13-8 ■ Cellular components of excitation-contraction (E-C) coupling and relaxation in skeletal muscle. An action potential initiated at the neuromuscular junction is normally the first event in E-C coupling in skeletal muscle. The action potential rapidly propagates over the sarcolemma and into the T-tubules. The voltage sensor in the dihydropyridine receptors (DHPRs) (+) moves in response to a depolarization of the T-tubule membrane. Voltage sensor movement opens the Ca^{2+} release channel (ryanodine receptor [RyR]) in the sarcoplasmic reticulum (SR) membrane, permitting Ca^{2+} to flow out of the SR into the cytosol to trigger contraction. The Ca^{2+} that is released from the SR is subsequently removed from the cytosol and is returned to the SR by Ca^{2+} pumps (SERCA) in the SR membrane.

In Cardiac Muscle, Communication Between the SR and Sarcolemmal Membrane Occurs at Dyads and Peripheral Couplings

In cardiac cells the T-tubule system is present, although less extensive than in skeletal muscle, and the T-tubules have a much larger diameter (see Figure 12-10). The SR in cardiac muscle is less regular and more sparse than in skeletal muscle. The sarcolemma is functionally coupled to the SR and, as in skeletal muscle, the cytoplasmic domains of RyR proteins span the narrow gap (<20 nm) between the two membranes. In cardiac muscle the functional interactions between the sarcolemma and the SR membrane occur either at a **dyad** formed between a T-tubule and a single flattened terminal cistern of the SR or at a **peripheral coupling** formed between the surface membrane and a subsarcolemmal cistern of the SR. At these sites of interaction the sarcolemmal DHPRs are close to the

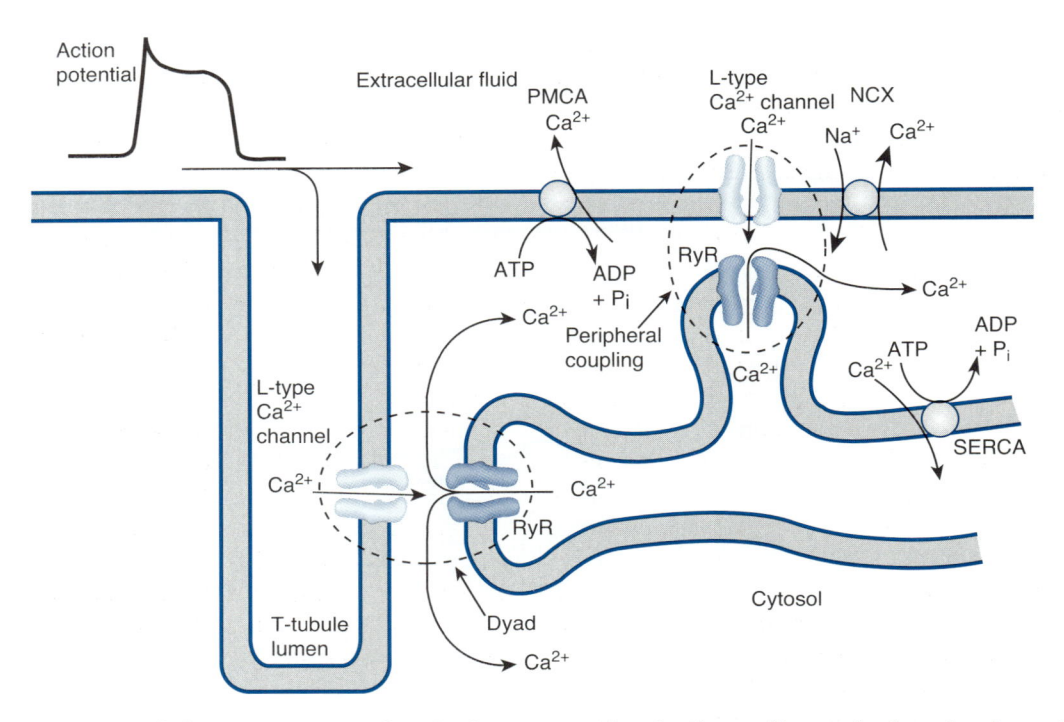

Figure 13-9 ■ Cellular components of excitation-contraction (E-C) coupling and relaxation in cardiac muscle. The cardiac action potential initiates E-C coupling in cardiac muscle. The action potential opens L-type Ca^{2+} channels in both surface and T-tubule membranes, and Ca^{2+} ions enter the cell through these open channels. At dyads and peripheral couplings (enclosed by dashed ellipses) the Ca^{2+} that enters through the L-type Ca^{2+} channel binds to, and thereby opens, RyR Ca^{2+} release channels in the sarcoplasmic reticulum (SR). About 80% of the Ca^{2+} required to activate contraction in cardiac muscle comes from the SR, and 20% comes from the extracellular space. Ca^{2+} is removed from the cells by the plasma membrane Ca^{2+} pump (PMCA) and Na^+/Ca^{2+} exchangers (NCX). The Ca^{2+} pump (SERCA) in the SR membrane returns Ca^{2+} from the cytosol to the SR. Normally, about 5% of the Ca^{2+} is removed by PMCA, 15% by NCX, and 80% by SERCA. A small change in the balance of these transporters can significantly change the $[Ca^{2+}]_{SR}$ and thereby alter the force of contraction of the heart (see Chapter 11).

RyRs in the SR, but these proteins do not exhibit the high degree of regular spatial organization observed in skeletal muscle.

In Cardiac Muscle, Excitation-Contraction Coupling Requires Extracellular Ca^{2+} and Ca^{2+} Entry Through L-Type Ca^{2+} Channels

The activation of cardiac contraction requires *both* Ca^{2+} release from the SR and Ca^{2+} entry from the extracellular space across the surface membrane (Figure 13-9); removal of extracellular Ca^{2+} abolishes cardiac contraction. The sarcolemma of cardiac cells contains L-type voltage-gated Ca^{2+} channels that open during the cardiac action potential. The Ca^{2+} ions that enter the cell through these L-type Ca^{2+} channels are directly involved in the activation of contraction in the heart. In the heart, L-type Ca^{2+} channels activate rapidly (in about 2 to 3 msec). This is fast enough to allow Ca^{2+} influx through the L-type Ca^{2+} channels to be directly involved in activating contraction.

In cardiac cells the inward Ca^{2+} current (I_{Ca}) is also crucial in activating contraction by triggering the release of Ca^{2+} from the SR. The RyRs in cardiac muscle are activated by Ca^{2+} ions that enter the cell through L-type Ca^{2+} channels. This mechanism, which is known as **Ca^{2+}-induced Ca^{2+} release (CICR),** appears to be the main mechanism of E-C coupling in cardiac cells (Box 13-5). The close association between DHPRs (L-type Ca^{2+} channels) in the sarcolemma and RyR Ca^{2+} release channels in the SR membrane suggests a functional coupling between these proteins, as illustrated in Figure 13-10. Depolarization of the sarcolemma opens an L-type Ca^{2+} channel, which permits Ca^{2+} entry. This results in a local increase in $[Ca^{2+}]_i$ that activates a number of RyR Ca^{2+} release channels in the immediate vicinity of the L-type Ca^{2+} channel. The Ca^{2+} release through the RyR Ca^{2+} release channels can be visualized as **"Ca^{2+} sparks"** (Box 13-6). The sum of a large number of these Ca^{2+} release events results in a global rise in $[Ca^{2+}]_i$ that activates contraction.

The Ca^{2+} That Enters the Cell During the Cardiac Action Potential Must Be Removed to Maintain a Steady State

When $[Ca^{2+}]_i$ increases during contraction, TnC and three Ca^{2+} transport proteins all compete for Ca^{2+} ions. The transporters are the plasma membrane Ca^{2+}-ATPase (PMCA), the Na^+/Ca^{2+} exchanger in the sarcolemma, and SERCA. Some of the excess Ca^{2+} ions in the cytoplasm are transported out of the cell by the Na^+/Ca^{2+} exchanger and PMCA, although PMCA plays a minor role. The remainder of the Ca^{2+} is taken up into the SR by SERCA pumps. Thus *both the Na^+/Ca^{2+} exchanger and SERCA* act to lower $[Ca^{2+}]_i$, cause the relaxation of cardiac muscle, and maintain long-term Ca^{2+} balance.

Cardiac Contraction Can Be Regulated by an Alteration in $[Ca^{2+}]_i$

The force of contraction of cardiac muscle can be regulated by physiologically relevant mechanisms that change the level of $[Ca^{2+}]_i$. In Chapter 11 we already learned that partial inhibition of the Na^+ pump with cardiac glycosides indirectly results in an increase in the amount of Ca^{2+} stored in the SR and thus the amount of Ca^{2+} released during depolarization. In another example of physiological regulation, activation of β-adrenergic receptors in the cardiac sarcolemma increases the open probability of the L-type Ca^{2+} channel (see Chapter 8). This increases I_{Ca} during the action potential, thereby causing a larger force to develop because of the larger, elevation of $[Ca^{2+}]_i$.

■ ACTIVATION OF SMOOTH MUSCLE DIFFERS IN FUNDAMENTAL WAYS FROM EXCITATION-CONTRACTION COUPLING IN SKELETAL AND CARDIAC MUSCLES

Smooth Muscles Are Highly Diversified

In Chapter 12 we learned that contraction in smooth muscles, as in skeletal and cardiac muscles, is triggered by a rise in $[Ca^{2+}]_i$. The mechanisms by which smooth muscles are activated differ, however, from those in skeletal and cardiac muscles and even vary considerably among the many diverse types of smooth muscles. Some smooth muscles (e.g., intestinal and vascular smooth muscles) are extensively innervated by **sympathetic or parasympathetic neurons.** These neurons do not form specialized junctions comparable to the neuromuscular junctions of skeletal muscle. Instead, the autonomic neurons have numerous small swellings **(varicosities)** along their axons. Synaptic vesicles containing packets of neuro-

BOX 13-5

In Cardiac Muscle, But Not Skeletal Muscle, Ca^{2+}-Induced Ca^{2+} Release Is the Primary Mechanism of Excitation-Contraction Coupling

A comparison of the voltage dependence of Ca^{2+} current (I_{Ca}), $[Ca^{2+}]_i$, and the activation of contraction provides some of the key evidence that Ca^{2+}-induced Ca^{2+} release (CICR) plays an important role in excitation-contraction (E-C) coupling in cardiac muscle cells. As the membrane potential moves in the positive direction from the resting level, I_{Ca} increases, reaches a maximum, and then decreases in amplitude (see Chapter 8 and Figure B-1). I_{Ca} increases because the number of open voltage-gated Ca^{2+} channels increases as the membrane is depolarized. At still more positive potentials, it decreases because of a reduction in the driving force ($V_m - E_{Ca}$). In cardiac muscle, $[Ca^{2+}]_i$ and cell shortening have a voltage dependence that is similar to I_{Ca} (Figure B-1, A): they reach a maximum value at about the same voltage and then decrease in size as the membrane potential becomes more positive. The fact that $[Ca^{2+}]_i$, and cell shortening are correlated with the amplitude of I_{Ca} is part of the evidence that CICR is the primary mechanism of E-C coupling in cardiac muscle. In skeletal muscle, which does not depend on CICR for E-C coupling, the voltage dependence of $[Ca^{2+}]_i$ and tension do not mirror the voltage dependence of I_{Ca} (Figure B-1, B). Although $[Ca^{2+}]_i$ and tension increase as the membrane potential moves in the positive direction from the resting potential, they do not decrease with the additional increase in membrane potential that reduces I_{Ca} (Figure B-1, B).

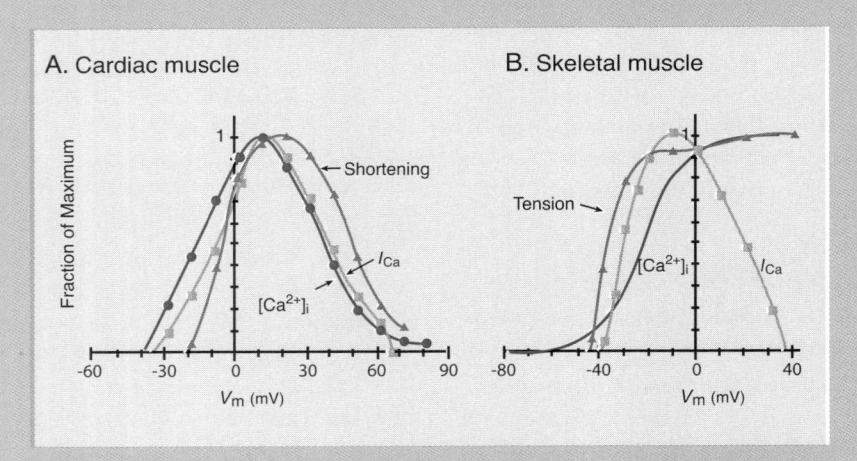

Figure B-1 ■ The voltage dependence of inward Ca^{2+} current (I_{Ca}), $[Ca^{2+}]_i$, and contraction (shortening or tension) are compared in cardiac and skeletal muscle. A, Each parameter was measured in voltage clamp experiments on isolated ventricular muscle cells. Each set of values was normalized and plotted as a function of membrane potential (V_m). B, I_{Ca}, $[Ca^{2+}]_i$, and tension were measured in voltage clamp experiments on skeletal muscle cells. (Modified from Bers DM: *Excitation-contraction coupling and cardiac contractile force*, Dordrecht, The Netherlands, 1991, Kluwer.)

Excitation-Contraction Coupling in Muscle

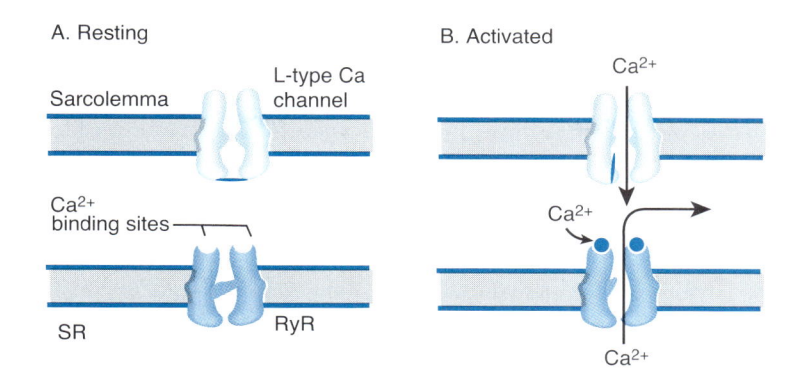

Figure 13-10 ■ Functional coupling between L-type Ca^{2+} channel and ryanodine receptor (RyR)/Ca^{2+} release channel in cardiac muscle. At the dyads and peripheral couplings between the sarcolemma and sarcoplasmic reticulum (SR) membrane, L-type Ca^{2+} channels in the sarcolemma are located directly opposite RyR Ca^{2+} release channels in the SR. A, In the resting state the gates on both channels are closed. B, During the cardiac action potential, L-type Ca^{2+} channels are opened, allowing Ca^{2+} ions to enter the cell. Ca^{2+} ions bind to sites on RyRs and open the Ca^{2+} release channels, allowing Ca^{2+} to flow from the SR into the cytosol. Although two binding sites are shown on the RyR, the precise stoichiometry has not been determined.

BOX 13-6

Ca^{2+} Sparks Are Localized Increases in $[Ca^{2+}]_i$ Triggered by the Opening of a Single L-Type Ca^{2+} Channel in Cardiac Muscle

The level of $[Ca^{2+}]_i$ in living cells can be measured by use of fluorescent Ca^{2+} indicator dyes. One such indicator, Fluo-3, becomes brightly fluorescent only when it binds Ca^{2+}. When Ca^{2+}-dependent indicator fluorescence is monitored in single cardiac cells with a laser-scanning confocal microscope, *localized* increases in $[Ca^{2+}]_i$ can be observed as small bursts of light that are called *Ca^{2+} sparks*. In resting cardiac cells, Ca^{2+} sparks occur spontaneously at a relatively low frequency: they increase in frequency with membrane depolarization. The Ca^{2+} sparks appear to result from the transient opening of a small, tight cluster of ryanodine receptor Ca^{2+} release channels. A comparison of the properties (e.g., the voltage dependence) of Ca^{2+} sparks with the properties of L-type Ca^{2+} channels reveals that a Ca^{2+} spark can be triggered by the Ca^{2+} entering through a single, open nearby L-type Ca^{2+} channel. The global increase in $[Ca^{2+}]_i$ that occurs during the cardiac action potential is the result of the synchronized triggering of myriad Ca^{2+} sparks throughout the cell.

---

transmitter molecules are clustered in the varicosities, which are the sites of transmitter release. There are a variety of neurotransmitters, including purines, peptides, and amino acids, as well as norepinephrine (NE) and acetylcholine (ACh). The distance between a varicosity and the closest smooth muscle cell can vary from about 15 to 150 nm or more (1 nm = 10^{-6} mm). When released, the transmitters diffuse to the surface of nearby smooth muscle cells, where they bind to transmitter-specific receptors. These receptors tend to be clustered in smooth muscle cell plasma membrane regions (microdomains) close to the neuronal varicosities.

The Density of Innervation Varies Greatly Among Different Types of Smooth Muscles

Some blood vessels are densely innervated by sympathetic neurons. The gastrointestinal (GI) tract has its own **enteric nervous system** that includes sympathetic and parasympathetic neurons and sensory neurons. This is needed to coordinate the contractions of the circular and longitudinal smooth muscle layers in order to regulate the complex motility of the gastrointestinal tract known as **peristalsis.** Peristalsis is responsible for mixing the contents of the intestinal lumen and for propelling this material along the GI tract. Failure of the neuronal ganglion cells of the colon to develop *(aganglionic colon)* results in intestinal obstruction, the absence of defecation, and *megacolon* (massive distention of the colon and abdomen) early in infancy (Hirschsprung's disease; Box 13-7).

At the other extreme are some smooth muscles, such as uterine smooth muscle, that have little or no innervation. In this case, as well as in instances of dense neuronal innervation, the smooth muscles can be activated by circulating and locally released hormones. The pregnant uterus at term (i.e., the time of delivery at the end of fetal gestation), for example, is activated by the posterior pituitary gland hormone *oxytocin,* by locally released *prostaglandins,* and by several other substances. These agents, too, act on specific plasma membrane receptors to initiate contraction.

Stretch or increased wall pressure may also activate contraction in some smooth muscles, perhaps in part by opening *stretch-activated, cation-permeable channels.* For example, increased intraluminal pressure slightly depolarizes vascular smooth muscle cells, increases Ca^{2+} entry, and activates contraction in small arteries;

BOX 13-7

Hirschsprung's Disease (Aganglionic Megacolon) Is Due to the Failure of Colon Ganglion Cells to Develop

Congenital aganglionic megacolon (Hirschsprung's disease) is manifested, usually in newborns or young infants, as a massive distention of the colon. This is the result of the absence of ganglion cells in a small, distal segment of the colon. This segment of the colon is therefore unable to undergo reflex dilation and remains constricted when the more proximal, normally innervated segments are distended. As a consequence of this intestinal obstruction, fecal material piles up and greatly distends the proximal segments.

The failure of some ganglion cells of the colon to develop occurs with an incidence of about 1 in 5000 live births. At least half of the cases can be attributed to defects in the genes that code for a tyrosine kinase receptor (RET) or endothelin 3 (EDN3) or its receptor, the endothelin B receptor (EDNRB). The endothelins are a family of oligopeptide hormones; the prototype, EDN1, was identified as a secretion of the endothelium. EDN1 and EDN3 promote vascular constriction. EDN3 is also a neurotrophic factor (i.e., a substance that promotes the survival and development of nerve cells). EDN3 is synthesized by glial cells. During development of the embryo, RET, EDN3, and EDNRB are all required for the migration of neural crest–derived cells to the intestinal wall and their subsequent development into the colon ganglion cells of the enteric nervous system.

the detailed mechanisms are still incompletely understood. This pressure-activated, sustained vascular constriction is known as **myogenic tone** (Figure 13-11). This is needed to maintain a relatively constant blood flow even when blood pressure varies.

Some Smooth Muscles Are Normally Activated by Depolarization

Some smooth muscles (e.g., intestinal smooth muscles) are "excitable": activation of contraction is triggered by action potentials or by rhythmic changes in membrane potential. These types of smooth muscle are often referred to as **phasic smooth muscles.** The depolarization opens L-type voltage-gated Ca^{2+} channels, and the entering Ca^{2+} then triggers Ca^{2+} release from the SR via RyRs (i.e., CICR; see the earlier discussion of cardiac muscle). In this case Ca^{2+} entry is essential for triggering contraction, as in cardiac muscle.

In many instances the smooth muscle cells are connected to one another by low-resistance gap junctions. These junctions couple cells electrically so that depolarization can be propagated from cell to cell (as in the heart). This enables many cells to act in a coordinated fashion, as a *syncytium*, to alter organ lumen diameter or volume. Smooth muscles that function in this way are known as *single-unit smooth muscles* (e.g., intestinal smooth muscles). In contrast, smooth muscles in which the individual myocytes (muscle cells) act independently are called *multiunit smooth muscles* (e.g., the iris diaphragm of the eye).

Some Smooth Muscles Are Normally Activated by Agents That Induce Little or No Depolarization

Types of smooth muscle that usually do not generate action potentials are known as **tonic smooth muscles.** These smooth muscles also express L-type voltage-gated Ca^{2+} channels, but

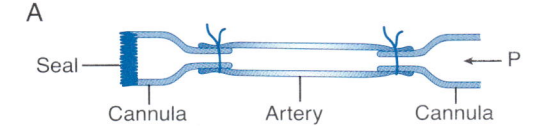

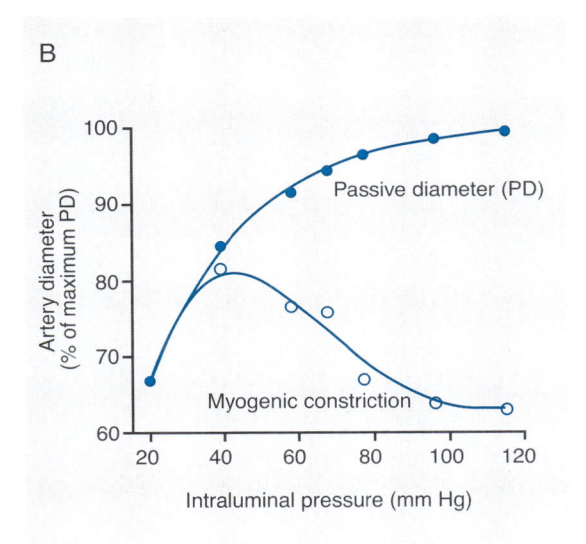

Figure 13-11 ■ Myogenic tone in isolated, cannulated, and pressurized mouse small mesenteric arteries. A, Small artery, cannulated at both ends to obtain the data in B. One cannula is sealed, and pressure (P) is applied at the other cannula. B, Pressure-diameter relationship. *Solid circles,* Passive (external) diameter (PD) measured as a function of intraluminal pressure in Ca^{2+}-free medium; PD at 120 mm Hg is taken as the maximum PD. *Open circles,* Relative diameter (i.e., relative to maximum PD) as a function of pressure in normal medium containing 2.5 mM Ca^{2+}. Myogenic tone is the vasoconstriction observed in the Ca^{2+}-containing solution, relative to that in Ca^{2+}-free solution, at pressures above 40 mm Hg. (Courtesy J. Zhang and M.P. Blaustein.)

they have few if any voltage-gated Na^+ channels. These types of smooth muscle (e.g., vascular smooth muscles) often have relatively small resting potentials (e.g., −55 to −40 mV). Some Ca^{2+} channels are open at these potentials. The number of open channels of course depends directly on the membrane potential. Small changes in the membrane potential (e.g., mediated by opening or closing of K^+ channels) may significantly alter Ca^{2+} entry by altering the number of open Ca^{2+} channels. Such variations in Ca^{2+} entry may in turn modulate the strength of the tonic contraction that is usually observed under "resting" (or quasi-steady-state) conditions in these muscles (Figure 13-11). Thus incremental changes in membrane potential may lead to graded changes in tonic contraction (Figure 13-12).

A major mechanism of activation of tonic smooth muscles is called **pharmacomechanical coupling.** In contrast to electrical (E-C) coupling, which involves depolarization, pharmacomechanical coupling involves the activation of smooth muscles by various stimulatory agonists that often have little or no effect on the membrane potential. These agonists are usually neurotransmitters or hormones; some examples are NE, ACh, serotonin, histamine, nitric oxide (NO), vasopressin, angiotensin, and oxytocin.

Specificity is governed by the fact that different smooth muscles have different com-

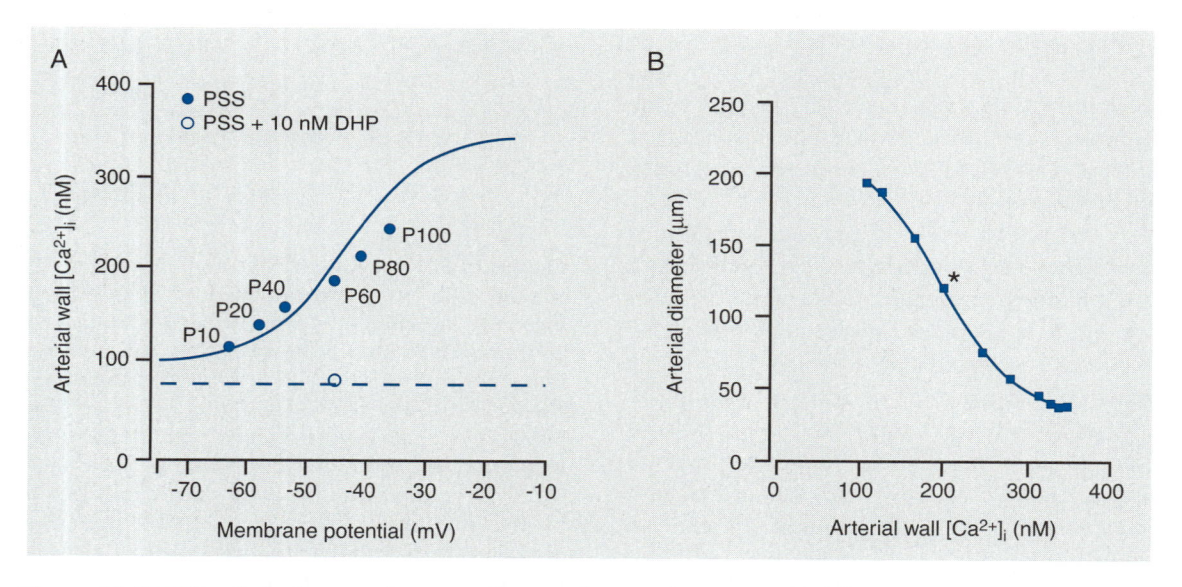

Figure 13-12 ■ Graded changes in smooth muscle membrane potential cause graded changes in $[Ca^{2+}]_i$ and, consequently, contraction. A, Relationship between spatially averaged arterial wall $[Ca^{2+}]_i$ and arterial myocyte membrane potential. The intraarterial pressure was varied between 10 and 100 mm Hg, as indicated (P10 to P100), where 60 mm Hg is the normal, in vivo pressure. Both $[Ca^{2+}]_i$ and membrane potential (V_m) were measured at each pressure. *PSS*, Normal physiological salt solution; *DHP*, dihydropyridine blocker of voltage-gated Ca^{2+} channels, nisoldipine. B, Relationship between arterial wall $[Ca^{2+}]_i$ and artery diameter. The arterial pressure was maintained at 60 mm Hg, and V_m was altered by varying $[K^+]_o$ (asterisk indicates the normal resting condition). The change in V_m affected both $[Ca^{2+}]_i$ and diameter, as illustrated. The relationship between $[Ca^{2+}]_i$ and V_m under these isobaric (constant pressure) conditions is shown as the solid line in A. The data were obtained in isolated small cerebral arteries with myogenic tone (see Figure 13-11, *A*). (Modified from Knot HJ, Nelson MT: *J Physiol* 508:199, 1998.)

plements of **agonist receptors.** In most cases a variety of different agonists can act on a single cell type. Some transmitters or hormones antagonize contraction and relax smooth muscles. In the intestine, for example, ACh activates contraction whereas NE promotes relaxation. On the other hand, NE directly activates arterial smooth muscle contraction while ACh promotes relaxation by acting on the vascular endothelium that lines the lumen of blood vessels. ACh triggers the secretion of NO by the endothelial cells. NO, by stimulating the intracellular production of cyclic guanosine monophosphate (cGMP), relaxes the adjacent arterial smooth muscle. As discussed in Chapter 12, cGMP promotes smooth muscle relaxation by reducing the sensitivity of the contractile proteins to Ca^{2+} (see Box 12-2). Indeed, this is the basis of NO's role in promoting penile erection, as well as the mechanism of action of sildenafil (Viagra) in treating erectile dysfunction (Box 13-8). It is also the basis of action of nitroglycerin and the organic nitrates, which have long been used to treat *angina pectoris,* the chest pain associated with obstructed coronary arteries (Box 13-8). This may be contrasted with the relief of angina pectoris by L-type Ca^{2+} channel blockers that dilate arteries by reducing Ca^{2+} entry.

In pharmacomechanical coupling an agonist binds to its specific plasma membrane (PM) receptor. Then, as a result of receptor activation and a cascade of chemical reactions, the cytosolic

---

BOX 13-8

Nitric Oxide, Nitroglycerin, Organic Nitrates, and Sildenafil (Viagra) Promote Vasodilation by Activating a Cyclic Guanosine Monophosphate–Dependent Protein Kinase (G-Kinase)

Nitric oxide (NO) is one of the products of the oxidation of arginine to citrulline by the enzyme NO synthase, which is found in endothelial cells, neurons, and certain other cell types. NO is a highly reactive, short-lived (several seconds) hormone-neurotransmitter. In blood vessels, for example, NO rapidly diffuses from the endothelial cells to the smooth muscle cells. There NO binds to the heme group of a soluble cytosolic guanylyl cyclase and activates this enzyme, which catalyzes the synthesis of cyclic guanosine monophosphate (cGMP) from guanosine triphosphate. The elevated cGMP level then stimulates a G-kinase. The G-kinase catalyzes the phosphorylation of RhoA. The net result (see Box 12-2) is the activation of myosin light chain phosphatase. This phosphatase dephosphorylates the myosin light chain and thereby decreases the sensitivity of the smooth muscle contractile apparatus to Ca^{2+}. In blood vessels this induces vasodilation and promotes blood flow.

Drugs such as nitroglycerin and isosorbide dinitrate release NO, which activates soluble guanylyl cyclase. Because of the resulting vasodilation, these agents can be effective in relieving the chest pain (angina pectoris) caused when coronary artery vasospasm (transient vasoconstriction) reduces blood flow and oxygen delivery to the cardiac muscle.

The action of cGMP is terminated when it is hydrolyzed by the enzyme phosphodiesterase. The action of cGMP can be greatly prolonged and amplified by inhibition of the cGMP phosphodiesterase. Sildenafil (Viagra) is such an inhibitor; it therefore enhances the NO–cGMP signaling pathway. In so doing, sildenafil relaxes the vascular smooth muscle of the corpus cavernosum and thereby enables it to fill with blood and induce an erection (enlargement and stiffening) of the penis.

second messenger, inositol-1,4,5-trisphosphate (IP_3), is formed (Box 13-9). In addition, the activated PM receptor usually induces the transient opening of a poorly understood class of Ca^{2+} channels (so-called **receptor-operated channels, or ROCs**) that mediate Ca^{2+} entry, leading to the initiation of contraction. The main result of agonist-receptor binding, however, is the production of IP_3.

Inositol-1,4,5-Trisphosphate Activates the Release of Ca^{2+} from Smooth Muscle Sarcoplasmic Reticulum

The IP_3 formed at the cytoplasmic face of the PM diffuses to nearby SR, where it binds to its receptor (IP_3R) in the SR membrane. This opens a channel that is part of the receptor (analogous to the Ca^{2+} release channel that is part of the RyR in skeletal and cardiac muscle). As a result, Ca^{2+} is released from the SR and enters the cytosol. The elevated $[Ca^{2+}]_i$ then promotes smooth muscle contraction through the activation of myosin light chain kinase (see Chapter 12).

Smooth muscles also possess RyRs, but their physiological role is less clear than in skeletal and cardiac muscles. The elevated $[Ca^{2+}]_i$, generated as a result of Ca^{2+} entry through the PM and release from the SR via IP_3R, may trigger further release of SR Ca^{2+} via RyR to help maintain the elevated $[Ca^{2+}]_i$. However, some of the Ca^{2+} released through the RyR may be directed into the narrow cytosolic space between the SR and the adjacent PM. Some of this Ca^{2+} may open Ca^{2+}-activated K^+ channels that hyperpolarize the cells and promote relaxation. Thus an elevated $[Ca^{2+}]_i$ concentration not only leads to force generation, but also can act through the Ca^{2+}-activated K^+ channel-mediated *negative feedback* mechanism to limit force generation.

The SR Ca^{2+} stores that are depleted by release of Ca^{2+} through IP_3R and RyR channels must be replenished. In addition to resequestration of the released Ca^{2+} by the SERCA in the SR membrane, special PM channels are opened as a result of SR store depletion. These **store-operated channels (SOCs)** permit Ca^{2+} entry from the extracellular fluid. This Ca^{2+} is then rapidly transported into the SR by the SERCA pumps. The molecular structure of the SOCs and the mechanism by which depletion of SR Ca^{2+} stores opens these channels are still controversial.

Long-Term Ca^{2+} Balance Is Maintained by Ca^{2+} Extrusion Mechanisms That Compensate for the Ca^{2+} Entry During Smooth Muscle Activation

A variety of smooth muscle Ca^{2+} entry mechanisms were discussed in the preceding sections of this chapter. Much of the entering Ca^{2+} is rapidly pumped into the SR by SERCA pumps. Indeed, activated smooth muscle cells frequently exhibit net gain of Ca^{2+} over short periods. Sustained net gain of Ca^{2+} would, however, lead to Ca^{2+} overload in the smooth muscle cells. Therefore, in the long term, Ca^{2+} entry must be exactly balanced by Ca^{2+} exit. The two Ca^{2+} extrusion mechanisms in smooth muscle cells, as in other cell types, are the PMCA and the Na^+/Ca^{2+} exchanger (see Chapters 10 and 11). Although the precise roles of these two transport systems are uncertain, the Na^+/Ca^{2+} exchanger apparently plays an indirect but key role in regulating the Ca^{2+} concentration in the SR compartments adjacent to the PM. The various smooth muscle Ca^{2+} transport mechanisms are diagrammed in Figure 13-13. It should be apparent that the maintenance of tonic contractions is governed by the interactions of (1) the mechanisms that deliver Ca^{2+} to the cytosol, (2) the mechanisms that remove Ca^{2+} from the cytosol (Figure 13-13), and (3) the mechanisms that regulate the Ca^{2+} sensitivity of the contractile machinery (see Box 12-2).

Excitation-Contraction Coupling in Muscle

> **BOX 13-9**
>
> ### Activation of Many Plasma Membrane Receptors Results in the Synthesis of Inositol-1,4,5-Trisphosphate
>
> Many agonist receptors are plasma membrane proteins containing seven transmembrane helices. These receptors are coupled to guanosine triphosphate (GTP)-binding proteins: the small monomeric GTP-binding proteins such as Ras and Rho, as well as the heterotrimeric G-proteins, such as G_q and G_s, which consist of alpha, beta, and gamma (α, β, and γ) subunits. In their inactive state the G-proteins all have a guanosine diphosphate (GDP) molecule bound in the nucleotide binding site of the α subunit. When the appropriate agonist binds to and activates its receptor (see Figure B-1, which shows norepinephrine activation of the alpha$_1$-adrenergic receptor [α_1AR]), the activated receptor promotes the exchange of GTP for GDP on the α subunit of $G_{q,\alpha}$. GTP binding activates $G_{q,\alpha}$, which dissociates from the β and γ subunits and activates membrane-associated phospholipase C (PLC). Active PLC cleaves phosphatidyl inositol-4,5-bisphosphate (PIP$_2$), which is present in the cytoplasmic leaflet of the plasma membrane, into inositol-1,4,5-trisphosphate (IP$_3$) and diacylglycerol (DAG; Figure B-1). The IP$_3$ binds to its receptor (IP$_3$R), which, like the ryanodine receptor (RyR), is a Ca^{2+} release channel on the sarcoplasmic or endoplasmic reticulum membrane. Opening this channel releases Ca^{2+} into the cytosol. The DAG activates protein kinase C (PKC).
>
> Figure B-1 ■ The agonist receptor–G protein–phosphoinositide cascade. The diagram shows the sequence of events that occurs between the binding of an agonist (norepinephrine [NE]) to its plasma membrane receptor (in this case an alpha$_1$-adrenergic receptor, or α_1AR) and the release of sarcoplasmic reticulum Ca^{2+} and activation of contraction. Ca^{2+} released from the sarcoplasmic reticulum binds to calmodulin (CaM), and this activates myosin light chain kinase (MLCK), which phosphorylates myosin light chain and initiates the formation of actin-myosin cross-bridges.

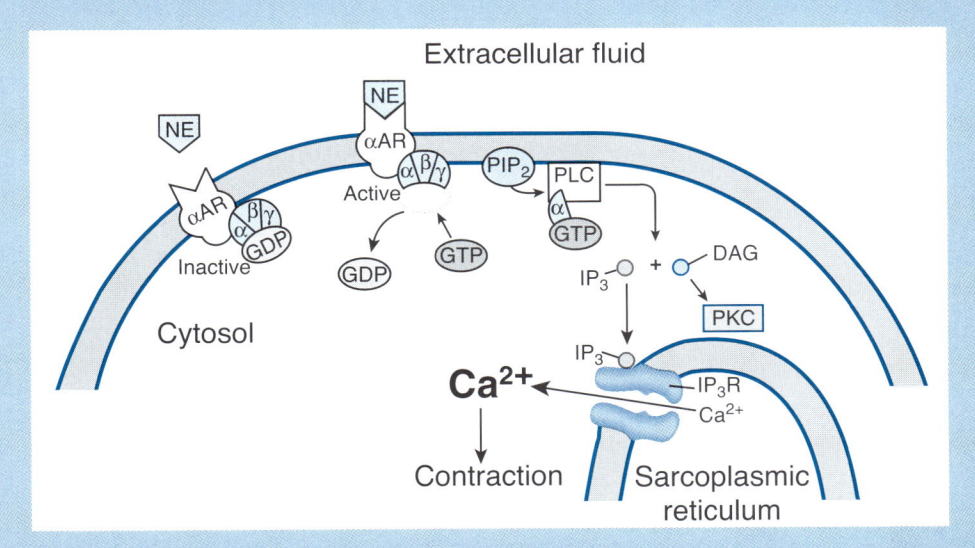

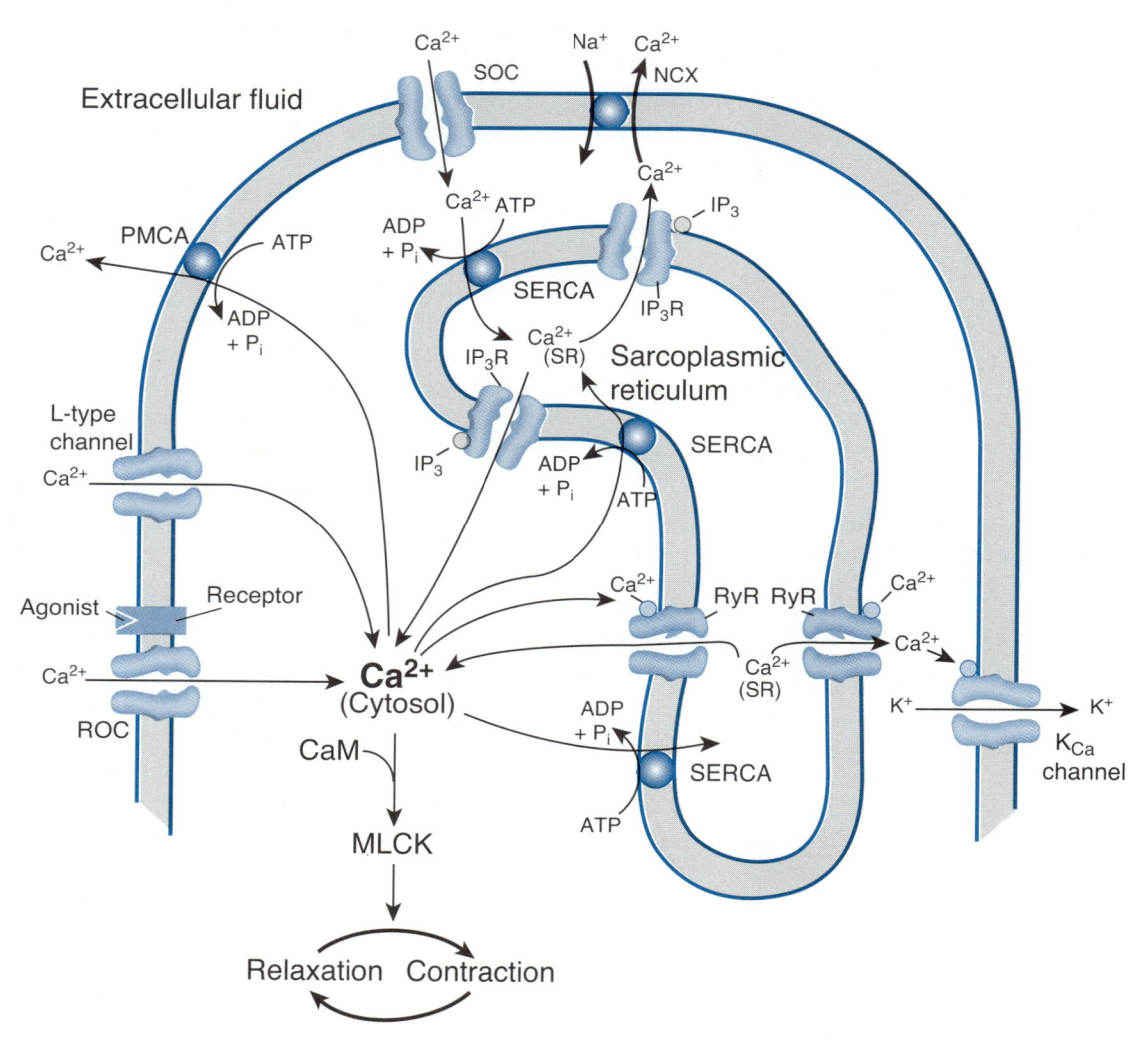

Figure 13-13 ■ The various transport systems that participate in the regulation of $[Ca^{2+}]_i$ in smooth muscle cells. Ca^{2+} can enter the cells through L-type voltage-gated channels, receptor-operated channels (ROCs), store-operated channels (SOCs), and Na^+/Ca^{2+} exchangers (NCX). Ca^{2+} is extruded from the cells by the plasma membrane Ca^{2+} pump (PMCA) and NCX. The Ca^{2+} pump in the sarcoplasmic reticulum membrane (SERCA) also removes Ca^{2+} from the cytosol. Much of the Ca^{2+} within the sarcoplasmic reticulum (SR) is bound to calsequestrin or calreticulin (not shown), two Ca^{2+}-binding proteins that buffer the free Ca^{2+} concentration in the lumen of the SR. Ca^{2+} is released from the SR stores through two types of channels, those that are opened by IP_3 (i.e., the IP_3 receptors, or IP_3Rs), and ryanodine receptors (RyRs) that are opened by elevated Ca^{2+} and mediate Ca^{2+}-induced Ca^{2+} release (CICR).

SUMMARY

1. Skeletal muscles are activated by depolarization of the muscle surface membrane (sarcolemma). This depolarization is usually in the form of an action potential. The process by which depolarization of the surface membrane causes contraction is termed excitation-contraction (E-C) coupling.
2. Force generation by skeletal muscle is voltage dependent. Thus E-C coupling in skeletal muscle involves a voltage sensor in the sarcolemma that couples depolarization to contraction.
3. The force transient produced by a skeletal muscle cell in response to a single action potential is called a twitch. Contractures are long-lasting mechanical responses produced by depolarizations that last several seconds.
4. A triad is a specialized junction in skeletal muscle consisting of a T-tubule that is flanked by terminal cisterns of the SR.
5. At the triads, Ca^{2+} release channels, or ryanodine receptors, are located in the SR membrane in precise register with clusters of dihydropyridine receptors (DHPRs) located in the T-tubule membrane. DHPRs are functional L-type Ca^{2+} channels.
6. Depolarization of the T-tubule is required for E-C coupling in skeletal muscle. Depolarization causes movement of the voltage sensor in the DHPRs. The voltage sensor appears to be mechanically linked to the opening of Ca^{2+} release channels.
7. All of the Ca^{2+} required for contraction in *skeletal muscle* is stored in the SR.
8. The relaxation of skeletal muscle occurs as Ca^{2+} is returned to the SR by SERCA. Nearly all of the Ca^{2+} that is released from the SR during a contraction is pumped back into the SR by SERCA.
9. In cardiac muscle, the functional couplings between SR and external membranes are dyads and peripheral couplings. At these couplings, DHPRs are located close to Ca^{2+} release channels.
10. In cardiac muscle the mechanism by which the action potential is coupled to the opening of Ca^{2+} release channels involves Ca^{2+}-induced Ca^{2+} release (CICR). The Ca^{2+} ions that enter the cell through L-type Ca^{2+} channels activate the RyRs in the immediate vicinity of the channel.
11. The activity of both the Na^+/Ca^{2+} exchanger and SERCA lower $[Ca^{2+}]_i$ and cause the relaxation of cardiac muscle.
12. Smooth muscles are diverse and are activated in different ways. Some are extensively innervated by the autonomic nervous system and are activated by neurotransmitters released from the varicosities along the nerve axons and at the nerve endings.
13. The intestine has its own intrinsic "enteric" nervous system to coordinate the contractions of the circular and longitudinal smooth muscle layers during peristalsis.
14. Some smooth muscles (e.g., uterine smooth muscle) are poorly innervated. Contractions of these smooth muscles are regulated by circulating and locally released hormones.
15. Stretch or increase in wall pressure may also directly activate some smooth muscles, such as those in the arterial wall.
16. Phasic smooth muscles are activated by depolarization; brief or rhythmic changes in membrane potential trigger the opening of voltage-gated L-type Ca^{2+} channels. The resulting Ca^{2+} entry is required to activate contraction.
17. Tonic smooth muscles have relatively small resting potentials (about -55 to -40 mV) and contraction can be regulated by small changes in membrane potential. Contraction can also be activated by Ca^{2+} release from SR stores in a process called pharmacomechanical coupling, which involves little or no change in membrane potential.

18. The specificity of agonist action is governed by the different agonist receptors expressed by the various types of smooth muscle cells.
19. Agonists that activate smooth muscle cells usually trigger the production of inositol-1,4,5-trisphosphate (IP_3) in the cytosol. The IP_3 binds to its receptor on the SR, opening a Ca^{2+} channel that is a part of the receptor. The consequent efflux of Ca^{2+} into the cytosol initiates contraction.
20. A rise in $[Ca^{2+}]_i$ may promote further release of SR Ca^{2+} via ryanodine receptors but may also promote relaxation by opening Ca^{2+}-dependent K^+ channels that hyperpolarize the smooth muscle cells (a form of negative feedback).
21. Maintained contraction in tonic smooth muscles is controlled by the balance between Ca^{2+} entry into, and removal from, the cytosol, as well as by the mechanisms that regulate the Ca^{2+} sensitivity of the contractile apparatus.

■ KEY WORDS AND CONCEPTS

- Contracture
- Excitation-contraction coupling
- Voltage sensor
- Twitch
- Dihydropyridine receptors (DHPRs)
- Sarcoplasmic or endoplasmic reticulum Ca^{2+} pump (SERCA)
- Ryanodine receptor (RyR)
- Ca^{2+} release channel
- Calsequestrin
- Triad
- Terminal cistern
- Dyads and peripheral couplings in cardiac muscle
- Ca^{2+}-induced Ca^{2+}-release (CICR)
- Ca^{2+} sparks
- Sympathetic and parasympathetic neurons
- Axonal varicosities
- Enteric nervous system
- Peristalsis
- Myogenic tone
- Tonic and phasic smooth muscles
- Pharmacomechanical coupling
- Agonist receptors
- Second messenger
- Inositol-1,4,5-trisphosphate
- Receptor-operated channels (ROCs)
- Store-operated channels (SOCs)

STUDY PROBLEMS

1. E-C coupling is similar in skeletal and cardiac muscle in some respects, but different in others. For example, a depolarization of the surface membrane (e.g., by an action potential) initiates E-C coupling in both types of muscle. Describe other similarities and differences.
2. In skeletal muscle only about half of the Ca^{2+} release channels in the SR are opposed by (and presumably linked to) tetrads of DHPRs in the T-tubules. These Ca^{2+} release channels are opened by a mechanical link between the voltage sensor in the DHPR and the gating mechanism of the Ca^{2+} release channel. During E-C coupling, what do you think happens to the Ca^{2+} release channels that are not opposed by DHPRs? Do you think they are nonfunctional? Or might they be opened via a different mechanism?
3. What general types of mechanisms influence smooth muscle contraction by altering (a) the availability of Ca^{2+} or (b) the sensitivity of the contractile apparatus to Ca^{2+}? (c) Why do you suppose so many types of mechanisms are available for regulating contraction in smooth muscles? (d) What are the possible clinical (therapeutic) implications?

■ BIBLIOGRAPHY

Bennett MR: Autonomic neuromuscular transmission at a varicosity, *Prog Neurobiol* 50:505, 1996.

Bers DM: *Excitation-contraction coupling and cardiac contractile force,* Dordrecht, The Netherlands, 1991, Kluwer.

Block BA, Imagawa T, Campbell KP, Franzini-Armstrong C: Structural evidence for direct interaction between the molecular components of the transverse tubule/sarcoplasmic reticulum junction in skeletal muscle, *J Cell Biol* 107:2587, 1988.

Bryant HJ, Harder DR, Pamnani MB, Haddy FJ: In vivo membrane potentials of smooth muscle cells in the caudal artery of the rat, *Am J Physiol Cell Physiol* 249:C78, 1985.

Chandler WK, Rakowski RF, Schneider MF: Effects of glycerol treatment and maintained depolarization on charge movement in muscle, *J Physiol* 254:285, 1976.

Hodgkin AL, Horowicz P: Potassium contractures in single muscle fibres, *J Physiol* 153:386, 1960.

Knot HJ, Nelson MT: Regulation of arterial diameter and wall [Ca^{2+}] in cerebral arteries of rat by membrane potential and intravascular pressure, *J Physiol* 508:199, 1998.

Murphy RA: Smooth muscle. In Berne RM, Levy MN, Koeppen BM, Stanton BA, editors: *Physiology*, ed 4, St Louis, 1998, Mosby.

Rüegg JC: *Calcium in muscle contraction*, ed 2, Berlin, 1992, Springer-Verlag.

Sanchez JA, Stefani E: Kinetic properties of calcium channels of twitch muscle fibres of the frog, *J Physiol* 37:1, 1983.

Somlyo AP, Somlyo AV: Signal transduction and regulation in smooth muscle, *Nature* 372:231, 1994.

CHAPTER 14

Mechanics of Muscle Contraction

Objectives:

1. Understand how a skeletal muscle twitch and a tetanus are generated.
2. Understand how the force generated by a muscle can be varied.
3. Understand the mechanical properties of muscle as described by the length-tension relationship and the force-velocity relationship.
4. Understand the roles of the three main types of phasic skeletal muscle.
5. Understand how the mechanical properties of skeletal muscle, cardiac muscle, and smooth muscle differ.
6. Understand the diversity of smooth muscle types.
7. Understand how the kinetic properties of some smooth muscles contribute to their ability to generate tonic contractions or "tone."

In Chapters 12 and 13 we described the sliding filament mechanism of contraction and the mechanism by which contraction is coupled to activation of the cell. In this chapter we consider the mechanical properties of muscle contraction in terms of force development and shortening.

■ THE TOTAL FORCE GENERATED BY A SKELETAL MUSCLE CAN BE VARIED BY SEVERAL MECHANISMS

Whole Muscle Force Can Be Increased by Recruitment of Motor Units

Skeletal muscle is normally activated through its innervation by α motor neurons. An individual α motor neuron may innervate just a few muscle fibers (cells) in extraocular muscles or as many as several thousand muscle fibers in large limb and trunk muscles. A single α motor neuron, together with all of the muscle cells it innervates, is referred to as a **motor unit**. The motor neurons release acetylcholine (ACh) at the neuromuscular junctions (see Chapter 8). A single motor neuron action potential normally releases sufficient ACh at each neuromuscular junction to trigger an action potential in all the muscle fibers it innervates. Consequently, all the muscle cells in a motor unit contract synchronously when the motor neuron generates an action potential. Thus the motor unit is the functional force-generating unit in whole muscle. The primary mechanism by which the central nervous system increases whole muscle force is by recruiting (i.e., simultaneously activating) motor units. Thus the amount of force generated by whole muscle is directly related to the number of motor units that are activated.

A Single Action Potential Produces a Twitch Contraction

A single action potential in a skeletal muscle cell triggers Ca^{2+} release from the sarcoplasmic reticulum (SR; see Chapter 13) to increase $[Ca^{2+}]_i$, and thus causes a **twitch** contraction. A comparison of the time course of $[Ca^{2+}]_i$ elevation and force development during a twitch is shown in Figure 14-1, A. Shortly after the action potential, $[Ca^{2+}]_i$ rapidly rises; the Ca^{2+} ions bind to troponin C (TnC) and activate actin-myosin cross-bridges. The resultant increase in external force develops over a slower time course than the rise in $[Ca^{2+}]_i$ (Figure 14-1, A).

Force development is slow because the activated contractile elements must first stretch **elastic elements,** and this process takes time. In skeletal muscle, force is not transmitted directly to the bones but must first stretch elastic elements (e.g., tendons) that are arranged in **series** with the contractile elements and bones. A major effect of the series elastic elements is to cause a delay between the activation of actin-myosin cross-bridges and the development of force by the muscle. The following

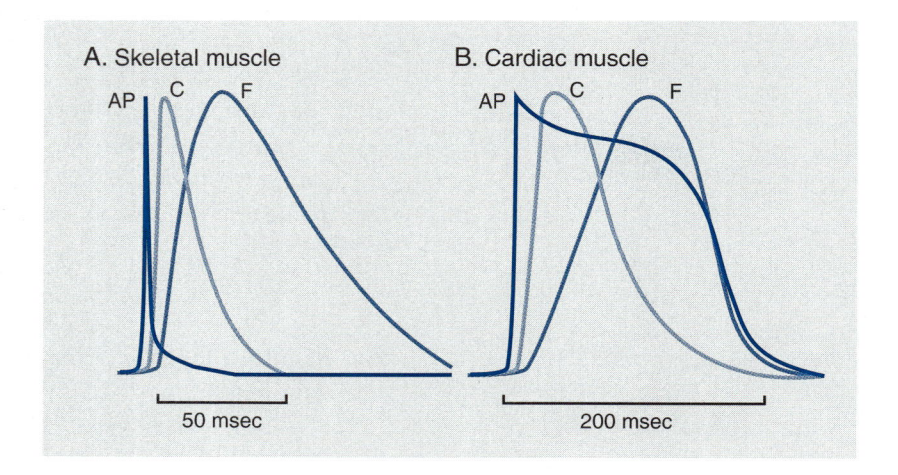

Figure 14-1 ■ Relative time course of the sarcolemmal action potential, average rise in $[Ca^{2+}]_i$ concentration, and force development in skeletal and cardiac muscle. A, A single stimulus applied to skeletal muscle evokes an action potential (*AP*), which causes Ca^{2+} to be released from the sarcoplasmic reticulum (see Chapter 13). $[Ca^{2+}]_i$ (*C*) rises rapidly after the action potential and reaches a level that saturates troponin C (TnC) binding sites, permitting actin-myosin cross-bridges to form. Because of the presence of elastic elements in the muscle, force development (*F*) occurs at a much slower rate than the rise in $[Ca^{2+}]_i$ and the subsequent activation of the contractile elements. B, Force (*F*), $[Ca^{2+}]_i$ (*C*), and action potential (*AP*) are shown for a single activation of cardiac muscle. The duration of the force transient is much longer than in skeletal muscle because Ca^{2+} channels remain open during the long-duration action potential, allowing prolonged Ca^{2+} entry to the cytoplasm. (A redrawn from Palade P, Vergara J: *J Gen Physiol* 79:679, 1982. B from Langer G, editor: *Calcium and the heart,* New York, 1990, Raven Press.)

Mechanics of Muscle Contraction

> **BOX 14-1**
>
> ### *A Mechanical Model of Muscle Includes a Spring in Series with the Contractile Elements*
>
> Skeletal muscle can be modeled as a system consisting of three mechanical components (Figure B-1). A viscous contractile element (CE) is in series with an elastic element (SE), represented by a spring. A parallel elastic element (PE) is in parallel with CE and SE. The series elastic element resides both in the tendons and in regions of the myosin molecules. The sarcolemma, intracellular components of the cytoarchitecture (e.g., titin), and extracellular connective tissue are part of the parallel elastic element. Several pieces of evidence support this model. The presence of a series elastic element explains the delay that occurs between the activation of the contractile elements and the development of external force: the series elastic element must be stretched before force can be applied to an external load. Furthermore, if a muscle is rapidly stretched immediately after stimulation and before it begins to develop tension, it develops more force than if it had not been stretched. The rapid stretch extends the series elastic element, so that the shortening of the contractile elements will pull on the external load sooner. When resting muscle is stretched to relatively long sarcomere lengths, the resting tension increases. This maintained resting tension is evidence of a parallel elastic element because without a parallel elastic element the nonelastic contractile elements would passively stretch and eliminate any steady-state tension.
>
> **Figure B-1** ■ Three-component mechanical model of skeletal muscle. A parallel elastic element is in parallel with a series combination of the contractile element and the series elastic elements. The elastic elements are modeled as springs, which develop tension when stretched according to the relationship $F = k \times \Delta x$, where F is the force, Δx is the change in length of the spring, and k is the spring constant. A stiffer, or stronger, spring has a larger spring constant. When the contractile element shortens, the series elastic element must be stretched before external force is developed. Resting tension is supported by the parallel elastic element alone because the contractile elements are not elastic.

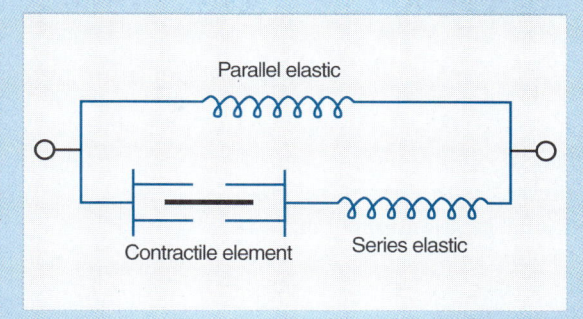

analogy helps to explain this effect: You hold in your hand a taut, but not stretched, rubber band that is attached to a weight resting on a table. As you raise your hand, the weight is not lifted immediately because the rubber band must first be stretched. As the rubber band is stretched (i.e., the length is increased), a force is developed in the rubber band, which pulls against the attached weight. The development of this force takes time, and the more elastic the rubber band, the longer the delay in lifting the weight (Box 14-1).

Sufficient Ca^{2+} is released by a single action potential to saturate all the TnC binding sites. These sites are saturated for only a brief time because $[Ca^{2+}]_i$ reaches a peak and then begins to fall rapidly as the Ca^{2+} is pumped back into the SR. Therefore the muscle does not develop its maximum *possible* force during a twitch because Ca^{2+} dissociates from TnC (as $[Ca^{2+}]_i$

declines) before the series elastic elements are completely stretched. If $[Ca^{2+}]_i$ remains elevated for a longer period, however, muscle force will continue to increase. This occurs physiologically if a second action potential is evoked before $[Ca^{2+}]_i$ has returned to the resting level. Note that contractile force can also be enhanced by increasing the amount of Ca^{2+} stored in the SR. This is an important mechanism for altering contractile force in the heart (see below), but not in skeletal muscle.

Repetitive Stimulation Produces Fused Contractions

The maximum force generated by skeletal muscle in response to two consecutive stimuli depends on the interval between the stimuli (Figure 14-2). If the two stimuli are separated by more than 100 msec, both stimuli produce twitch contractions (Figure 14-2, *A*). If the second stimulus is given before the first twitch relaxes completely, the force from the second twitch is added to the force from the first (Figure 14-2, *B*) and the resultant peak force is larger than the force generated by a single stimulus. This occurs because the second stimulus rereleases Ca^{2+} from the SR before all of the Ca^{2+} released by the first stimulus dissociates from TnC. Thus more TnC sites remain saturated for a longer period. This gives the contractile elements more time to stretch the series elastic elements and thus generate more external force. If the interval between the two stimuli is short enough, the second twitch becomes completely

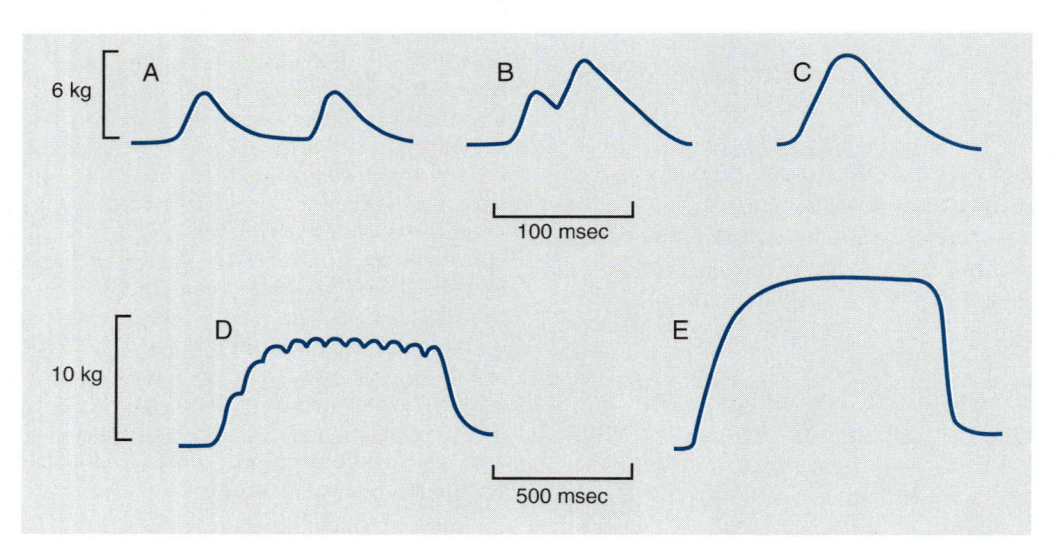

Figure 14-2 ■ Summation of force during high-frequency stimulation in mammalian gastrocnemius muscle. The force generated by a whole skeletal muscle in response to repetitive stimulation is shown. A, When a pair of stimuli is separated by about 100 msec, the muscle responds with two separate twitches of equal size. B, When the interval between the stimuli is reduced to about 50 msec, the force from the second twitch is added to the force from the first. C, With a short enough interval between stimuli, a single contraction with a smooth rising phase is generated. D, A train of stimuli at a rate of 24 per second generates a partial tetanus. E, A complete tetanus is generated by a stimulus frequency of 115 per second. The 100-msec time scale and 6-kg force scale apply to A, B, and C, and the 500-msec time scale and 10-kg force scale apply to D and E. (Redrawn from Coopers S, Eccles JC: *J Physiol* 69:377, 1930.)

Mechanics of Muscle Contraction

fused with the first, generating a single force transient with a smooth rising phase (Figure 14-2, *C*). If a train of stimuli is applied at a frequency of 20 to 40 per second, a partially fused contraction results (Figure 14-2, *D*). This is called a semifused tetanus, with the term **"tetanus"*** used to describe a relatively large contraction that results from a high-frequency train of action potentials in skeletal muscle. The tetanus becomes completely fused at higher rates of stimulation (80 to 100 stimuli per second; Figure 14-2, *E*). Thus force generation in skeletal muscle is regulated through two mechanisms: (1) control of the action potential frequency of the α motor neuron and (2) control of the number of α motor neurons (and consequently the number of motor units) activated.

■ SKELETAL MUSCLE MECHANICS IS CHARACTERIZED BY TWO FUNDAMENTAL RELATIONSHIPS

The mechanical properties of muscle can be characterized by two fundamental relationships: the **length-tension curve** and the **force-velocity relationship.** Note that the terms "tension" and "force" have the same meaning in muscle physiology and are used interchangeably. The experimental apparatus diagrammed in Figure 14-3 can be used to determine these relationships either for a single muscle fiber or for whole muscle. In this experimental setup, two important mechanical variables are measured as a function of time: contractile force and muscle length. The initial length of the muscle and the attached load can both be varied.

When muscle is activated and filaments begin to slide, two types of mechanical events can

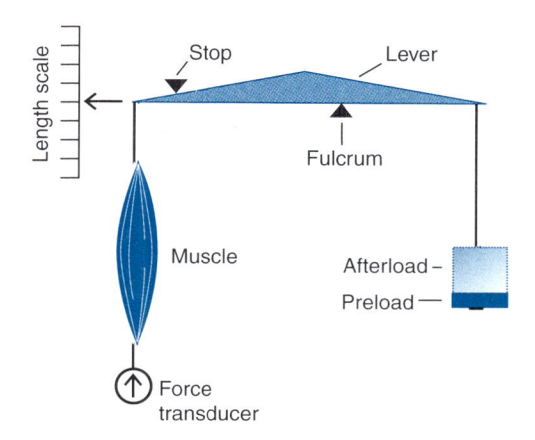

Figure 14-3 ■ **Apparatus used to study the mechanical properties of muscle. One end of an isolated muscle is attached to a force transducer, which measures total force. The other end is attached to a lever, which is used to measure shortening. Weights attached to the opposite end of the lever are used to set the initial muscle length and to provide loads against which the muscle will contract. Variations in the "preload" weight are used to adjust the initial muscle length. With the preload in place, a mechanical stop is adjusted to prevent further stretch of the muscle when the "afterload" is added. Before stimulation of the muscle the force transducer measures the passive force and the vertical position of the lever is a measure of the muscle length. On activation of the contractile machinery by stimulation, the muscle begins to develop active force. If the force developed by the muscle exceeds the force resulting from the attached load (preload plus afterload), the muscle will begin to shorten.**

occur. The muscle can generate force as it pulls on the tendons, or the muscle can shorten. If the force generated by the muscle is too small to lift the attached load, the muscle will not shorten (Figure 14-4, *A*). In this **isometric contraction** the muscle generates force at a *constant* length. The magnitude of the force varies with the length of the muscle in a manner that is charac-

---

*Tetanus toxin, from the bacterium *Clostridium tetani*, causes tetanic convulsions by blocking inhibitory synaptic receptors in the spinal cord. The resultant disinhibition greatly increases action potential frequency in α motor neurons.

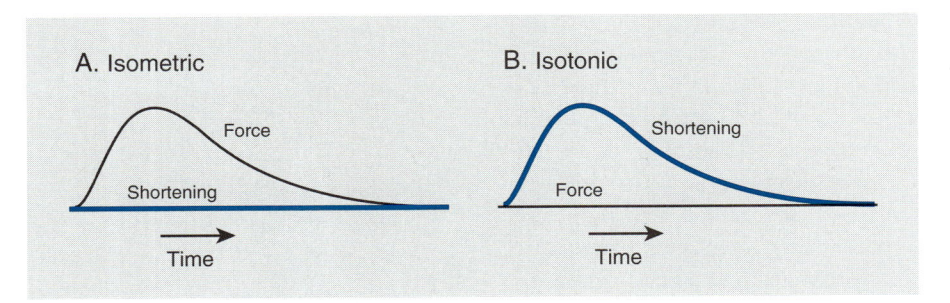

Figure 14-4 ■ Isometric and isotonic contractions. A, The maximum force generated by the muscle is not enough to lift the load. Thus no shortening occurs (*blue line*) and the muscle generates force (*black line*) at a constant length. This is an isometric contraction. B, With no load attached the muscle does not need to generate force to overcome a load and thus begins to shorten immediately. This is an isotonic contraction, which in general refers to a period of muscle shortening at constant force.

---

terized by the length-tension curve (Figure 14-5). If the muscle is activated with no weight attached, the contraction will result in shortening with no force generation (Figure 14-4, *B*). This is an example of an **isotonic contraction**, in which the muscle shortens while generating a constant amount of force. Macroscopic movement and force generation are the result of summing numerous molecular power strokes that are generated by interactions between individual actin and myosin molecules. The force and movement generated by a single actin-myosin cross-bridge have been measured (Box 14-2).

The Relationship Between Initial Muscle Length and Force Can Be Understood in Terms of the Sliding Filament Mechanism

The amount of force generated by skeletal muscle varies with the length to which a muscle is stretched. This fundamental property of muscle was studied by A.F. Huxley and colleagues, who varied the initial length of single muscle cells and measured the maximum isometric tetanic force generated by a muscle cell at fixed length. Some force (tension) is required to stretch relaxed muscle. The relationship between this **passive tension** and muscle length is shown in Figure 14-5. When the muscle is stimulated to contract, the total tension increases. The difference between the total tension generated by contracting muscle and the passive tension in relaxed muscle is the **active tension** (Figure 14-5). The active length-tension relationship demonstrates that there is an **optimal length** (L_0) at which tension is maximal. In skeletal muscle the range of optimal lengths is from 2.0 to 2.2 µm per sarcomere (Figure 14-5).

The active length-tension relationship can be understood in terms of the sliding filament mechanism. When the muscle is at a length of 2.0 to 2.2 µm per sarcomere, the active force is maximal (Figure 14-5, *B* and *C*). This sarcomere length corresponds to optimal overlap between thick and thin filaments. At this length, the maximum number of cross-bridges can form. As the muscle is stretched from 2.2 to 3.65 µm per sarcomere, the active force decreases because of the decreased overlap between thick and thin filaments (Figure 14-5, *A* and *B*). As a result, fewer cross-bridges can form on activation and therefore the maximum tetanic force at that

Mechanics of Muscle Contraction

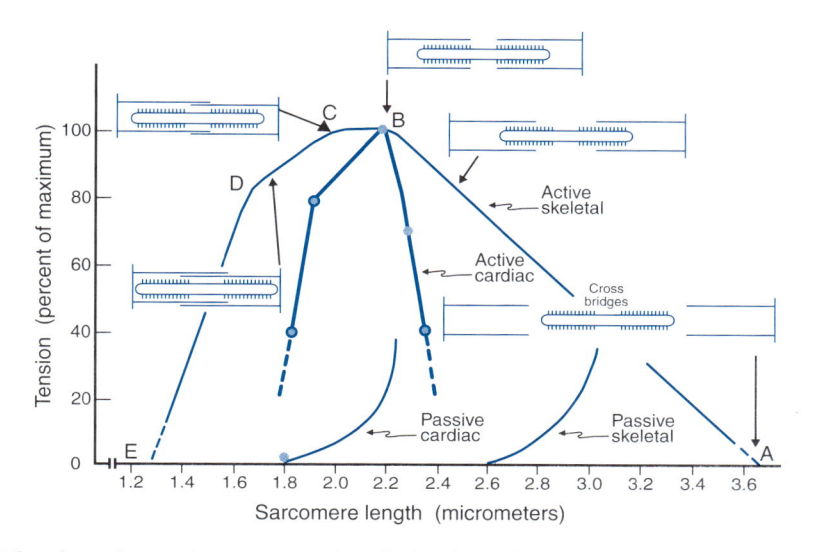

Figure 14-5 ■ The length-tension curves in skeletal and cardiac muscle are similar. Actively developed isometric tension and passive, resting tension are plotted as a function of sarcomere length for skeletal and cardiac muscle. The diagrams of the myofilaments show the extent of overlap between thick and thin filaments at five specific sarcomere lengths in skeletal muscle. In skeletal muscle, maximum tension occurs at sarcomere lengths between 2.0 and 2.2 μm (between points *B* and *C*). Tension decreases between 2.2 and 3.65 μm of sarcomere length (between points *A* and *B*) because there is a decrease in the overlap between thick and thin filaments. Tension decreases below 2.0 μm sarcomere length, in part because of a double overlap of thin filaments (between points *C* and *D*). In cardiac muscle, active tension falls steeply with sarcomere lengths greater or less than 2.2 μm. The increase in passive tension occurs at much shorter sarcomere lengths in cardiac muscle than in skeletal muscle. (Redrawn from Gordon AM, Huxley AF, Julian FJ: *J Physiol* 184:143, 1966; and Braunwald E, Ross J Jr, Sonnenblick EH: *Mechanisms of contraction of the normal and failing heart*, Boston, 1976, Little, Brown.)

---

length is reduced. At sarcomere lengths less than 2.0 μm, force declines for at least two reasons (Figure 14-5, *C* to *E*). A double overlap of thin filaments is present, which allows cross-bridges to form in the wrong orientation, and filament geometry may be disrupted as thick filaments hit the Z line and actin filaments are forced to move away from the thick filaments.

Thus the shape of the active length-tension relationship is precisely predicted by the sliding filament model of contraction. This result leads to the important conclusion that *the active force generated by a muscle is proportional to the number of attached cross-bridges*.

The Velocity of Shortening Decreases as Force Increases in Isotonic Contractions

The force-velocity relationship for a given muscle can also be determined by use of the apparatus shown in Figure 14-3. The force of contraction and the length changes are measured during contractions with different weights attached. When the muscle generates sufficient force to lift the weight, a partly

> **BOX 14-2**
>
> ### The Force and Displacement Generated by a Single Actin-Myosin Interaction Can Be Measured with an Optical "Trap"
>
> In the optical "trap" experimental technique, myosin molecules are bound to a small silica bead, which is then fixed to a glass coverslip. A single actin filament is attached at each end to a plastic bead. The bead is held in place, or trapped, at the focal point of a laser. The operator can move the bead by moving the laser focal point and can change the force with which the bead is held in place by varying the intensity of the laser. Thus the position of the actin filament and the force with which it is held in place can be varied. The actin filament is moved close to the myosin-coated bead, permitting single actin-myosin interactions to occur. When the actin filament is allowed to move freely during a single cross-bridge cycle, the displacement generated by that single interaction is about 10 nm (nm = 10^{-9} m). If the actin filament is prevented from moving by continuous variation of the laser intensity, the isometric force generated by a single cross-bridge can be shown to be about 5×10^{-12} Newtons. (The Newton is a unit of force and is equal to 1 kg $\times$ m/sec^2. If a 1-Newton force is applied to a 1-kg mass, it would impart an acceleration of 1 m/sec^2.)

isometric, partly isotonic contraction occurs (Figure 14-6). After activation the muscle begins to develop force isometrically until the muscle force is equal to the force required to lift the attached weight. At that point, force development stops and the muscle begins to shorten isotonically. With a small weight attached, the velocity of shortening (i.e., the rate of change of muscle length with time) is relatively fast (Figure 14-6). With a larger weight attached, more time is spent developing force, leaving less time for isotonic shortening. As a result, the velocity of shortening is slower. The overall force-velocity relationship, which is constructed by measuring a series of contractions against different loads, is shown in Figure 14-7. The maximum velocity of shortening (V_0) occurs with no load.

At the molecular level the rate of muscle shortening reflects the rate of cross-bridge cycling. Thus V_0 is a reflection of the maximum rate of cross-bridge cycling. Cross-bridge cycling requires myosin ATPase activity (see Chapter 12); therefore V_0 is also directly proportional to the myosin ATPase activity. The inverse relationship between load and shortening velocity can be understood with the help of Figure 14-8. Shortening is caused by rotation of the myosin head; the force generated by this rotation is opposed by the load. If the load is relatively small, myosin head rotation meets little resistance and occurs at a relatively high rate. In addition, many myosin heads are unattached and available for cycling. Together, these factors produce a relatively fast shortening velocity. In contrast, if the load is large, head rotation meets stiff opposition and the rotation speed is slow. Furthermore, many more cross-bridges are attached in this case and fewer are available for recycling. Thus shortening velocity is slow.

■ THERE ARE THREE MAIN TYPES OF PHASIC SKELETAL MUSCLE MOTOR UNITS

The main criteria used to classify motor units are speed of contraction and susceptibility to fatigue. Three main motor unit types have been described: **type FF (fast-twitch, fatigable), FR (fast-twitch, fatigue-resistant),** and **S (slow-twitch, fatigue-resistant).** Both FF and FR

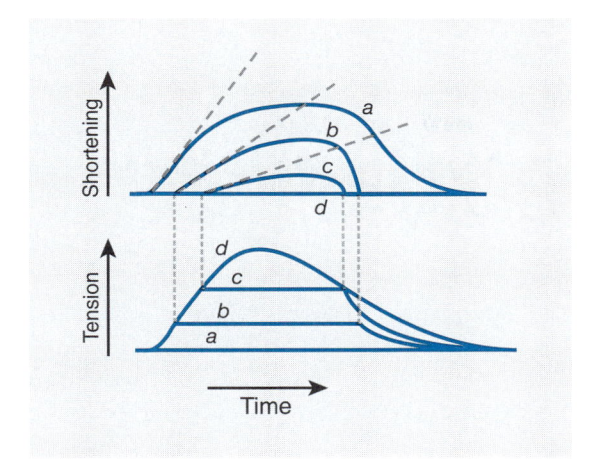

Figure 14-6 ■ Partly isometric, partly isotonic contractions. When a contracting muscle can generate enough force to lift an attached load, the contraction has an isometric component and an isotonic component. This figure shows superimposed traces of four contractions of skeletal muscle obtained with the apparatus shown in Figure 14-3. In the presence of an afterload, upon stimulation the muscle begins to develop tension isometrically *(lower traces)*. When the muscle tension exceeds the attached load, tension remains constant and the muscle starts to shorten isotonically *(upper traces)*. The maximum velocity of shortening is measured from the slope of a line *(dashed line)* that is tangent to the shortening curve just after shortening has begun. The maximum velocity of shortening is fastest with no load and becomes smaller as the load is increased.

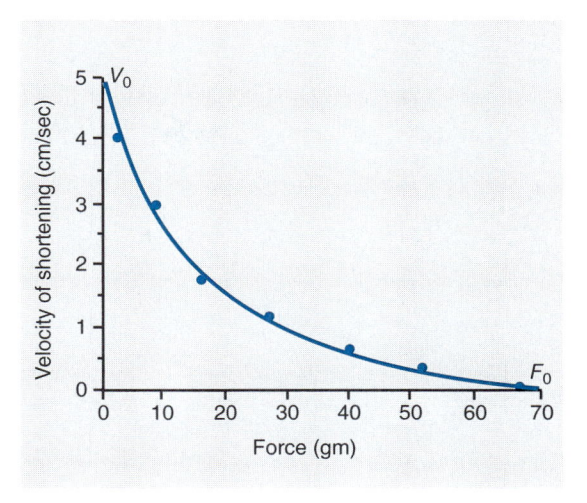

Figure 14-7 ■ The force-velocity relationship in skeletal muscle. The velocity of shortening during an isotonic contraction is plotted as a function of the force generated by the muscle during the isotonic shortening. The maximum velocity of shortening (V_0) occurs with no load (this would be an isotonic contraction). When the attached load is equal to the maximum force produced by the muscle (F_0), the muscle does not shorten (this would be an isometric contraction). (Redrawn from Hill AV: *Proc R Soc Lond B* 126:136, 1938.)

motor units have twitch contraction times (time to peak twitch force) of 10 to 40 msec, whereas S units take from 60 to over 100 msec to develop peak twitch force. The contraction time is directly related to the myosin ATPase activity. The myosin isoforms present in FF and FR muscle fibers have a higher ATPase activity than the isoform present in S fibers. FF motor units generate the largest tetanic forces; S motor units generate the smallest forces; and FR motor units are intermediate. Several factors contribute to the variation in force output across motor unit types. These include the *innervation ratio* (i.e., the number of muscle fibers innervated by the motor neuron) and the force output of individual muscle fibers, which depends in part on the average cross-sectional area of the individual muscle fibers.

The response of the different types of motor units to repetitive tetanic stimulations is shown in Figure 14-9. The decrease in force that occurs with repetitive trains of tetanic stimuli is called **fatigue.** This property can be quantitated with the *fatigue index,* which is defined as the ratio of the tetanic force after 2 minutes of repetitive

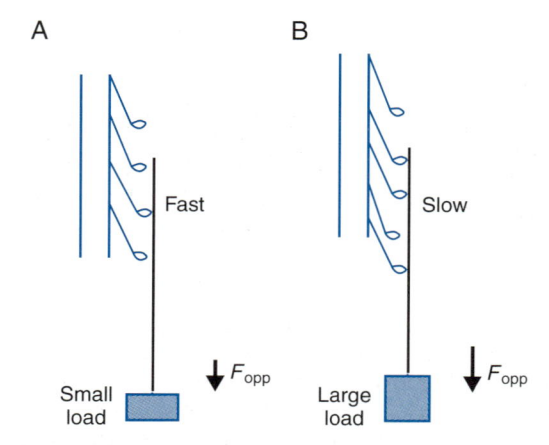

Figure 14-8 ■ Myosin head rotation occurs at a slower rate with a larger load attached to the muscle. The load attached to an isotonically contracting muscle represents a force (F_{opp}) that opposes myosin head rotation. **A**, When the muscle is contracting isotonically against a small load, many cross-bridges are unattached and available for cycling. Myosin head rotation occurs rapidly because little resistance is present. **B**, At larger loads, head rotation is slower because the opposing force is larger. (Redrawn from Berne RM, Levy MN, Koeppen BM, Stanton BA, editors: *Physiology*, ed 4, St Louis, 1998, Mosby.)

stimulation to the force generated by the first tetanus. The fatigue index of FF motor units is typically less than 0.25, whereas in FR and S motor units it is greater than 0.75. Although fatigue is a well-characterized phenomenon, the underlying cellular mechanisms remain obscure.

Whole muscle usually contains mixtures of the three types of motor units. For example, the medial gastrocnemius (calf) muscle of the cat contains FF, FR, and S motor units. The recruitment order of these motor units follows the "size principle": the motor units that generate the smallest force are recruited first, followed by larger and larger motor units as the requirement for additional force increases. This size-ordered recruitment confers certain mechanical advantages on the operation of the whole muscle (Box 14-3).

■ THE FORCE GENERATED BY CARDIAC MUSCLE IS REGULATED BY VARIOUS MECHANISMS THAT CONTROL $[Ca^{2+}]_i$

Cardiac Muscle Generates Long-Duration Contractions

The contraction of cardiac muscle is initiated by an action potential that ultimately causes Ca^{2+} to be released from the SR (see Chapter 13). A comparison of the time course of the action potential, changes in $[Ca^{2+}]_i$, and force development in cardiac muscle is shown in Figure 14-1, *B*. One of the obvious differences between the cardiac muscle force transient (Figure 14-1, *B*) and the skeletal muscle twitch contraction (Figure 14-1, *A*) is the longer duration of the cardiac contraction. In the heart, Ca^{2+} release from the SR is triggered by Ca^{2+} entry through voltage-gated Ca^{2+} channels that open during the action potential (see Chapter 13). Prolonged Ca^{2+} entry during the long-duration cardiac action potential causes $[Ca^{2+}]_i$ to be elevated for a relatively long time compared with skeletal muscle, resulting in a longer contraction.

Contractions in healthy cardiac muscle are always of the "twitch-type," such as the one shown in Figure 14-1, *B*. The summation of twitch forces with repetitive stimulation that occurs during a tetanus in skeletal muscle cannot occur in the heart. The reason is that the cardiac action potential has approximately the same duration as the force transient (Figure 14-1, *B*). Thus, even at the shortest possible interval between cardiac action potentials, the force transient from the first action potential has returned to the resting level and summation cannot occur. This behavior and the electrical communication between cardiac myocytes through gap junctions are crucial in enabling the coordinated constriction

Mechanics of Muscle Contraction

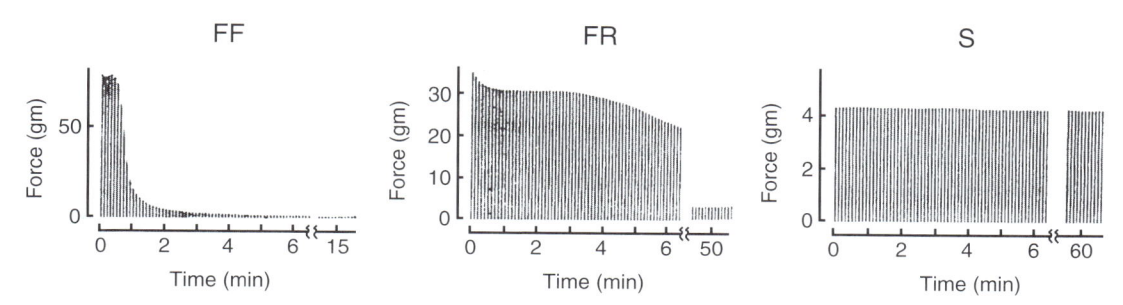

Figure 14-9 ■ Response of fast-twitch, fatigable (FF); fast-twitch, fatigue-resistant (FR); and slow (S) motor units to repetitive tetanic stimulations. Individual motor neurons were stimulated at a rate of 40 pulses per second for 330 msec to produce a tetanic contraction in a single motor unit, and the tetanic stimulation was repeated every second for up to 60 minutes. This figure shows the change in tetanic force during these repetitive tetanic stimulations. In FF motor units the tetanic force decreases rapidly: after 1 minute the force has dropped to 25% of its initial value. Tetanic force declines much more slowly in FR motor units: after 5 minutes of stimulation, the force has dropped only 30%. These motor units do eventually fatigue, and after 50 minutes of stimulation the force is a low percentage of its initial value. In contrast, the tetanic force in S motor units does not decrease even after 60 minutes of stimulation. Note that FF units generate the greatest force but are the most easily fatigable. In contrast, S units generate the smallest force but are essentially completely fatigue resistant. (From Burke RE, Levine DN, Tsairis P, Zajac FE: *J Physiol* 234:723, 1973.)

The Total Force Developed by Cardiac Muscle Is Related to the Level of [Ca^{2+}]$_i$ Attained During Activation

The force of contraction of cardiac muscle can be altered by numerous factors that are both intrinsic and extrinsic to the cardiac muscle cell. The major intrinsic factor is the length-tension relationship, which is described in the next section. Many extrinsic factors affect cardiac contractility by altering [Ca^{2+}]$_i$. For example, β-adrenergic agonists increase the inward Ca^{2+} current and thus increase cardiac contractility (see Chapter 8). This is referred to as a **positive inotropic effect**.* L-type Ca^{2+} channel blockers (see Chapter 8) reduce Ca^{2+} entry and thus decrease contractility (a negative inotropic effect). Cardiac glycosides reduce the Na$^+$ gradient, which reduces Ca^{2+} extrusion via the Na$^+$/Ca^{2+} exchanger and thereby increases [Ca^{2+}]$_{SR}$ (see Chapter 11). Activation then results in higher [Ca^{2+}]$_i$ and enhanced contractility (a positive inotropic effect).

■ THE MECHANICAL PROPERTIES OF CARDIAC AND SKELETAL MUSCLE ARE SIMILAR, BUT THERE ARE SIGNIFICANT QUANTITATIVE DIFFERENCES

Isolated Cardiac Muscle and Skeletal Muscle Have Similar Length-Tension Relationships

The length-tension relationship in isolated cardiac muscle is similar to that observed in skeletal muscle (Figure 14-5). The active isometric force is maximal when the initial sarcomere length is

---

*In the heart, an inotropic effect is a change in contractility, whereas a chronotropic effect is a change in heart rate.

BOX 14-3

Size-Ordered Recruitment of Motor Units Provides Mechanical Advantages in the Operation of Whole Muscle

The medial gastrocnemius (calf) muscle in the cat is a mixture of fast-twitch, fatigable (FF); fast-twitch, fatigue-resistant (FR); and slow (S) motor units. Ordered motor unit recruitment occurs strictly by the size of the force generated by each motor unit; a nonlinear relationship exists between total muscle force and the fraction of motor units activated (Figure B-1). The first units to be recruited are type S, which generate small, slow contractions and are fatigue resistant. These mechanical properties are advantageous during sustained activity at low force levels, such as maintaining posture. If an action requires more force, FR units are recruited next. FR motor units contract quickly, generate moderate force, and are relatively resistant to fatigue. These properties are advantageous for a sustained activity requiring moderate force, such as running. Together, FR and S motor units constitute 60% of the pool but generate only about 25% of the maximum force. Larger forces require activation of FF motor units. These motor units generate large forces rapidly, but they fatigue quickly and are used infrequently. They are recruited when a short burst of strenuous activity is required, as in galloping or jumping.

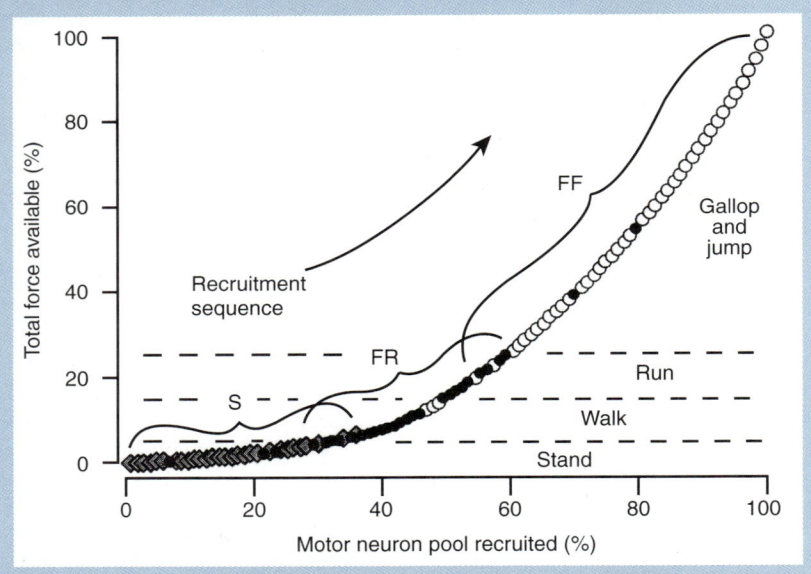

Figure B-1 ■ Size-ordered recruitment of motor units in the gastrocnemius muscle. The total force available from the medial gastrocnemius muscle (the chief muscle of the calf of the leg) is plotted as a function of the percentage of the motor neuron pool recruited under the assumption that the order of recruitment is strictly by size. The initial 30% of the pool is dominated by type S (slow) units, the next 30% is dominated by FR (fast-twitch, fatigue-resistant) units, and the final 40% is dominated by FF (fast-twitch, fatigable) units. The diamonds, filled circles, and open circles represent S, FR, and FF motor units, respectively. (From Karpati G, Hilton-Jones D, Griggs RC, editors: *Disorders of voluntary muscle,* Cambridge, Eng, 2001, Cambridge University Press.)

Mechanics of Muscle Contraction

~2.2 μm. At this sarcomere length in cardiac muscle the overlap of thick and thin filaments is optimal, which enables the maximum number of cross-bridges to form. As in skeletal muscle, the active force decreases at both longer and shorter sarcomere lengths.

Although the length-tension relationships in skeletal and cardiac muscle are similar, there are at least two important differences. In cardiac muscle, changes in filament overlap account only partly for the changes in active tension that occur with changes in sarcomere length. At muscle lengths below L_0 (i.e., the ascending limb of the length-tension curve), an increase in muscle length increases the Ca^{2+} sensitivity of the myofilaments, which partially accounts for the increase in active tension. The second difference between skeletal and cardiac muscle is related to the passive tension. Cardiac muscle is stiffer than skeletal muscle. Thus, when cardiac muscle is passively stretched beyond L_0, the passive tension increases to high levels (Figure 14-5). This prevents sarcomere length from exceeding about 2.3 μm and prevents the decreased overlap of thick and thin filaments that would otherwise occur at longer sarcomere lengths. Consequently, healthy cardiac muscle functions almost exclusively on the ascending limb of the length-tension curve.

The Force of Contraction of the Intact Heart Varies as a Function of Its Initial (End-Diastolic) Volume

The length-tension relationship observed in isolated cardiac muscle also applies to cardiac muscle fibers in the intact heart. The relationship between ventricular pressure (which is a direct function of the force generated by ventricular myocytes) and the ventricular end-diastolic volume (which is a measure of the initial length of the myocyte) is shown in Figure 14-10. The curve labeled *Diastole* shows the relationship between the ventricular pressure

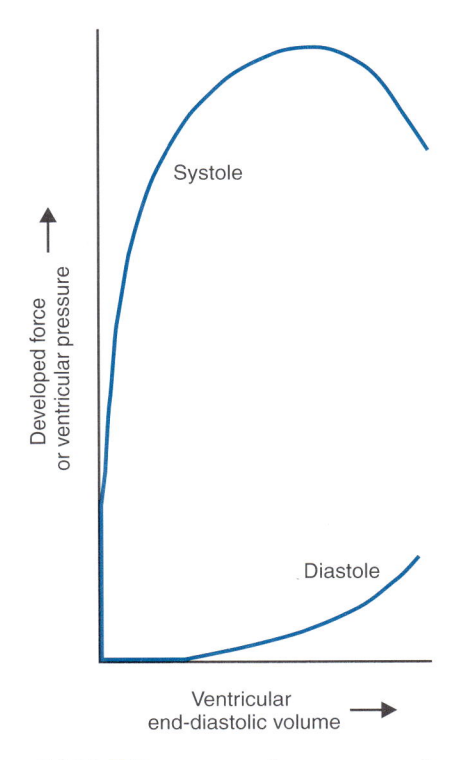

Figure 14-10 ■ Pressure-volume curve in the heart. The curve labeled *Diastole* shows the relationship between the ventricular pressure and the ventricular volume in a relaxed heart (i.e., during diastole). The curve labeled *Systole* shows the relationship between peak systolic ventricular pressure during contraction as a function of end-diastolic volume. (From Berne RM, Levy MN, Koeppen BM, Stanton BA, editors: *Physiology*, ed 4, St Louis, 1998, Mosby.)

and the intraventricular volume in a relaxed heart (i.e., during diastole). This is analogous to the passive length-tension curve in isolated cardiac muscle (Figure 14-5). The curve labeled *Systole* shows the maximum pressure developed by the ventricle during contraction (systole) for each level of filling. This is the **Frank-Starling relationship,** which is analogous to the active length-tension relationship of isolated cardiac muscle (Figure 14-5). One of the important features of this relationship, in terms of cardiac performance, is that an increase in ventricular filling pressure (i.e., passive tension) will increase the end-diastolic volume of the ventricle and thereby increase cardiac output (Berne and Levy, 2001). The normal heart operates on the ascending limb of the Frank-Starling relationship (Figure 14-10), which corresponds to the ascending limb of the active length-tension relationship (Figure 14-5).

The Velocity of Shortening in Cardiac Muscle Is Slower Than in Skeletal Muscle

The maximum velocity of shortening during isotonic contractions in cardiac muscle occurs at zero load, as in skeletal muscle. As the load increases, the shortening velocity decreases until a load is reached at which the muscle can no longer shorten and the contraction is isometric (Figure 14-11). Although the shape of the curve is similar to that for skeletal muscle (Figure 14-7), the maximum velocity of shortening (V_0) is slower in cardiac muscle. In cardiac muscle a positive inotropic intervention, such as stimulation of β-adrenergic receptors with norepinephrine, increases the velocity of shortening at all loads and increases the isometric contraction force (Figure 14-11).

■ THE DYNAMIC PROPERTIES OF SMOOTH MUSCLE CONTRACTION DIFFER MARKEDLY FROM THOSE OF SKELETAL AND CARDIAC MUSCLE

Three Key Relationships Can Be Used to Define the Kinetic Properties of Smooth Muscle Function

In smooth muscle, as in skeletal and cardiac muscles, many critical aspects of contractile function can be described by the three relationships mentioned previously: the temporal sequence that relates cell activation to $[Ca^{2+}]_i$ elevation and force development, the force-velocity relationship, and the length-tension

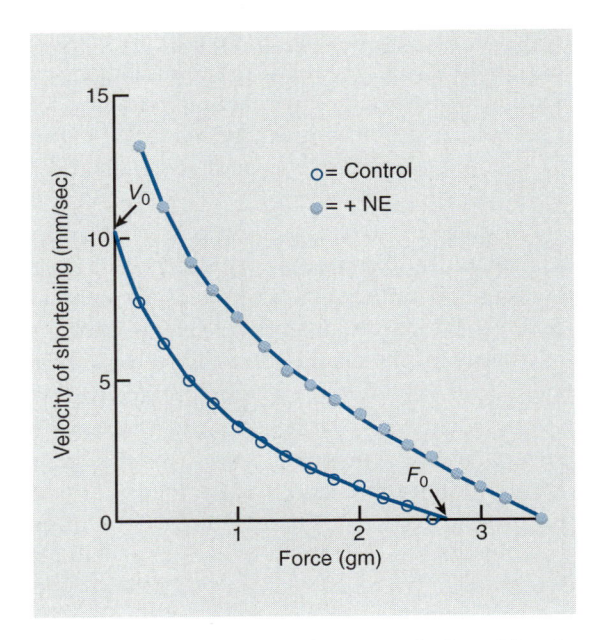

Figure 14-11 ■ Force-velocity relationship in cardiac muscle. The velocity of shortening during isotonic contractions in isolated cardiac muscle decreases as the load force increases. The addition of norepinephrine (+*NE*) increases the velocity of shortening at all loads. (From Braunwald E, Ross J Jr, Sonnenblick EH: *Mechanisms of contraction of the normal and failing heart*, Boston, 1976, Little, Brown.)

relationship. Nevertheless, some key quantitative differences in these relationships distinguish smooth muscles from skeletal and cardiac muscles.

The Length-Tension Relationship in Smooth Muscles Is Consistent with the Sliding Filament Mechanism of Contraction

As in skeletal muscle, there is an optimal "resting" length (L_0) at which the greatest amount of active force can be developed (Figure 14-12). When smooth muscles are stretched beyond this optimal length, the maximum active

Mechanics of Muscle Contraction

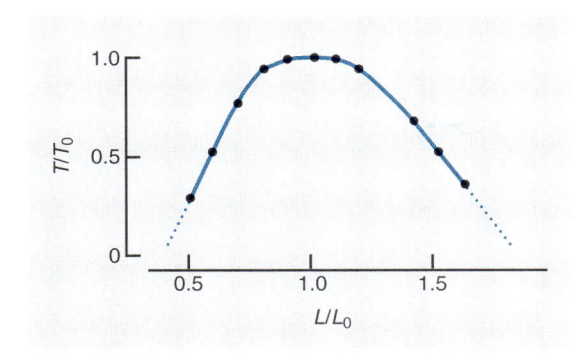

Figure 14-12 ■ The smooth muscle length-tension curve for a rat small mesenteric artery. The length (L) refers to the internal circumference of the artery. L_0 is the length at which maximum active tension is developed. T is the tension (force) at any length, and T_0 is maximum tension developed at the optimal length (L_0). (Modified from Mulvany MJ, Warshaw DM: *J Gen Physiol* 74:85, 1979.)

force that can be developed declines. When smooth muscles are permitted to shorten to less than the optimal length, the maximum developed tension also declines (Figure 14-12). (Note that for smooth muscle, the term "stress" rather than "force" is often used, where **Stress = Force/Cross-sectional area.**)

The shape of the smooth muscle length-tension relationship, as well as its similarity to that of skeletal muscle (Figure 14-5), implies that the sliding filament mechanism of muscle contraction also applies to smooth muscle. For several reasons, however, the smooth muscle length-tension relationship cannot be correlated directly with sarcomere length, as it is in skeletal muscle (Figure 14-5). First, as noted in Chapter 12, the myofibrils and thus the sarcomeres are not all arrayed in parallel and in register in smooth muscle. Therefore the type of experiment used to demonstrate the relationship between sarcomere length and tension development in skeletal muscle (Figure 14-3) cannot be performed in comparable fashion in smooth muscle. Second, as discussed in Chapter 12, smooth muscle contractile force can be altered by an increase or decrease in the Ca^{2+} sensitivity of the contractile apparatus without a change in $[Ca^{2+}]_i$ or myosin light chain (MLC) phosphorylation. Third, the ability of smooth muscle cells to generate *tonic* force and to adapt to various "initial" lengths complicates the effort to correlate active tension with smooth muscle "sarcomere" length in a manner that is implied by the length-tension relationship.

Studies at the molecular level, which are not subject to the complications just described, reveal that smooth muscle actin-myosin interactions are similar to those in skeletal muscle. With phosphorylated smooth muscle myosin molecules (the molecular motors) tethered to a synthetic support (e.g., a tiny bead), single actin filaments can be moved along the myosin heads as a result of ATP-dependent actin attachment-displacement-detachment cycles (see Figure 12-9). Thus there is no doubt that the basis of force development in smooth muscle, as in skeletal muscle, is the sliding of thin actin filaments along the thick myosin filaments.

The Velocity of Shortening Is Much Lower in Smooth Muscle Than in Skeletal Muscle

Despite the similarity in the mechanisms of force generation in smooth muscle and skeletal muscle, some critical kinetic differences exist. This is exemplified by the force-velocity relationship illustrated in Figure 14-13. The shapes of the skeletal and smooth muscle curves are similar (Figure 14-13, *A* and *B*). However, over the entire range of forces, from zero force (i.e., $F = 0$, so that the muscle shortens when there is no load) to maximal force (just sufficient to prevent shortening at $F = F_0$), the velocity of contraction of tonic smooth muscle is less than one tenth that of skeletal muscle. This is true even when the smooth muscle MLC is maximally phosphorylated. Recall that phosphorylation of

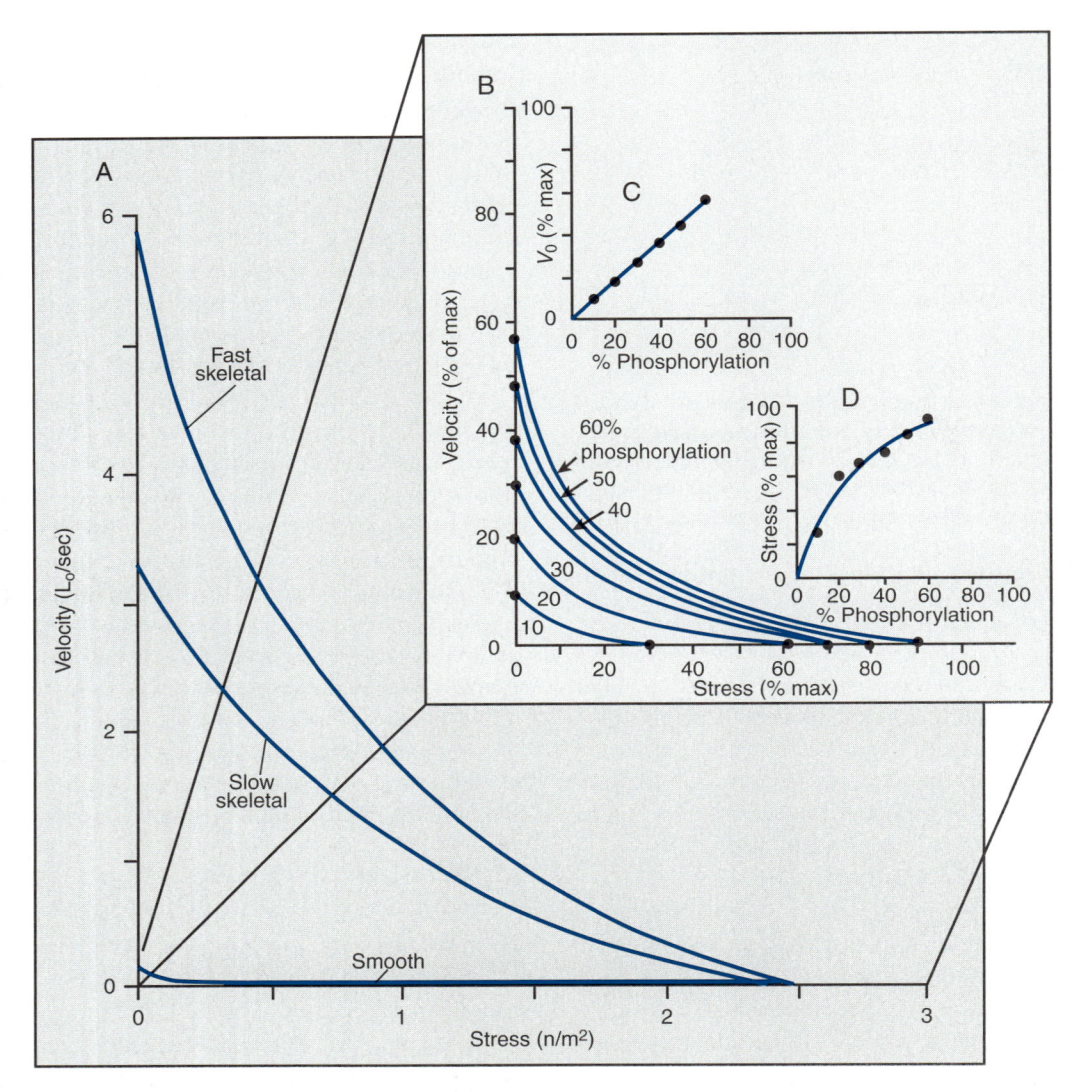

Figure 14-13 ■ Smooth muscle stress-velocity relationship; comparison with skeletal muscle. A, Relationship between the shortening velocity (in muscle lengths per second [L_0/sec]) and stress (in Newtons/m²) for human fast and slow skeletal muscles and smooth muscle. B, Shortening velocity is expressed as a percent of the maximum unloaded shortening velocity (i.e., stress = 0). Note that the shape of the curve is similar to those for skeletal muscle in A. C, Relationship between the percentage of myosin light chain (MLC) phosphorylation and the unloaded shortening velocity, V_0 (i.e., the ordinate intercepts in B). D, Relationship between the percentage of MLC phosphorylation and the percentage of maximal developed stress (i.e., the *X*-intercepts in graph B). (Redrawn from Berne RM, Levy MN, editors: *Principles of physiology,* St Louis, 1990, Mosby.)

Mechanics of Muscle Contraction

MLC is the "switch" that activates contraction of smooth muscles (see Chapter 12).

When smooth muscle cells are maximally activated and $[Ca^{2+}]_i$ is maximally elevated, about 60% of the MLC is phosphorylated. This level of phosphorylation is associated with maximal steady force development (Figure 14-13, D). Interestingly, smooth muscles and skeletal muscles generate about the same amount of maximal active force per unit cross-sectional area (i.e., stress). This seems surprising in view of the large difference in shortening velocities and the fact that smooth muscles contain only about one fifth as much myosin as do skeletal muscles. How can these latter observations be explained? One possibility is that the smooth muscle myosin motor might generate much more force than can the myosin motor of skeletal muscle. Alternatively, the explanation may lie in the structural arrangement of the contractile apparatus. These ideas are explored in subsequent sections.

■ SOME PROPERTIES OF SPECIFIC TYPES OF SMOOTH MUSCLES CAN BE RESOLVED BY A STUDY OF INDIVIDUAL MYOSIN MOTORS

Analysis of Single Actin and Myosin Molecule Interactions Has Resolved the Question of How Smooth and Skeletal Muscles Generate the Same Amount of Stress Despite Very Different Shortening Velocities

Formation of a single actin-myosin cross-bridge leads to a **unitary displacement step** of the actin by ~5 nm (1 nm = 10^{-9} m) along either skeletal muscle myosin or smooth muscle myosin. In other words, the unitary displacement step is the same length in both types of muscle. At the molecular level, shortening (i.e., filament sliding) velocity is defined as the length of the unitary displacement step (d) divided by the length of time (t_s) that the myosin head remains attached to actin (see Figure 14-16); that is, velocity = d/t_s. Thus, with identical unitary displacement steps, the lower shortening velocity of smooth muscle than skeletal muscle (Figure 14-13, A) appears to be due to differences in the *step duration*: t_s is much longer in smooth muscle.

The force that a muscle produces under isometric conditions can also be described at the molecular level. This force is related to both the **unitary force** (F_{uni}; see Figure 14-16) generated by a single actin-myosin cross-bridge and its **duty cycle ratio**, where this ratio (t_s/t_{cycle}) is defined as the fraction of the total cross-bridge cycle time (t_{cycle}; see Figure 14-16) that myosin is attached to actin and generating force (t_s). Interestingly, both skeletal and smooth muscle myosins are able to generate similar unitary force per attached cross-bridge (~1 to 3 × 10^{-12} Newtons; see Box 14-2). In contrast, the duty cycle ratio (see Figure 14-16) for tonic smooth muscle myosin is 4-fold greater than in skeletal muscle. This difference in the duty cycle ratio of the actin-myosin interaction appears to account for the ability of smooth muscle to generate comparable stress to skeletal muscle despite having only one fifth as much myosin. Smooth muscle's lower shortening velocity and enhanced force generation (per mole of myosin) are therefore due to differences in the kinetics of the cross-bridge cycle. The rate-limiting transition step in the cross-bridge cycle is the cross-bridge detachment (i.e., the rate at which the myosin head detaches from actin): the slower the detachment, the slower the filament sliding (and contraction). This influences both shortening velocity and force generation. The slower detachment rate in smooth muscle also contributes to smooth muscle's high duty cycle ratio. This results in a larger fraction of smooth muscle than skeletal muscle myosin heads being attached to actin and generating force at any moment in time.

> **BOX 14-4**
>
> ### Myosin Isoform Expression Determines the Rate of Cross-Bridge Cycling
>
> Comparisons between tonic and phasic smooth muscles reveal that tonic smooth muscle cells express higher levels of LC17a, the acidic isoform of the 17-kiloDalton (kDa) essential myosin light chain (MLC). A single gene encodes the smooth muscle myosin heavy chain (MHC), but alternative splicing at the N-terminal (SM-A, SM-B) results in the expression of two variants. Tonic smooth muscles express higher levels of the MHC isoform that lacks a seven–amino acid insert (SM-A) in the N-terminal myosin motor domain. Conversely, phasic smooth muscles express the MHC that contains the seven–amino acid insert (SM-B). The cross-bridge cycling rates are slower in myosins in which the SM-A isoforms are expressed. For example, studies of single myosin molecular motors reveal that the average cross-bridge attachment time is twice as long in myosins that contain the SM-A isoform as in those that contain the SM-B isoform.

The Kinetic Properties of the Cross-Bridge Cycle Depend Largely on the Myosin Isoforms Expressed in the Cells

The more rapid shortening velocity of **phasic** (e.g., esophageal) **smooth muscle**, as compared with **tonic** (e.g., vascular) **smooth muscle**, can be explained by a seven–amino acid insert in the myosin heavy chain (Box 14-4). This influences the rate of cross-bridge cycling.

Pathological conditions (or even the "normal" aging process) may alter myosin isoform expression and thus the kinetic properties of smooth muscles. For example, obstruction of the urethra, as may occur in benign prostatic hypertrophy (BPH; Box 14-5), causes a slowing of urinary bladder smooth muscle contraction and incomplete emptying of the urinary bladder. These effects of urinary tract obstruction may be attributed to a change in myosin heavy chain isoform expression in the bladder smooth muscle, as well as to bladder tissue hyperplasia (increase in tissue mass as a result of an increase in cell number) (Box 14-5).

Myosin Light Chain Phosphorylation Determines the Velocity of Smooth Muscle Shortening and the Amount of Stress Generated

In view of the key role of MLC phosphorylation in the activation of smooth muscle contraction (see Figure 12-12), it is not surprising that the velocity of shortening is directly proportional to the extent of MLC phosphorylation (Figure 14-13, C). The shortening velocity in the absence of a load (Force = 0) is, in fact, a measure of the maximal rate of cross-bridge cycling.

The amount of stress that can be generated is also a function of the level of MLC phosphorylation (Figure 14-13, D). Indeed, the stress provides a measure of the number of attached actin-myosin cross-bridges. The maximum number of cross-bridges is formed under isometric conditions, when maximum stress is developed. Thus, as in skeletal muscle, smooth muscle shortening velocity is determined by the rate of cross-bridge cycling and stress is a function of the number of attached cross-bridges. In smooth muscles but not skeletal muscles, however, both the cross-bridge cycling rate and the number of attached cross-bridges depend on MLC phosphorylation.

■ THE RELATIONSHIP AMONG $[Ca^{2+}]_i$, MYOSIN PHOSPHORYLATION, AND LIGHT CHAIN FORCE IN SMOOTH MUSCLES IS COMPLEX

The time courses of changes in $[Ca^{2+}]_i$, MLC phosphorylation, and mechanical force in a tonic smooth muscle during brief and sustained stimulation are compared in Figure 14-14. The response of the smooth muscle to a brief stimulation is similar to that of skeletal muscle

BOX 14-5

Prostate Gland Hypertrophy Obstructs Urine Outflow from the Urinary Bladder and Induces a Change in the Expression of Myosin Isoform in Bladder Smooth Muscle

A common form of urinary bladder outflow obstruction is observed in older men as a result of the age-related progressive enlargement of the prostate gland that surrounds the urethra. This condition, benign prostatic hypertrophy (BPH), is actually neither benign nor a hypertrophy (cell enlargement). The prostate enlargement is due primarily to hyperplasia (an increase in cell number), and it may cause serious problems such as acute urinary retention (i.e., a sudden inability to urinate), which requires immediate medical intervention.

The partial obstruction of urine outflow increases urinary bladder volume and tension and alters smooth muscle myosin heavy chain splicing. In addition to the N-terminal SM-A and SM-B isoforms (Box 14-4), there is alternative splicing at the C-terminus to produce SM1 and the shorter SM2. Thus, there are four heavy chain variants. Obstructed urine outflow downregulates the SM2 isoform, so that the SM2/SM1 ratio in the bladder smooth muscle is decreased. As a consequence, the depolarization-activated rate of bladder smooth muscle force generation and the amount of force development are reduced. This results in a weaker urine stream and slower and incomplete bladder emptying.

The significance of the changes in myosin isoform expression is that bladder smooth muscle (a phasic smooth muscle) in which the SM2/SM1 isoform ratio is decreased exhibits a slower velocity of shortening (i.e., a more tonic phenotype) than does the normal bladder smooth muscle. The combination of this change in kinetics, the partial physical obstruction of the urethra, and the hypertrophy of the bladder wall (so that the concentration of myosin per gram of bladder tissue is reduced) contributes to the observed changes in bladder function and micturition (urination).

The effects of urethral obstruction are reversible. Removal of the urethral obstruction (in the case of prostate hypertrophy, surgical extirpation of some prostate tissue) leads to an increase in the SM2/SM1 ratio, improves the urinary stream, and promotes more complete emptying of the urinary bladder.

---

after a single action potential, but on a somewhat slower time scale. Brief stimulation of the smooth muscle evokes a rapid, transient rise in $[Ca^{2+}]_i$. This is followed, after a short delay, by phosphorylation of myosin and, after a further delay, by a transient increase in mechanical force. The force reaches a peak at about the time that $[Ca^{2+}]_i$ has nearly recovered to its resting level, and the phosphorylation and force also then slowly return to their resting levels.

When a tonic smooth muscle such as arterial smooth muscle is activated by a large, prolonged stimulus, $[Ca^{2+}]_i$ transiently rises to a peak synchronously in all cells (Figures 14-14, *B*, and 14-15, *A* to *C*). $[Ca^{2+}]_i$ then declines and begins to oscillate, but the oscillations are asynchronous from cell to cell (Figure 14-15, *A* and *B*, shows the behavior of single cells). Thus, while $[Ca^{2+}]_i$ averaged over many cells appears to maintain a steady level substantially above the resting level (Figure 14-15, *C*, and see Figure 14-14, *B*), in fact $[Ca^{2+}]_i$ in individual cells fluctuates markedly (Figure 14-15).

Tonic Smooth Muscles Can Maintain Tension with Little Consumption of ATP

One of the characteristic features of tonic smooth muscles, such as those in the walls of arteries or the lower esophageal sphincter, is their ability to remain at least partly contracted for very long periods. This tonic smooth muscle contraction is maintained despite minimal consumption of ATP and thus a low cross-bridge cycling rate. How is this possible?

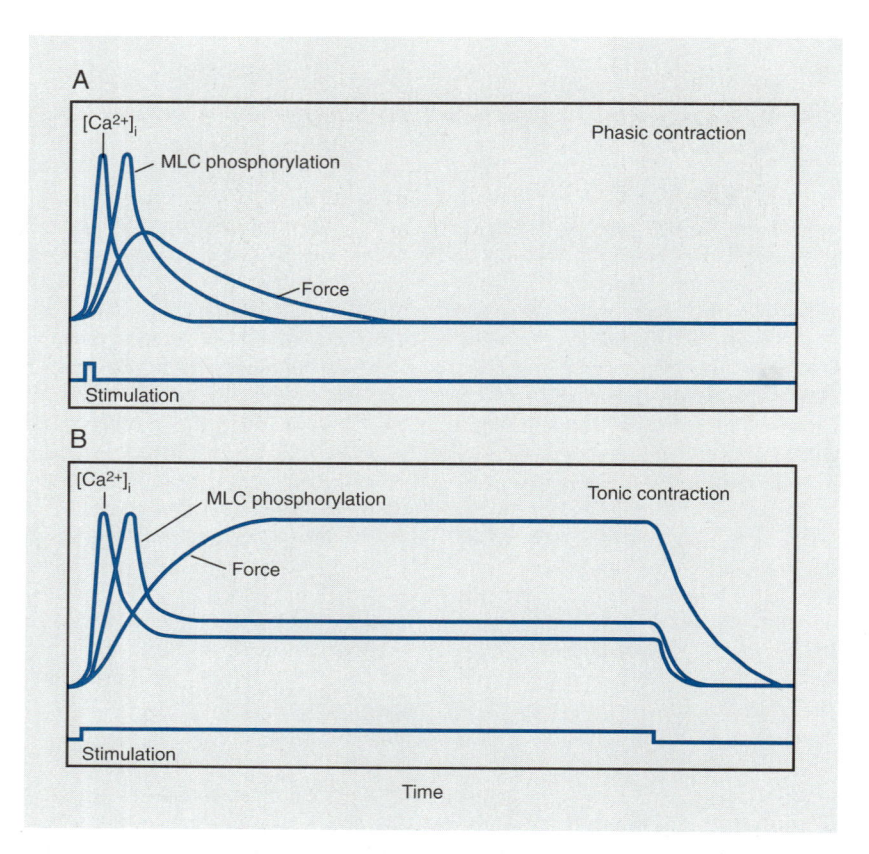

Figure 14-14 ■ Relative time course of average $[Ca^{2+}]_i$ elevation, myosin light chain (MLC) phosphorylation, and force development in smooth muscle with, A, a brief (phasic) stimulus and, B, a sustained (tonic) stimulus. The $[Ca^{2+}]_i$ corresponds to the spatially averaged $[Ca^{2+}]_i$ in the arterial wall (i.e., including a large number of smooth muscle cells or myocytes). In tonic smooth muscle such as artery smooth muscle, with prolonged stimulation (B), $[Ca^{2+}]_i$ and MLC phosphorylation rise to peak levels and rapidly decline to much lower, sustained levels, while force rises to a maximum sustained level. (Modified from Berne RM, Levy MN, editors: *Principles of physiology*, St Louis, 1990, Mosby.)

ATP is consumed during active cross-bridge cycling as a result of the myosin ATPase (see Figures 12-9 and 12-12). Skeletal muscle is about 4-fold more *efficient* than arterial smooth muscle, where **the efficiency is the amount of mechanical work** (i.e., shortening with a load) **that can be performed per mole of ATP consumed**. In contrast, arterial smooth muscle is at least 300-fold more *economical* than skeletal muscle in terms of using ATP to *maintain* stress. **The economy of the contraction is defined as the amount of stress that can be maintained at a given rate of ATP consumption.** A possible mechanism for maintaining this tone in smooth muscle depends on the low rate of dissociation of ADP from attached cross-bridges with a dephosphorylated MLC (Box 14-6 and Figure 14-16).

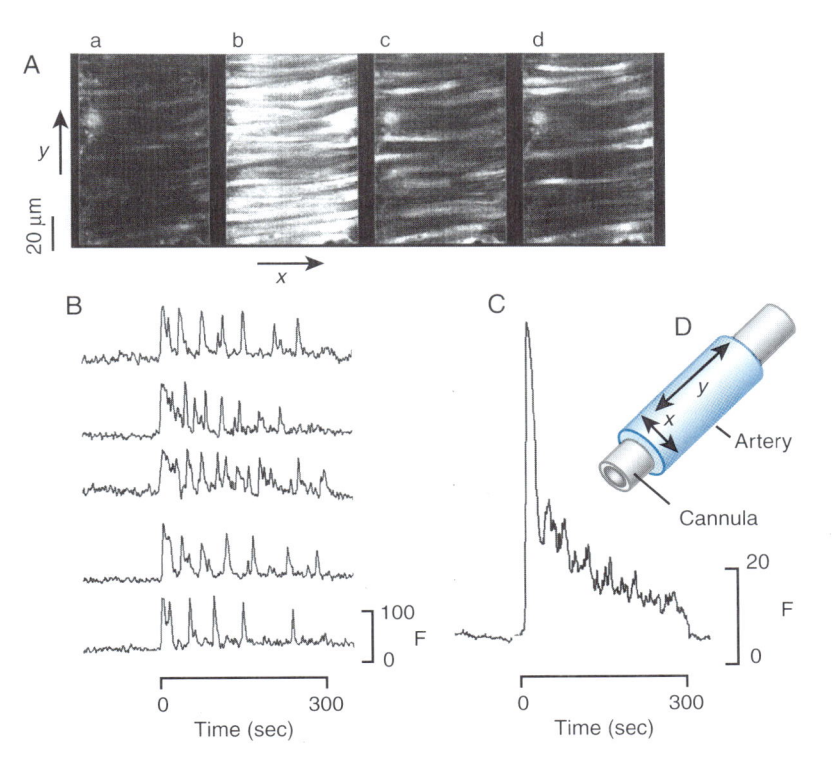

Figure 14-15 ■ Comparison of $[Ca^{2+}]_i$ elevation in individual arterial smooth muscle cells and the average change in $[Ca^{2+}]_i$ in a large group of smooth muscle cells. The increase in $[Ca^{2+}]_i$ was evoked by a relatively high, sustained concentration (5 μM) of the $α_1$-adrenergic receptor agonist phenylephrine (PE) in a rat small (250 μm diameter) mesenteric artery. The artery was stretched on a glass cannula (D) to prevent vasoconstriction. The myocytes form a single circular layer in the artery wall around the lumen. The lumen runs vertically (y-axis, here) and is perpendicular to the long axis of the cells (x-axis here). The artery was loaded with a Ca^{2+}-sensitive fluorescent dye whose brightness (F) increases with $[Ca^{2+}]_i$. Fluorescence is very low when $[Ca^{2+}]_i$ is at the resting level of about 0.1 μM (100 nM). Fluorescence increases markedly when $[Ca^{2+}]_i$ rises to its peak (about 1 to 5 μM). A, Fluorescent images of the arterial myocytes in one wall of the artery before (*a*) and during (*b-d*) PE application; *b* is 20 sec after PE addition, and *c* and *d* are about 50 and 100 sec later. About 25 myocytes are visible in *b*, which shows that $[Ca^{2+}]_i$ rose synchronously in virtually all cells shortly after PE was introduced. B, Time course of fluorescence changes in five representative cells. C, Time course of the spatially averaged changes in fluorescence over the entire area imaged in A (this curve is comparable to the $[Ca^{2+}]_i$ curve in Figure 14-14, *B*). The PE was present during the 5 min indicated by the bars at the bottom of B and C. (From Zhang W-J, Balke CW, Wier WG: *Cell Calcium* 29:327, 2001.)

BOX 14-6

Maintenance of Force with Low Levels of ATP Hydrolysis Can Be Explained by Slow Detachment of Cross-Bridges Containing Dephosphorylated Myosin Light Chain

A critical question in smooth muscle physiology is, "How is force maintained in tonic smooth muscles with so little consumption of ATP?" Smooth muscle myosins with a phosphorylated myosin light chain (MLC) continuously cycle and consume ATP (see Chapter 12). When the MLC becomes dephosphorylated while the cross-bridges are still attached, however, the detachment rate is greatly slowed. Thus force can be maintained without continued detachment and reattachment of the actin-myosin cross-bridges and concomitant hydrolysis of ATP. This slowed cycling rate is apparently due primarily to a large increase in the affinity of myosin for adenosine diphosphate (ADP) and a reduction in affinity for ATP that occur when the attached cross-bridges are dephosphorylated. The force is maintained because the actin cannot detach from the myosin until ADP dissociates and ATP binds to the myosin.

Perspective: Smooth Muscles Are Functionally Diverse

The preceding discussion indicates the wide range of properties exhibited by smooth muscles. Urinary bladder smooth muscle is an example of a phasic smooth muscle that is relatively relaxed most of the time; the bladder muscle relaxes as the bladder fills with urine. This smooth muscle then contracts when neuronally activated to empty the bladder. Most gastric and intestinal smooth muscles, which are also phasic, usually contract rhythmically, so that they are rarely fully relaxed.

Among the tonic smooth muscles, sphincters such as the lower esophageal sphincter occupy the opposite end of the spectrum. This sphincter is closed (i.e., the smooth muscle is contracted) most of the time; the smooth muscle relaxes during brief periods to permit a food bolus to move from the lower esophagus into the stomach. Arterial smooth muscle, another tonic muscle, is usually partially contracted and may further contract or relax to alter local blood flow.

To carry out their diverse activities, the many different smooth muscles must express different myosin isoforms and different complements of agonist receptors, ion channels, and ion carriers and pumps. These membrane proteins not only play key roles in conferring the cell-specific properties, but also may be targets for drug development for rational therapy.

■ SUMMARY

1. Shortly after a single action potential in a skeletal muscle cell, $[Ca^{2+}]_i$ rises, causing a transient, twitch contraction. Contractile force develops over a much slower time course than the rise in $[Ca^{2+}]_i$ because elastic elements must be stretched before external force can be generated.
2. A single α motor neuron and all the skeletal muscles it innervates are collectively referred to as a motor unit. The amount of force generated by whole muscle can be increased by recruiting motor units.
3. Muscle force can also be increased by stimulating the muscle repetitively.
4. When skeletal muscle is activated and filament sliding begins, the muscle can generate force, or it can shorten, or both can occur. In an isometric contraction the muscle generates force at a constant length. In an isotonic contraction the muscle shortens while generating a constant amount of force. Most contractions are part isometric and part isotonic.
5. Skeletal muscle mechanics are character-

Mechanics of Muscle Contraction

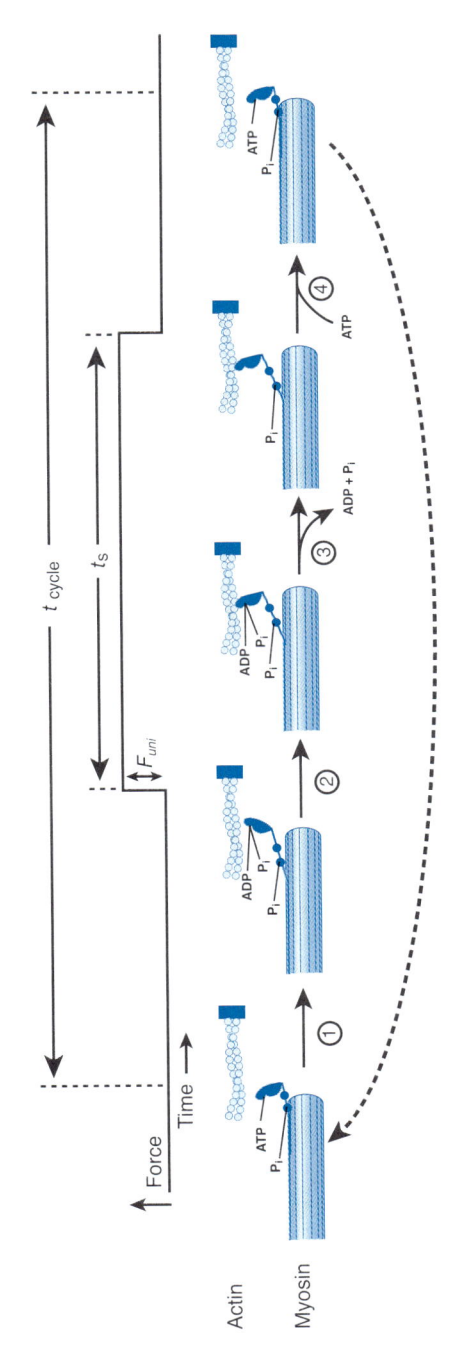

Figure 14-16 ■ Steps in the attachment and detachment of an actin-myosin cross-bridge in smooth muscle. The lower portion of the figure illustrates the steps in the cycle; a myosin with a phosphorylated myosin light chain is shown. Starting with ATP bound to the unattached myosin, in step 1 the ATP is hydrolyzed to adenosine diphosphate (ADP) + phosphate (P_i). This recocks the myosin head and enables step 2, the attachment of the myosin head to actin (i.e., the formation of the cross-bridge) and generation of force (the "power stroke") as the myosin head bends back (to the left in this diagram). In step 3, the rate-limiting step, the ADP and P_i dissociate. This dissociation is much slower in smooth muscle myosins than in skeletal muscle myosins and is even slower in smooth muscles if P_i dissociates from the myosin light chain while the cross-bridge is still attached (see Boxes 14-4 and 14-6). Step 4, ATP binding, which is rapid, leads to cross-bridge detachment. The cycle is then repeated. The line at the top shows the portion of the cycle (t_s) during which force is developed.

ized by two relationships: the length-tension curve and the force-velocity relationship.
6. There is an optimal length (L_0) of skeletal muscle at which active tension is maximal. Active tension declines at shorter and longer lengths.
7. The relationship between active length and tension is consistent with the sliding filament mechanism. Active force is maximal at L_0, where overlap between thick and thin filaments is maximal. At longer lengths the overlap decreases and active force declines because fewer cross-bridges can form.
8. The active force generated by a muscle is proportional to the number of attached cross-bridges.
9. During isotonic shortening the velocity of shortening is inversely related to the load. The maximum velocity of shortening (V_0) occurs with no load.
10. The rate of muscle shortening reflects the rate of cross-bridge cycling, and V_0 is directly proportional to myosin ATPase activity.
11. The three main motor unit types are fast-twitch, fatigable (FF); fast-twitch, fatigue-resistant (FR); and slow (S).
12. The time to peak twitch force is 20 to 40 msec in FF and FR motor units and 60 to over 100 msec in S units. Twitch contraction time is highly correlated with myosin ATPase activity.
13. FF motor units generate the largest tetanic forces, S motor units generate the smallest forces, and FR motor units are intermediate.
14. Cardiac muscle generates long-duration "twitch-type" contractions, which are caused by prolonged Ca^{2+} entry through voltage-gated Ca^{2+} channels that open during the action potential.
15. The total force generated by cardiac muscle is directly related to the level of $[Ca^{2+}]_i$ attained during the contraction. A positive inotropic effect is caused by agents that elevate $[Ca^{2+}]_i$.
16. Cardiac and skeletal muscle cells have similar length-tension relationships.
17. The maximum velocity of shortening is much slower in cardiac muscle than in skeletal muscle.
18. The kinetic properties of smooth muscle contraction can be defined in terms of three relationships: the temporal sequence that relates cell activation to the rise in $[Ca^{2+}]_i$ and force development; the force-velocity relationship; and the length-tension relationship.
19. Like skeletal muscle, smooth muscle has an optimal "resting" length at which active tension is maximal; active tension declines at shorter and longer lengths. This is consistent with the sliding filament model of contraction.
20. Smooth muscles and skeletal muscles generate about the same amount of active force per unit cross-sectional area (= "stress"). Nevertheless, smooth muscle shortening velocity is about 10-fold slower than skeletal muscle shortening velocity.
21. Single actin-myosin cross-bridges formed by smooth muscle and skeletal muscle myosin molecules generate similar unitary forces and have similar unitary displacement steps during a single cross-bridge cycle. The duration of force maintenance by cross-bridges formed by smooth muscle myosin is about eight times longer than the duration of skeletal muscle cross-bridges.
22. In smooth muscle, but not skeletal muscle, the cross-bridge cycling rate and the number of attached cross-bridges depend on MLC phosphorylation. Maximum stress is developed when the maximum number of cross-bridges are formed under isometric conditions.
23. The velocity of smooth muscle shortening

Mechanics of Muscle Contraction

is directly proportional to the extent of MLC phosphorylation. In the absence of a load, shortening velocity is a measure of the maximal rate of cross-bridge cycling.

24. Shortening velocity also depends on the myosin isoform. Phasic smooth muscles shorten more rapidly than tonic smooth muscles because of differences in myosin isoform expression.

25. Pathological conditions may alter myosin isoform expression and thus the speed of shortening. An example is the slowing of urinary bladder smooth muscle contraction when the urethra is partially obstructed.

26. The brief contractions observed in phasic smooth muscles, as well as in tonic smooth muscles after brief stimulation, are associated with transient increases in $[Ca^{2+}]_i$, MLC phosphorylation, and, with a time delay, tension development.

27. During prolonged stimulation of tonic smooth muscles, $[Ca^{2+}]_i$ oscillates after the initial transient rise, while MLC phosphorylation, after an initial peak, declines to a much lower steady level. During this time, tension rises slowly to a high, sustained level (= tonic tension or "tone").

28. Smooth muscle tone is maintained with little consumption of ATP because of the slow cross-bridge cycling rate. This is due to a slow rate of dissociation of ADP from attached cross-bridges when MLC becomes dephosphorylated.

29. The varied mechanical properties of smooth muscles reflect their diverse functions.

■ KEY WORDS AND CONCEPTS

- Motor unit
- Twitch
- Series elastic elements
- Tetanus
- Length-tension curve
- Force-velocity relationship
- Isometric and isotonic contractions
- Active and passive tension
- Optimal length (L_0)
- Fast-twitch, fatigable (FF); fast-twitch, fatigue-resistant (FR); slow (S) motor units
- Fatigue
- Positive inotropic effect
- Frank-Starling relationship
- Stress = Force per unit cross-sectional area
- Phasic smooth muscles
- Tonic smooth muscles
- Muscle efficiency = amount of mechanical work performed per mole of ATP consumed
- Economy of contraction = stress maintained at a given rate of ATP consumption

STUDY PROBLEMS

1. Consider the partly isometric, partly isotonic contraction shown in the figure below (similar to the ones shown in Figure 14-6), in which the initial muscle length is 2.8 µm per sarcomere. On this figure, identify the following four phases of the contraction: isometric force development, isotonic shortening, isotonic relaxation, and isometric relaxation. Then, on the skeletal muscle length-tension curve (see Figure 14-5), indicate each of these phases of the contraction.

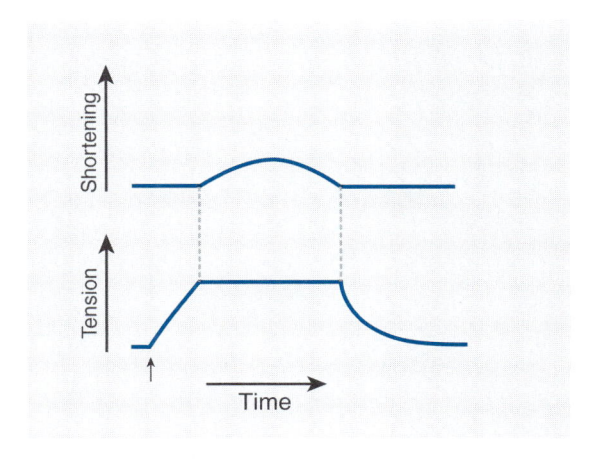

Graphs show the time course of the change in tension *(lower trace)* and the muscle shortening *(top trace)* during a partly isometric, partly isotonic contraction.

2. Stimulation of β-adrenergic receptors on ventricular myocytes increases contractility in these cells, by increasing the maximum force at all muscle lengths along the ascending limb of the length-tension curve. What effect would this increase in contractility have on the change in ventricular volume following contraction?
3. Compare the primary mechanisms used to change the amount of force generated by whole skeletal muscle with those used by cardiac ventricular muscle.
4. How do the mechanisms that control shortening velocity and cross-bridge cycling rate enable some smooth muscles to maintain tone without fatigue? Why is this an important property that is observed in many smooth muscles, but is undesirable in skeletal or cardiac muscles?

■ BIBLIOGRAPHY

Arafat HA, Kim GS, DiSanto ME, et al: Heterogeneity of bladder myocytes in vitro: modification of myosin isoform expression, *Tissue Cell* 33:219, 2001.

Babu GJ, Warshaw DM, Periasamy M: Smooth muscle myosin heavy chain isoforms and their role in muscle physiology, *Micros Res Tech* 50:532, 2000.

Blinks JR, Rudel R, Taylor SR: Calcium transients in isolated amphibian skeletal muscle fibres: detection with aequorin, *J Physiol* 277:291, 1978.

Braunwald E, Sonnenblick EH, Ross J: Mechanisms of cardiac contraction and relaxation. In Braunwald E, editor: *Heart disease: a textbook of cardiovascular medicine*, ed 4, Philadelphia, 1992, Saunders.

Burke RE: The structure and function of motor units. In Karpati G, Hilton-Jones D, Griggs RC, editors: *Disorders of voluntary muscle,* Cambridge, Eng, 2001, Cambridge University Press.

Burke RE, Levine DN, Tsairis P, Zajac FE: Physiological types and histochemical profiles in motor units of the cat gastrocnemius, *J Physiol* 234:723, 1973.

Gordon AM, Huxley AF, Julian FJ: The variation in isometric tension with sarcomere length in vertebrate muscle fibers, *J Physiol* 184:143, 1966.

Guilford WH, Warshaw DM: The molecular mechanics of smooth muscle myosin, *Comp Biochem Physiol B Biochem Molec Biol* 119:451, 1998.

Hill AV: The heat of shortening and the dynamic constants of muscle, *Proc R Soc Lond B* 126:136, 1938.

Miriel VA, Mauban JR, Blaustein MP, Wier WG: Local and cellular Ca^{2+} transients in smooth muscle of pressurized rat resistance arteries during myogenic and agonist stimulation, *J Physiol* 518:815, 1999.

Morano I: Tuning smooth muscle contraction by molecular motors. *J Mol Med* 81:41, 2003.

Murphy RA: Muscle cells of hollow organs, *News Physiol Sci* 3:124, 1988.

Murphy RA: Smooth muscle. In Berne RM, Levy MN, Koeppen BM, Stanton BA, editors: *Physiology*, ed 4, St Louis, 1998, Mosby.

Rovner AS, Fagnant PM, Lowey S, Trybus KM: The carboxy-terminal isoforms of smooth muscle myosin heavy chain determine thick filament assembly properties, *J Cell Biol* 156:113, 2002.

Tyska MJ, Warshaw DM: The myosin power stroke, *Cell Motility Cytoskel* 51:1, 2002.

Epilogue

This book provides a conceptual view of the currently understood molecular mechanisms responsible for maintaining cellular solute and solvent homeostasis. We also discuss the mechanisms responsible for generation and conduction of electrical signals and for muscular contraction. To appreciate how far the study of cellular physiology has come during the last half century, consider that 50 years ago not one of the mechanisms described in this book was understood at the molecular level. The cellular physiological processes were then known only at the phenomenological (descriptive) level. For example, in the 1950s electrical signals were just starting to be recognized in terms of "ionic conductances" and transport processes were identified only on the basis of solute and water fluxes. The sliding filament mechanism of muscle contraction was proposed in 1954.

The subject of cellular physiology was revolutionized by the identification of the specific proteins responsible for transport phenomena. The application of molecular biological methods led to advances involving the cloning, expression, and molecular manipulation of these proteins. Structural analyses of the proteins by x-ray crystallography, exemplified by the potassium ion channels and the sarcoplasmic and endoplasmic reticulum Ca^{2+} pump, are providing detailed information about the precise mechanisms by which these molecules are gated, as well as the ways in which they transfer solutes across a membrane.

The importance of understanding molecular mechanisms is illustrated by a brief history of the physiology of gastric acid secretion and the therapeutics of gastric hyperacidity (heartburn), peptic ulcers, and gastric reflux disease, as introduced in Chapter 11. The clinical problem was known to the early Greeks and Romans (e.g., Diocles of Carystos and Aurelius Cornelius Celsus), who recognized sour eruptions and epigastric hunger pains. The "modern" era began with the English physician and physiological chemist Prout, who demonstrated in 1824 that the stomach secretes hydrochloric acid. In the mid–nineteenth century the Austrian physician Rokitansky and the French physician Cruveilhier first prescribed chalk and alkaline substances to treat gastric ulcers. Numerous newer antacid formulations such as Tums and Maalox came into widespread clinical use during the twentieth century. These "first-generation" therapeutic agents were the mainstay of pharmacological therapy for peptic ulcers, heartburn, and gastroesophageal reflux. An important side effect of this therapy is the alkalinization of the urine, which greatly increases the tendency to form kidney stones.

The Russian physician Pavlov demonstrated that the vagus nerve plays a key role in the neural control of gastric secretion (1902). Subsequently, the French physician Latarjet treated peptic ulcers by surgical ablation of the branch of the vagus nerve that innervates the stomach (vagotomy) (1921). This procedure was not immediately accepted but came into more frequent use when it was reintroduced by the Chicago surgeon and physiologist Dragstedt (1943). Vagotomy is a major surgical procedure that, although it relieves ulcer pain and reduces gastric acidity, is accompanied by some unpleasant gastrointestinal side effects. These include nausea and the feeling of fullness in the stomach as a result of gastric retention. Thus the use of vagotomy in the therapy of peptic ulcer disease has been abandoned.

Knowledge of the details of neural control of gastric acid secretion, specifically the involvement of histamine as a neurotransmitter that activates parietal cells via histamine type 2 (H_2) receptors, is relatively recent. Black and colleagues first described H_2 receptors in 1972. This mechanistic discovery led to the development, in the 1970s, of H_2-receptor blockers such as cimetidine (Tagamet) and ranitidine (Zantac). These "second-generation" compounds became a mainstay in the treatment of gastric hyperacidity. The H_2 antagonists are effective and well tolerated, and they have few side effects. They do not, however, totally suppress gastric acid secretion, and because they are short acting, they are usually administered twice daily.

The discovery of the parietal cell proton pump (H,K-ATPase) by Forte and Sachs and their colleagues in the 1970s resulted in the development, by Wallman and associates, of specific proton pump inhibitors such as omeprazole (Prilosec) and lansoprazole (Prevacid). These "third-generation" therapeutic agents were introduced into clinical use in the late 1980s. They are particularly effective because they directly block the acid secretion mechanism, are well tolerated, and have few side effects. Moreover, they are long acting and can be administered in a single daily dose.

The preceding historical synopsis highlights the rationale for studying cellular physiological mechanisms as a basis for understanding therapeutics and current clinical practice. The aim is to develop the most specific therapies with the fewest side effects. Indeed, with basic molecular mechanisms being elucidated at an accelerating rate, we can expect the understanding of cellular physiology and its clinical applications to advance at an ever increasing pace.

BIBLIOGRAPHY

Black JW, Duncan WAM, Dunant CJ, et al: Definition and antagonism of histamine H_2-receptors, *Nature* 236:385, 1972.

Harvey SC: Gastric antacids and digestants. In Goodman LS, Gilman AG, editors: *The pharmacological basis of therapeutics*, ed 4, New York, 1970, Macmillan.

Hoogerwerf WA, Pasricha PJ: Agents used for control of gastric acidity and treatment of peptic ulcers and gastroesophageal reflux disease. In Hardman JG, Limbird LE, editors: *Goodman & Gilman's The pharmacological basis of therapeutics,* ed 10, New York, 2001, McGraw-Hill.

Modlin IM: From Prout to the proton pump—a history of the science of gastric acid secretion and the surgery of peptic ulcer, *Surg Gynecol Obstet* 170:81, 1990.

Sachs G: The gastric proton pump: the H^+,K^+-ATPase. In Johnson LR, editor: *Physiology of the gastrointestinal tract*, ed 2, New York, 1987, Raven Press.

APPENDIX A

A Mathematical Refresher

■ EXPONENTS

Definition of Exponentiation

Multiplying the number 3 by itself four times gives

$$3 \times 3 \times 3 \times 3 = 81$$

which can be written more simply with the shorthand notation

$$3^4 = 81$$

The shorthand notation 3^4 is read as "3 raised to the 4th power" or, more simply, "3 to the 4th power." The number 3 in the above example is usually referred to as the "base," and the number 4 is called the "exponent." In the natural sciences the most frequently used base is an irrational number* given the symbol e. The number e is referred to as the base of the "natural" exponential function; the reason for this will become apparent in a later section. The value of e to three decimal places is 2.718.

The most general representation of exponentiation is

$$a^m = c$$

where a and m can be arbitrary numbers. A few numerical examples are

$$2^{13} = 8192; \quad 7^3 = 343; \quad 3.7^4 = 187.4161;$$
$$10^{3.32} = 2089.2961...; \quad \text{and} \quad 2.13^{4.71} = 35.21015...$$

The first three examples above are readily verified by hand calculation. The last two examples could also be verified by hand with the information we will provide shortly, but the task is incomparably easier with the use of a calculator.

Multiplication of Exponentials

The rule for multiplying exponentials by combining exponents follows from the definition of exponentials:

---

*An irrational number is just a number that cannot be written as a fraction. The square root of 2 ($\sqrt{2}$) and the number pi (π) are examples of irrational numbers.

$$a^m \times a^n = a^{(m+n)} \quad [1]$$

This rule is easily verified by checking an example:

$$3^2 \times 3^4 = (3 \times 3) \times (3 \times 3 \times 3 \times 3) = 3^6 = 3^{(2+4)}$$

Meaning of the Number 0 as Exponent

All of the other properties of exponentials follow directly from the rule for combining exponents. First, the rule allows us to deduce what a to the 0th power (a^0) means. To make the point concrete, take $a = 3$. Equation [1] allows us to write

$$3^2 \times 3^0 = 3^{(2+0)} = 3^2$$

This expression is true if, and only if, $3^0 = 1$. In general, any non-0 number raised to the 0th power is equal to 1:

$$a^0 = 1 \text{ (as long as } a \neq 0) \quad [2]$$

The reason for excluding 0 from the definition will be clear shortly.

Negative Numbers as Exponents

So far we have dealt with positive exponents. What does a negative exponent mean? Equation [1] also allows us to deduce the answer. If we again use $a = 3$ as the base, Equation [1] implies that

$$3^2 \times 3^{-2} = 3^{[2+(-2)]} = 3^0 = 1$$

This expression is true if, and only if, $3^{-2} = 1/3^2$. In general,

$$a^{-m} = \frac{1}{a^m} \text{ (as long as } a \neq 0) \quad [3]$$

Division of Exponentials

The definition in Equation [3] extends the rule for combining exponents (Equation [1]) to include division of exponentials:

$$\frac{a^m}{a^n} = a^m \times a^{-n} = a^{(m-n)} \quad [4]$$

We now see why in the definition of the 0th power (Equation [2]), the base a could not be 0. That is because $a = 0$ in Equation [4] would force a division of 0 by 0—an operation that has no meaning.

Exponentials of Exponentials

Knowing how to combine exponents allows us to see what happens when an exponential is raised to another power, for example, $(7^2)^3$:

$$(7^2)^3 = 7^2 \times 7^2 \times 7^2 = 7^{(2+2+2)} = 7^6$$

In general,

$$(a^m)^n = a^{(m \times n)} \quad [5]$$

Fractions as Exponents

So far, only exponents that are whole numbers have been discussed. We now investigate the case in which the exponent is a fraction (i.e., $a^{m/n}$). Again, taking a concrete example in which $a = 7$, we ask what is meant by $7^{1/2}$. Applying the multiplication rule (Equation [1]) gives

$$7^{1/2} \times 7^{1/2} = 7^{(1/2 + 1/2)} = 7^1 = 7$$

which immediately shows that $7^{1/2} = \sqrt{7}$ (the square root of 7). In general, a to the $1/n$ is the nth root of a:

$$a^{\frac{1}{n}} = \sqrt[n]{a} \quad [6]$$

A direct consequence of combining Equations [6] and [4] is that

$$a^{\frac{m}{n}} = a^{(m \times \frac{1}{n})} = (a^m)^{\frac{1}{n}} = \sqrt[n]{a^m} = (a^{\frac{1}{n}})^m = (\sqrt[n]{a})^m \quad [7]$$

Since any rational decimal number can always be written as a fraction (e.g., 1.5 = 3/2, 0.47 = 47/100), decimal numbers in the exponent can be dealt with precisely as if they were fractions.

Equations [1] to [7] constitute essentially all the properties of exponentials that are important for computation. For convenience, all of these properties are summarized in Box A-1.

Appendix A

> **BOX A-1**
>
> **Properties of Exponentials**
>
> $$a^m \times a^n = a^{(m+n)}$$
>
> $$\frac{a^m}{a^n} = a^m \times a^{-n} = a^{(m-n)}$$
>
> $$a^0 = 1 \text{ (as long as } a \neq 0)$$
>
> $$a^{-m} = \frac{1}{a^m} \text{ (as long as } a \neq 0)$$
>
> $$(a^m)^n = a^{(m \times n)}$$
>
> $$a^{\frac{1}{n}} = \sqrt[n]{a}$$
>
> $$a^{\frac{m}{n}} = a^{(m \times \frac{1}{n})} = (a^m)^{\frac{1}{n}} = \sqrt[n]{a^m} = (a^{\frac{1}{n}})^m = (\sqrt[n]{a})^m$$

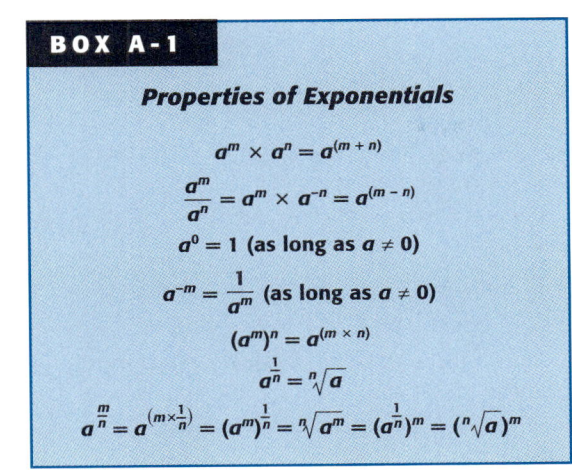

■ LOGARITHMS

Definition of the Logarithm

The logarithm can be thought of as an inverse way to look at the exponential process. The general way of representing a logarithm is

$$\log_a c = m$$

This expression is read as "the logarithm 'to the base a' of the number c is equal to m." The meaning of this expression is "m is the power to which a must be raised in order to get the number c." But this is really just another way of representing the exponential process $a^m = c$, which we had just examined (we may consider the logarithm the *inverse* of the exponential). The logarithm is the answer to the question, "To what power must a be raised to give the value c ($a^? = c$)?" The answer is the definition of the logarithm:

$$a^{\log_a c} = c$$

Examples corresponding to some of those in the previous section would be

$\log_2 8192 = 13$; $\log_7 343 = 3$; $\log_{3.7} 187.4161 = 4$;
$\log_{10} 2089.2961... = 3.32$ $\log_{2.13} 35.21015... = 4.71$

Historically, the number 10 is the most commonly used base for logarithms. For this reason, base-10 logarithms are referred to as "common logarithms." In the natural sciences the irrational number e is usually used as the base for logarithms. Just as the exponential function using e as the base is called the "natural" exponential function, a logarithm using the base e is called the "natural" logarithm and is given the symbol ln. Thus the natural logarithm of x is symbolized as ln$x$.

The definitions given above, along with the properties of exponentials, imply three rules governing calculations involving logarithms.

Logarithm of a Product

The logarithm of a product is given by

$$\log_a (b \times c) = \log_a b + \log_a c \qquad [8]$$

Examining the definition of a logarithm immediately shows where this rule comes from:

$$b = a^{\log_a b} \quad \text{and} \quad c = a^{\log_a c}$$

so

$$b \times c = a^{\log_a b} \times a^{\log_a c} = a^{(\log_a b + \log_a c)}$$

(the last step is a consequence of the rule for combining exponents—Equation [1]). Therefore

$$\log_a (b \times c) = \log_a b + \log_a c$$

Incidentally, the product rule (in conjunction with the rule for taking the logarithm of an exponential—Equation [9] below) also gives the logarithm of a quotient:

$$\log_a\left(\frac{b}{c}\right) = \log_a[b \times c^{-1}] = \log_a b + \log_a(c^{-1}) =$$
$$\log_a b + (-1) \log_a c = \log_a b - \log_a c$$

Logarithm of an Exponential

The logarithm of an exponential is given by

$$\log_a c^m = m \times \log_a c \qquad [9]$$

This rule is a consequence of the rule governing logarithm of a product (Equation [8]) combined with the definition of an exponential:

$$\log_a c^m = \log_a (c \times c \times \ldots \times c)_{m \text{ times}} =$$
$$(\log_a c + \log_a c + \ldots + \log_a c)_{m \text{ times}} = m \times \log_a c$$

A special case of the logarithm of an exponential occurs frequently and is sometimes given as a separate "rule":

$$\log_a\left(\frac{1}{c}\right) = \log_a c^{-1} = -1 \times \log_a c = -\log_a c \quad [10]$$

Changing the Base of a Logarithm

For any number c, its logarithms using two different bases, a and b, are related by the expression

$$\log_a c = (\log_a b) \times \log_b c \quad [11]$$

This rule is the result of combining the definition of a logarithm

$$c = b^{\log_b c}$$

with the rule for taking the logarithm of an exponential (Equation [9])

$$\log_a c = \log_a b^{(\log_b c)} = (\log_b c) \times \log_a b$$

which is the rule shown in Equation [11].

The rules of logarithms are summarized in Box A-2.

BOX A-2

Properties of Logarithms

$$\log_a (b \times c) = \log_a b + \log_a c$$
$$\text{or } \log_a \left(\frac{b}{c}\right) = \log_a b - \log_b c$$
$$\text{or } \log_a c^m = m \times \log_a c$$
$$\log_a \left(\frac{1}{c}\right) = -\log_a c$$
$$\log_a c = (\log_a b) \times \log_b c$$

SOLVING QUADRATIC EQUATIONS

Any equation that can be put into the form

$$ax^2 + bx + c = 0 \quad [12]$$

can be solved for the value of x through the *quadratic formula*:

$$x = \frac{-b \pm \sqrt{b^2 - 4ac}}{2a} \quad [13]$$

The $\pm$ sign means that x may take on two different values, one corresponding to using the + sign in the numerator, and one corresponding to using the − sign. Solving the quadratic equation $4x^2 - 9 = 0$ illustrates the technique. Comparing this equation with the general form of the quadratic equation given above shows the coefficients to be $a = 4$, $b = 0$, and $c = -9$. The two solutions that will satisfy the equation are given by the quadratic formula:

$$x = \frac{-(0) \pm \sqrt{0^2 - 4(4)(-9)}}{2(4)} = \frac{\pm\sqrt{+144}}{8} = \pm\frac{12}{8} = \pm\frac{3}{2}$$

So the two answers are $x = 3/2$ and $x = -3/2$ (or, $x = 1.5$ and $x = -1.5$).

DIFFERENTIATION AND DERIVATIVES

The Slope of a Graph and the Derivative

The derivative of a function at a particular point is most easily viewed as the "slope" of the function at that point. A slope is really just a rate of change of one variable relative to another. For a straight line, the slope, being the rate of change of y relative to x ($\Delta y/\Delta x$), is everywhere the same and is easy to compute, as shown in Figure A-1.

For functions with nonlinear graphs, determining the slope at a particular point on the curve is slightly more involved. Assume, for the moment, that the function of interest is the parabola, $y = x^2$, with the graph shown in Figure A-2. The general problem of the finding the slope of the parabola at any particular point (x, y) is to find the slope of the *tangent* line that just touches the parabola at that point.

Appendix A

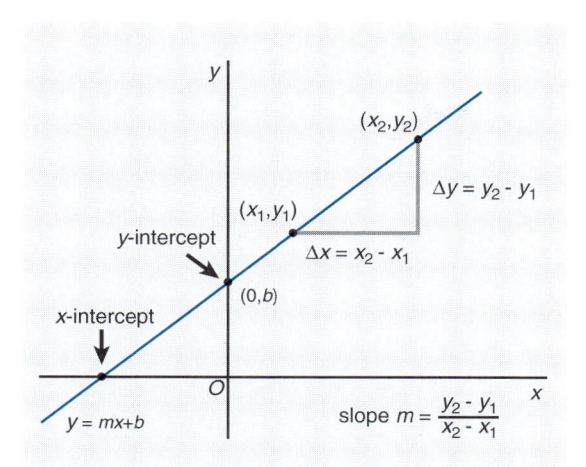

Figure A-1 ■ Graph of a line represented by the equation $y = mx + b$. The slope of the line is m, and b is the y-intercept; that is, the line crosses the y-axis at the point $(0, b)$. If two points lying on the line, (x_1, y_1) and (x_2, y_2), are known, the slope can be calculated: $m = \Delta y / \Delta x = (y_2 - y_1)/(x_2 - x_1)$.

The general features of the problem are shown in Figure A-2. To determine the slope of the parabola at the point (x, y), we can first pass a "test" line through a second, arbitrary point $(x + \Delta x, y + \Delta y)$. As Δx becomes smaller, so will Δy, and eventually the test line should *become* the tangent line as Δx approaches 0. Because the points (x, y) and $(x + \Delta x, y + \Delta y)$ both lie on the parabola $y = x^2$, we can write the two points as (x, x^2) and $(x + \Delta x, (x + \Delta x)^2)$, respectively. The slope of the line connecting these points must be

$$\text{slope} = \frac{\Delta y}{\Delta x} = \frac{y_2 - y_1}{x_2 - x_1} = \frac{(x + \Delta x)^2 - x^2}{(x + \Delta x) - x} =$$

$$\frac{(x^2 + 2x\Delta x + \Delta x^2)}{\Delta x} - x^2 = 2x + \Delta x$$

As Δx approaches 0, the slope, $\Delta y / \Delta x$, approaches $2x$. This means that at *any* arbitrary point on our parabola, the slope of the curve must be $2x$. This

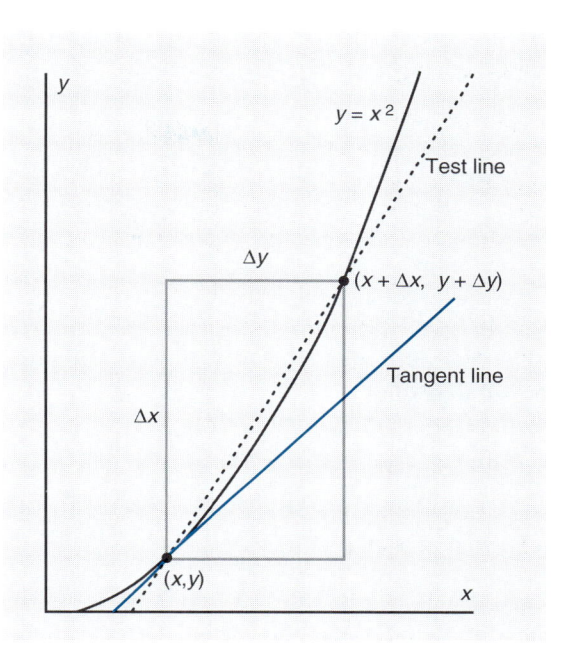

Figure A-2 ■ Graph of the parabola $y = x^2$. Two lines are also shown: (1) a tangent line (solid) that passes through one point, (x, y), on the parabola, and (2) a "test" line (dashed) that passes through (x, y), as well as a second point, $(x+\Delta x, y+\Delta y)$. As Δx (and thus Δy) grows ever smaller, the test line approaches the tangent line ever more closely. In the limit of infinitesimally small Δx (i.e., as $\Delta x \to 0$), the test line *becomes* the tangent line. At the point (x, y) the derivative of the function has a value equal to the slope of the tangent line.

slope of the curve (which is equal to the slope of the tangent line touching the curve) is the *derivative* of the curve and is given the symbol $\frac{dy}{dx}$. To summarize:

$$\text{as } \Delta x \to 0, \quad \frac{\Delta y}{\Delta x} \to \frac{dy}{dx}$$

Therefore the slope at *any* point on the parabola $y = x^2$ is given by its derivative

$$\frac{dy}{dx} = 2x$$

Thus, at the point (2,4) on the parabola, the slope is 2(2) = 4; at the point (5,25), the slope is 2(5) = 10.

The same approach can be used to find the derivative of any function. For functions that involve only x raised to some power ($y = x^n$), it is relatively easy to show that

$$\frac{dy}{dx} = n\, x^{(n-1)} \quad \text{for} \quad y = x^n \qquad [14]$$

The general process whereby we find the derivative of a function is called *differentiation*. A few examples of derivatives that follow from formula [14] are

$$\frac{d}{dx} x^7 = 7\, x^{(7-1)} = 7\, x^6$$

$$\frac{d}{dx} x^{-3} = -3\, x^{(-3-1)} = -3\, x^{-4}$$

or written in alternative form:

$$\frac{d}{dx}\left(\frac{1}{x^3}\right) = \frac{-3}{x^4}$$

$$\frac{d}{dx}(x^{0.5}) = 0.5\, x^{(0.5-1)} = -0.5\, x^{-0.5}$$

or written in alternative form:

$$\frac{d}{dx}(\sqrt{x}) = \frac{1}{2}\frac{1}{\sqrt{x}}$$

A simple extension of formula [14] (which can be demonstrated by the methods we have already used) expands our ability to differentiate functions:

$$\frac{d}{dx}(ax^n) = a\frac{d}{dx}x^n = a\, n\, x^{n-1}$$

In other words, multiplying an exponential function by a constant number a means that the derivative is also multiplied by the same factor. In general, for any function $f(x)$, if $\frac{df}{dx}$ is the derivative of the function, then

$$\frac{d}{dx}(a \times f) = a\frac{df}{dx} \quad \text{for } a = \text{constant number} \qquad [15]$$

Derivative of a Constant Number

A constant number, c, can be viewed as the function $y = c$, which is a straight horizontal line intersecting the y-axis at c. The derivative of this function should just be the slope of the horizontal line. But a horizontal line has slope 0 (i.e., regardless of the size of Δx, Δy is always 0, which means that the slope $\Delta y/\Delta x = 0$). This result means that the derivative of any constant number is 0:

$$\frac{d}{dx} c = 0 \quad \text{for } c = \text{constant number} \qquad [16]$$

Differentiating the Sum or Difference of Functions

Applying the "shrinking Δx" definition of the derivative gives us the following rules governing the differentiation of the sum or the difference of functions. Let $f(x)$ and $g(x)$ be different functions of x. If $y = f(x) + g(x)$,

$$\frac{dy}{dx} = \frac{d}{dx}[f(x) + g(x)] = \frac{d}{dx}f(x) + \frac{d}{dx}g(x) \qquad [17a]$$

And if $y = f(x) - g(x)$,

$$\frac{dy}{dx} = \frac{d}{dx}[f(x) - g(x)] = \frac{d}{dx}f(x) - \frac{d}{dx}g(x) \qquad [17b]$$

An Example Illustrating the Computation of a Derivative To illustrate all of the computational rules we have derived so far, consider differentiating the function

$$y = 7x^3 + \sqrt{x} - \frac{4}{x^3} + 19$$

This problem becomes easier if we rewrite the function using regular exponential notation to give

$$y = 7x^3 + x^{\frac{1}{2}} - 4x^{-3} + 19$$

We see that y is the sum and difference of four functions. The derivative can be obtained by differentiating each of the four parts in turn:

$$\frac{d}{dx}(7x^3) + \frac{d}{dx}\left(x^{\frac{1}{2}}\right) - \frac{d}{dx}(4x^{-3}) + \frac{d}{dx}(19) =$$

$$7(3x^{(3-1)}) + \frac{1}{2}x^{\left(\frac{1}{2}-1\right)} - 4(-3x^{(-3-1)}) + 0$$

to give the result

$$\frac{dy}{dx} = 21x^2 + \frac{1}{2}x^{(-\frac{1}{2})} + 12x^{-4}$$

What Makes the "Natural" Exponential Function Natural? Knowing how to find the derivative of a function, we can now investigate the natural exponential function $y = e^x$. What is the derivative of the natural exponential function? Proceeding as we had done for the parabola, the slope of the exponential function at some x is given by

$$\text{slope} = \frac{\Delta y}{\Delta x} = \frac{e^{(x+\Delta x)} - e^x}{\Delta x} = \frac{e^x e^{\Delta x} - e^x}{\Delta x} = \frac{e^x(e^{\Delta x} - 1)}{\Delta x}$$

[18]

As before, we try to obtain the derivative dy/dx by allowing Δx to approach 0. As Δx approaches 0, $e^{\Delta x}$ approaches $e^0 = 1$, and the term $(e^{\Delta x} - 1)$ approaches 0. Apparently, this would make the slope 0/0, which is meaningless. This approach clearly gives no real information about the behavior of the slope as Δx shrinks. A better way to examine the behavior of the slope as $\Delta x \to 0$ is needed. First, we look closely at the behavior of $e^{\Delta x}$ when Δx becomes small. Table A-1 summarizes our numerical investigation.

Table A-1 shows that numerically, as Δx gets progressively closer to 0, $e^{\Delta x}$ approaches $(\Delta x + 1)$. The slope expression (Equation [18]) can now be written as

$$\text{slope} = \frac{\Delta y}{\Delta x} = \frac{e^x(e^{\Delta x} - 1)}{\Delta x} = \frac{e^x[(\Delta x + 1) - 1]}{\Delta x}$$

$$= \frac{e^x \Delta x}{\Delta x} = e^x$$

when Δx becomes very small. So, as $\Delta x \to 0$, the slope expression no longer contains Δx, and becomes the derivative dy/dx:

$$\frac{d}{dx}e^x = e^x \qquad [19]$$

The essence of the natural exponential function is that the value of its derivative at any point is

TABLE A-1

Behavior of $e^{\Delta x}$ as $\Delta x \to 0$

Δx	$e^{\Delta x}$	$e^{\Delta x} - \Delta x$
0.1	1.1051709...	1.0051709...
0.05	1.0512710...	1.0012710...
0.01	1.0100501...	1.0000501...
0.005	1.0050125...	1.0000125...
0.001	1.0010005...	1.0000005...
0.0005	1.0000500...	1.0000001...
0.0001	1.0001000...	1.0000000...
0.00005	1.0000050...	1.0000000...
0.00001	1.0000100...	1.0000000...

the same as the value of the exponential function itself. Alternative ways of saying this are (1) the natural exponential function is its own derivative, or (2) differentiation of the natural exponential function gives back the natural exponential function. It is this property of the natural exponential function that makes it "natural."

Differentiating Composite Functions: the Chain Rule

Consider the function $y = x^6 - 1$, whose derivative we know to be $dy/dx = 6x^5$. One potentially different way of looking at this function is to think of it as $y = (x^2)^3 - 1$. In other words, we think of $y = u^3 - 1$, where $u = x^2$ (y is a function of u, but u is, in turn, a function of x). In this context, y is called a *composite* function. We can think of the derivative of the composite function y as having two parts: dy/du and du/dx:

$$y = u^3 - 1, \quad \frac{dy}{du} = 3u^2; \quad u = x^2, \quad \frac{du}{dx} = 2x$$

Multiplying the two parts together gives

$$\frac{dy}{du} \cdot \frac{du}{dx} = (3u^2)(2x) = (3(x^2)^2)(2x) = (3x^4)(2x) = 6x^5$$

which is what we had already determined at the outset. We thus infer the general property that when y is a function of u, and u is, in turn, a function of x,

$$\frac{dy}{dx} = \frac{dy}{du} \cdot \frac{du}{dx} \qquad [20]$$

This relationship is called the *chain rule* for the derivative of a composite function. It frequently occurs in the natural sciences that one function may be viewed as a function of another function. A less trivial example is

$$y = e^{-x^2}$$

In this case the function y is a composite function: $y = e^u$, $u = -x^2$. The derivative is easily found by recalling that the derivative of e^u is e^u and applying the chain rule:

$$\frac{dy}{dx} = \frac{dy}{du} \cdot \frac{du}{dx} = e^u(-2x) = e^{-x^2}(-2x) = -2xe^{-x^2}$$

Derivative of the Natural Logarithm Function

In the section on logarithms we stated that the logarithm can be considered the *inverse* of the exponentiation process. We now wish to find the derivative of a logarithmic function. We can do this by using the idea of the *inverse* of a function. The definition is logical; for example, if $y = e^x$, the inverse would be $x = e^y$. If we take the natural logarithm of both sides of the inverse function, we find

$$\ln x = \ln(e^y) = y(\ln e) = y(1) = y \quad \text{or} \quad y = \ln x$$

Thus the inverse of the natural exponential function is indeed the natural logarithm function. Differentiating the inverse function means

$$\frac{d}{dx} x = \frac{d}{dx} e^y$$

But

$$\frac{d}{dx} x = 1 \quad \text{and} \quad \frac{d}{dx} e^y = (e^y)\frac{dy}{dx} = (e^{\ln x})\frac{dy}{dx} = x\frac{dy}{dx}$$

(because $y = \ln x$ and $e^{\ln x} = x$), so

$$1 = x\frac{dy}{dx}$$

which means,

$$\frac{dy}{dx} = \frac{1}{x}$$

or more explicitly

$$\frac{d}{dx} \ln x = \frac{1}{x} \qquad [21]$$

With the techniques developed above, any function that has a derivative can be differentiated. Box A-3 summarizes basic knowledge of differentiation and derivatives.

BOX A-3

Common Derivatives and Their Properties

$$\frac{d}{dx} c = 0 \quad \text{for } c = \text{constant number}$$

$$\frac{dy}{dx} = n\, x^{(n-1)} \quad \text{for } y = x^n$$

$$\frac{d}{dx} e^x = e^x$$

$$\frac{d}{dx} \ln x = \frac{1}{x}$$

If a = constant number, $\dfrac{d}{dx}[a \times f(x)] = a\dfrac{d}{dx} f(x)$

$$\frac{d}{dx}[f(x) + g(x)] = \frac{d}{dx} f(x) + \frac{d}{dx} g(x) \quad \text{and}$$

$$\frac{d}{dx}[f(x) - g(x)] = \frac{d}{dx} f(x) - \frac{d}{dx} g(x)$$

$$\frac{dy}{dx} = \frac{dy}{du} \cdot \frac{du}{dx} \quad \text{if } y = f(u) \text{ and } u = g(x)$$

Appendix A

■ INTEGRATION: THE ANTIDERIVATIVE AND THE DEFINITE INTEGRAL

Indefinite Integral (Also Known as the Antiderivative)

The term "integration" has two meanings. First, it is a process whereby for a function $g(x)$, we find a function $f(x)$ such that

$$g(x) = \frac{d}{dx} f(x)$$

In other words, we find a function $f(x)$ whose derivative is the function $g(x)$. Because in this sense, integration is just the reverse of differentiation, the integration process is sometimes referred to as *antidifferentiation*. The function $f(x)$ is called either the *antiderivative* or the *indefinite integral* of $g(x)$. Symbolically, we represent the antidifferentiation process as

$$\int g(x)dx = f(x)$$

For example, if we have a function $g(x) = nx^{(n-1)}$, its antiderivative is x^n because we recognize that $f(x) = x^n$ is the function, when differentiated, that gives $g(x)$. However, because the derivative of a constant number (C) is zero, we realize that it is not the *only* function whose derivative is $g(x)$; indeed, any function $f(x) = x^n + C$, when differentiated, will give $g(x) = nx^{(n-1)}$. Therefore

$$\int nx^{(n-1)}dx = x^n + C$$

Because C may take on any value, this expression tells us that really an infinite number of functions are the antiderivative of $g(x) = nx^{(n-1)}$. The constant, C, is referred to as the *constant of integration*. Because there is no *unique* antiderivative for $g(x)$, the antiderivative is also known as the *indefinite* integral. The properties of indefinite integrals corresponding to the properties of derivatives listed in Box A-3 are summarized in Box A-4.

Definite Integral

The second type of integration is conceptually equivalent to finding the area under a curve

---

BOX A-4

Indefinite Integrals and Their Properties

$\int nx^{(n-1)}dx = x^n + C$ or $\int x^m dx = \frac{1}{m+1}x^{(m+1)} + C$

$\int af(x)dx = a\int f(x)dx$ for $a =$ constant number

$\int e^x dx = e^x + C$

$\int \frac{1}{x}dx = \ln x + C$

$\int [f(x) + g(x)]dx = \int f(x)dx + \int g(x)dx$
and $\int [f(x) - g(x)]dx = \int f(x)dx - \int g(x)dx$

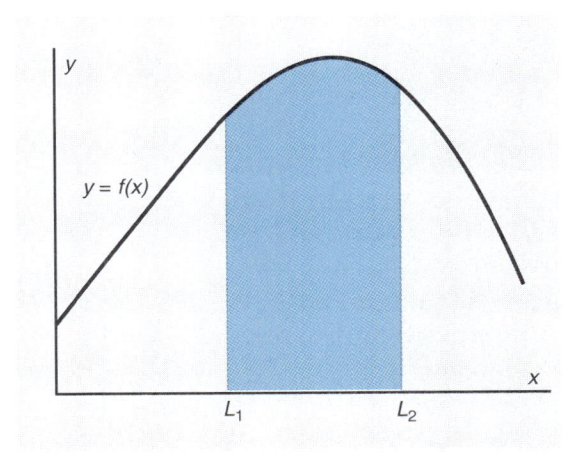

Figure A-3 ■ Graphic representation of the definite integral. The graph of the function $y = f(x)$ is shown. The definite integral $\int_{L_1}^{L_2} f(x)dx$ is the blue shaded area under the curve $y = f(x)$ between the limits L_1 and L_2.

(Figure A-3). The area under the curve $y = f(x)$ in Figure A-3 is symbolized by the integral

$$\text{Area} = \int_{L_1}^{L_2} f(x)dx$$

In this context the function $f(x)$ is called the *integrand* and the two numbers L_1 and L_2 are the *lower* and *upper* limits of integration, respectively. To take a concrete example: $y = f(x) = x^2$, and we wish to find out the area under the curve between $x = 3$ and $x = 7$. The definite integral is

$$\int_{x=3}^{x=7} x^2\, dx$$

This integral is evaluated in the following way. First we find the antiderivative of the integrand, which in the case of x^2 is $x^3/3$. Next we evaluate the antiderivative at the two integration limits and find the difference between them:

$$\int_{x=3}^{x=7} x^2\, dx = \left[\frac{1}{3}x^3\right]_3^7 = \frac{7^3}{3} - \frac{3^3}{3} = \frac{343}{3} - \frac{27}{3} = \frac{316}{3}$$

We note that whereas an indefinite integral is a function, the definite integral is always a number.

DIFFERENTIAL EQUATIONS

First-Order Equations with Separable Variables

Differential equations encountered in cellular physiology are ones wherein the rate of change of a variable is equal to some function:

$$\frac{dy}{dt} = f(t, y)$$

To solve the differential equation is to find the functional form of y. The easiest differential equations to solve are ones in which the independent and dependent variables (t and y, respectively, in the example) can be separated into separate groupings. For example, the equation

$$\frac{dy}{dt} = f(t) \qquad [22]$$

can be solved by separating the variables and integrating:

$$y = \int dy = \int f(t)\, dt \qquad [23]$$

A simple physical situation that can be described by a differential equation of this type (Equation [22]) might be a vertical cylinder of constant radius, r, that is being filled so that the volume of water in the cylinder is increasing at the rate of v. Assuming that at time $t = 0$ the cylinder was already filled to a height, h, what is the function that quantitatively predicts the height of liquid in the cylinder at any time? A volume, v, of water flowing into the cylinder will add a disk-shaped plug of liquid whose height is $v/\pi r^2$; therefore the rate of change of the height, y, is

$$\frac{dy}{dt} = \frac{v}{\pi r^2} \qquad [24]$$

This equation is easily solved by direct integration:

$$\int dy = \int \left(\frac{v}{\pi r^2}\right) dt$$

Knowing that the term in parentheses in the right-hand integral is just a constant, we can find the solution from Box A-4:

$$y = \left(\frac{v}{\pi r^2}\right) t + C \qquad [25]$$

C the constant of integration, can be determined from the knowledge that at time $t = 0$, the cylinder was already filled to a height of $y = h$ (knowledge that allows us to determine the value of the constant of integration is referred to as a *boundary condition*). Substituting this information back into Equation [25] gives $C = h$. The exact solution to differential Equation [24] is thus

$$y = \left(\frac{v}{\pi r^2}\right) t + h \qquad [26]$$

A graphical representation of the behavior of the liquid column as predicted by Equation [26] is shown in Figure A-4.

Exponential Decay

We now consider a differential equation that is frequently applicable in all natural sciences:

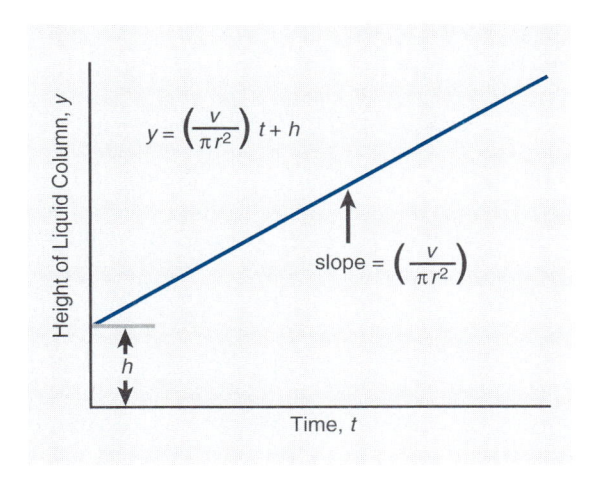

Appendix A

Figure A-4 ■ Graph of $y = (v/\pi r^2) \cdot t + h$ (Equation [26]). The equation is that of a straight line with slope = $v/\pi r^2$ and y-intercept = h.

$$\frac{dy}{dt} = -ky \qquad [27]$$

This equation basically says that the rate of decrease in some quantity, y, at a particular moment is directly proportional to the magnitude of y at that moment. This condition applies to loss of permeant solute from a compartment enclosed by a semipermeable membrane into a volume of fluid that is much larger than the volume of the compartment: the lower the solute concentration in the compartment, the fewer the number of molecules that can cross the membrane at any given moment, and the more slowly the concentration inside the compartment will change. Similarly, the condition applies in the case of radioactive decay, where the rate of decay (the rate of change of the quantity of radioactive atoms) is directly proportional to the number of radioactive atoms that are left (the fewer radioactive atoms there are, the fewer that can decay at any given moment).

Equation [27] can be solved by separating variables (collecting terms containing t with dt and collecting terms containing y with dy) and then integrating:

$$\int \frac{dy}{y} = \int -k\,dt$$

Again, the answer can be written down with the help of the integrals in Box A-4,

$$\ln y = -kt + C$$

and then rewritten in exponential notation,

$$y = e^{-kt} \cdot e^C$$

Using the boundary condition that at time $t = 0$, y had its initial value, y_0, we arrive at the exact solution of Equation [27]:

$$y = y_0 \cdot e^{-kt} \qquad [28]$$

Because the parameter, k, determines how fast y decreases, k is often referred to as the *rate constant*, which has dimensions of 1/time. The inverse of k ($1/k$), with dimensions of time, is known as the *time constant* (symbolized by the Greek letter τ). The larger the rate constant, k (or, the smaller the time constant, τ), the faster the value of y decreases. The behavior predicted by Equation [28] is shown in Figure A-5.

First-Order Linear Differential Equations

The last type of differential equation useful in this book is a first-order linear equation, which can always be put into the form

$$\frac{dy}{dt} + Py = Q \qquad [29]$$

where P and Q are functions of the dependent variable, t. This equation can be transformed into a separable equation if the entire equation is multiplied by a correctly chosen function, which is referred to as an *integrating factor*, φ:

$$\phi = e^{\int P\,dt} \qquad [30]$$

whose derivative is

$$\frac{d\phi}{dt} = e^{\int P\,dt}\, P = \phi P \qquad [31]$$

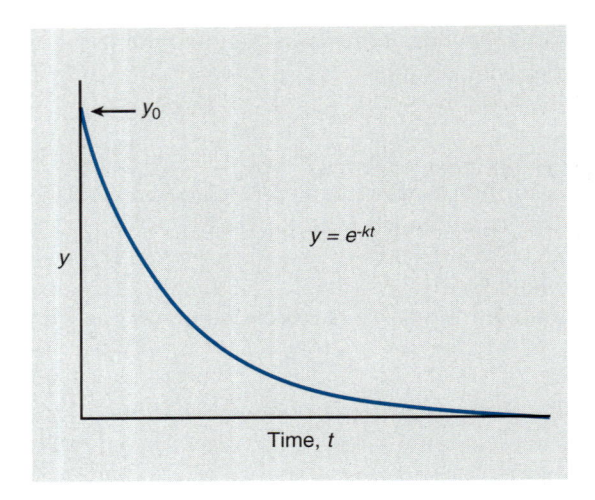

Figure A-5 ■ **Graph of the exponential decay, $y = y_0 e^{-kt}$. Initially ($t = 0$), $y = y_0$. As t increases, y asymptotically approaches 0.**

Multiplying Equation [29] by φ yields

$$\phi \frac{dy}{dt} + \phi P y = \phi Q$$

which is, in light of Equation [31],

$$\phi \frac{dy}{dt} + y \frac{d\phi}{dt} = \phi Q \quad [32]$$

Consulting the properties of derivatives (Box A-3), we recognize the left-hand side of Equation [32] as the derivative of a product function:

$$\frac{d}{dt}(\phi y) = \phi Q$$

This equation is now separable because the right-hand side, φQ, is a function of t exclusively and can be grouped with dt, whereas $d(\varphi y)$ is by itself. Separation of variables and integration yields

$$\phi y = \int \phi Q \, dt$$

which gives the solution to the differential Equation [29] as

$$y = \frac{1}{\phi} \int \phi Q \, dt \quad [33]$$

This solution is useful in a discussion of the electrical behavior of a biological membrane, which can be represented as an R-C circuit (Appendix C, Box C-3). The relevant differential equation there is

$$\frac{dV_m}{dt} + \frac{1}{RC} \cdot V_m = \frac{I_T}{C} \quad [34]$$

where V_m, R, and C are, respectively, the membrane voltage, membrane resistance, and membrane capacitance and I_T is the total current passing through the membrane. It is clear that Equation [34] is identical in form to Equation [29]; therefore the solution [33] applies. The integrating factor is

$$\phi = e^{\int \frac{1}{RC} dt} = e^{\frac{t}{RC}}$$

and the solution is

$$V_m = e^{-\frac{t}{RC}} \int e^{\frac{t}{RC}} \left(\frac{I_T}{C}\right) dt = e^{-\frac{t}{RC}} \left[\frac{I_T}{C} \cdot e^{\frac{t}{RC}} \cdot RC + Const\right]$$
$$= I_T R + Const \cdot e^{-\frac{t}{RC}}$$

where *Const.* is the constant of integration. A boundary condition helps to define the exact solution: at $t = 0$, $V_m = 0$; therefore $Const = -I_T R$. The exact solution is thus

$$V_m = I_T R \left[1 - e^{-\frac{t}{RC}}\right] \quad [35]$$

It is easy to verify through Equation [35] that (1) at very long times ($t \to \infty$), the membrane voltage will reach a steady-state value, $V_{m,\infty} = I_T R$, and (2) $R \times C$ has the dimensions of time and can be defined as the membrane time constant, τ_m. These two observations allow the solution to be written in a more compact form:

$$V_m = V_{m,\infty} \left[1 - e^{-\frac{t}{\tau_m}}\right] \quad [36]$$

APPENDIX B

Root-Mean-Squared Displacement of Diffusing Molecules

Initially there are N molecules, all at starting position 0. For any particular molecule (for our purposes, tagged with a label i), regardless of where the molecule is, it can move only either 1 step to the left (a distance of $-\delta$) or 1 step to the right (a distance of $+\delta$). This means that the location of any molecule i after n steps must be related to its immediately previous location (at $[n-1]$ steps) by either $+\delta$ or $-\delta$. In other words,

$$x_i(n) = x_i(n-1) \pm \delta \quad [1]$$

The first question we can ask is, "What is the average position of all of the molecules after all of them have taken n steps?" This is easy to calculate by simply adding up the positions of all of the molecules and then dividing by the total number of molecules, N. That is,

$$\text{Average position} = \frac{x_1(n) + x_2(n) + x_3(n) + \ldots + x_{N-2}(n) + x_{N-1}(n) + x_N(n)}{N} \quad [2]$$

Using the symbol $<x_i(n)>$ to represent the average position, and making use of summation notation, we can write the average position as

$$<x_i(n)> = \frac{\sum_{i=1}^{N} x_i(n)}{N} \quad [3]$$

Using the relationship between the position after n steps and the position after $(n-1)$ steps (Equation [1]) gives

$$<x_i(n)> = \frac{\sum_{i=1}^{N} [x_i(n-1) \pm \delta]}{N}$$

$$= \left\{ \frac{\sum_{i=1}^{N} x_i(n-1)}{N} \right\} + \left\{ \frac{\sum_{i=1}^{N} (\pm \delta)}{N} \right\} \quad [4]$$

In Equation [4] the first term enclosed in braces is just the average position after $(n-1)$ steps, $<x_i(n-1)>$. The second term in braces is the average of all the steps that all the molecules have just taken. Since the molecules moved randomly, essentially half of the steps must have size $+\delta$ and half must have size $-\delta$. This means that all the steps average to 0, so the second term in braces is equal to 0. Therefore Equation [4] simplifies to

$$<x_i(n)> = <x_i(n-1)> \quad [5]$$

Equation [5] says that the average position of all the molecules remains the same from one step to the next, regardless of how many steps have been taken.

The average position of the molecules is clearly not a very informative parameter. Nonetheless, we know that with time the molecules will progressively spread out in space (see Figure 2-4). How can we make this observation more quantitative? We can decide how to proceed by trying to understand why the average position (i.e., the average displacement from the initial point 0) is so uninformative. The reason is that since, on average, every $+\delta$ step must be balanced by a $-\delta$ step, the arithmetical average must always come out to be 0. One way to get around the fact that there are + and – steps is to square the displacements and *then* average them. Because any positive or negative number squared gives a positive number, averaging the squared displacements guarantees that the result would be non-0.

Squaring the displacements shown in Equation [1] yields

$$x_i^2(n) = [x_i(n-1) \pm \delta]^2$$
$$= [x_i(n-1) \pm \delta] \times [x_i(n-1) \pm \delta] \quad [6]$$

Actually multiplying out the last two terms gives

$$x_i^2(n) = x_i^2(n-1) \pm 2\delta x_i(n-1) + \delta^2 \quad [7]$$

Summing each term in Equation [7] for all N molecules and then dividing by N gives the average for each term:

$$\frac{\sum_{i=1}^{N} x_i^2(n)}{N} = \frac{\sum_{i=1}^{N} x_i^2(n-1)}{N} + \frac{\sum_{i=1}^{N} \pm 2\delta x_i(n-1)}{N} + \frac{\sum_{i=1}^{N} \delta^2}{N} \quad [8]$$

The term on the left side of the equal sign is the average squared displacement after n steps. The first term on the right is the average squared displacement after $(n-1)$ steps. By the argument we used earlier, that + and – displacements are equally likely, the second term on the right must be 0. Finally, the last term on the right is just adding δ^2 N times and then dividing by N again; the value must therefore be simply δ^2. After the above simplifications, Equation [8] turns into

$$<x_i^2(n)> = <x_i^2(n-1)> + \delta^2 \quad [9]$$

Knowledge about the distribution of molecules at time = 0 allows Equation [9] to be put into a much simpler and more useful form. At time = 0 (when 0 steps have been taken), all the molecules are clustered at position 0; the mean squared position or displacement must necessarily be 0. In symbols: $<x_i^2(0)> = 0$. Putting this back into Equation [9] gives

$$<x_i^2(1)> = <x_i^2(0)> + \delta^2 = \delta^2$$

In other words, the mean squared displacement after all the molecules have taken a *single* step ($n = 1$) of size δ is just $1\delta^2$. Using this new result in Equation [9] again gives

$$<x_i^2(2)> = <x_i^2(1)> + \delta^2 = 2\delta^2$$

In other words, the mean squared displacement after all the molecules have taken *two* steps ($n = 2$) of size δ is just $2\delta^2$. In fact, Equation [9] can be used iteratively to generate the mean squared displacement after *any* number of steps. The sequence of results generated in this way is thus

$<x_i^2(0)> = 0$ after 0 steps,
$<x_i^2(1)> = \delta^2$ after 1 step,
$<x_i^2(2)> = 2\delta^2$ after 2 steps,
$<x_i^2(3)> = 3\delta^2$ after 3 steps, etc.

Or, in general,

$$<x_i^2(n)> = n\delta^2 \quad \text{after } n \text{ steps} \quad [10]$$

Appendix B

This result is expressed in terms of the number of steps the molecules have taken. In reality, it is impossible to monitor all the steps that all the molecules actually take. Therefore it would be much more convenient to express the result in terms of *time* rather than the number of steps. If each step is taken in a time increment of Δt, then the elapsed time, t, after n steps is $t = n \times \Delta t$, which also means that $n = t/\Delta t$. These two facts allow us to put Equation [10] into the following form

$$<x_i^2(t)> = \left(\frac{t}{\Delta t}\right)\delta^2 = \left(\frac{\delta^2}{\Delta t}\right)t \quad [11]$$

If we define a "diffusion coefficient" or "diffusion constant," $D = (\delta^2/2\Delta t)$,* Equation [11] becomes

$$<x_i^2(t)> = 2Dt \quad [12]$$

Now, the average, or mean, *squared* displacement has weird dimensions of *length squared*. To get something that is more intuitively accessible, we can take the square root of both sides of Equation [12] to get the "root-mean-squared" (RMS) position or displacement, which again has dimensions of length:

$$\textbf{RMS displacement} = d_{RMS} = \sqrt{<x_i^2(t)>} = \sqrt{2Dt} \quad [13]$$

The RMS displacement is a measure of how "spread out" the initially clustered molecules become after some time has elapsed.

The RMS displacement derived above is for molecules diffusing along a single dimension. What happens in the more common case of molecules diffusing in two dimensions (e.g., along a membrane surface) or three dimensions (e.g., in solution)? Molecules cannot distinguish directions, so their diffusional behavior should be independent of direction. Figure B-1 shows that the Pythagorean theorem gives the answer:

$$\left(d_{RMS}^{2\text{-}D}\right)^2 = \left(d_x^{1\text{-}D}\right)^2 + \left(d_y^{1\text{-}D}\right)^2 \quad \text{or}$$
$$d_{RMS}^{2\text{-}D} = \sqrt{\left(d_x^{1\text{-}D}\right)^2 + \left(d_y^{1\text{-}D}\right)^2} \quad [14]$$

Since $d_{RMS} = \sqrt{2Dt}$ for any single dimension x, y, or z, substitution into Equation [14] gives the result for diffusion in two dimensions (2-D):

$$d^{2\text{-}D} = \sqrt{\left(d_x^{1\text{-}D}\right)^2 + \left(d_y^{1\text{-}D}\right)^2} = \sqrt{2Dt + 2Dt} = \sqrt{4Dt} \quad [15]$$

Similarly, for diffusion in three dimensions (3-D), the result is

$$d^{3\text{-}D} = \sqrt{6Dt} \quad [16]$$

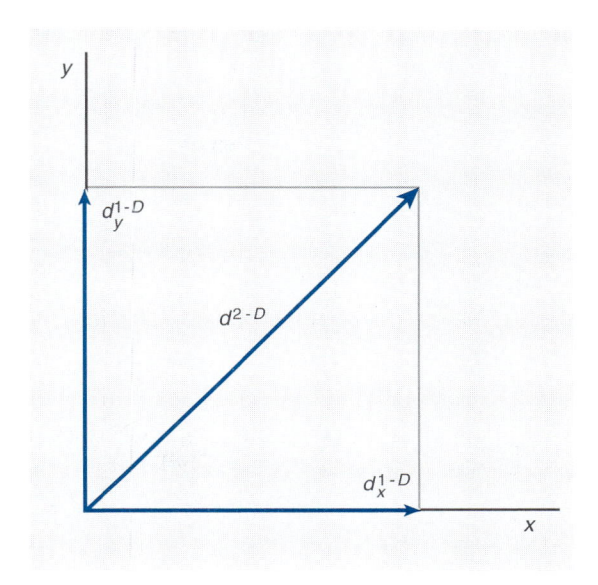

Figure B-1 ∎

---

*The thing to notice about the diffusion coefficient is that it embodies microscopic molecular properties (δ, the size of the step that a molecule can take, and Δt, the time over which such steps are taken). In addition, the diffusion coefficient has dimensions of length squared over time, as we had deduced from our discussion of Fick's First Law.

■ BIBLIOGRAPHY

Feynman RP, Leighton RB, Sands ML: *The Feynman lectures on physics*, vol 1, Reading, Mass, 1965, Addison-Wesley.

APPENDIX C

Summary of Elementary Circuit Theory

■ CELL MEMBRANES ARE MODELED WITH ELECTRICAL CIRCUITS

Knowledge of the behavior of elementary electrical circuits is extremely helpful for understanding the electrical activity of excitable cells because the membrane can be modeled with an electrical circuit. Figure C-1, *A*, is a schematic view of the structure of a biological membrane with a single open K^+-selective ion channel. This physical entity is electrically equivalent to the circuit shown in Figure C-1, *B*. The circuit consists of a resistor in series with a battery, and this combination is in parallel with a capacitor. The electrical behavior of most resting biological membranes is, in fact, indistinguishable from a circuit similar to that shown in Figure C-1, *B*. As a result, one application of such "equivalent circuits" is to obtain quantitative descriptions of important membrane electrical behavior. This approach is employed in Chapter 6 to describe such parameters as the length constant and the membrane time constant. The equivalent circuit is also helpful for describing current flow across membranes and the effect of current flow on the membrane potential. Equivalent circuits are used in Chapter 7 to help illustrate how the action potential is generated and propagated along an elongated structure such as an axon or a skeletal muscle cell.

■ DEFINITIONS OF ELECTRICAL PARAMETERS

Electrical Potential and Potential Difference

The potential difference between two points is the amount of work done per unit charge to move a unit of charge from one point to the other. The unit of measure of potential difference is the volt. Potential difference (often called voltage) reflects the electrostatic force exerted on a charge. We often use the term

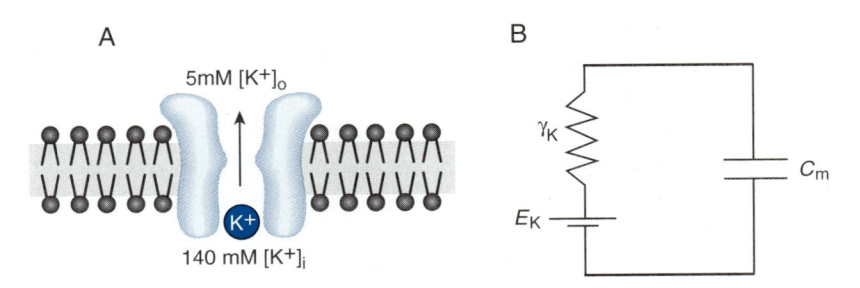

Figure C-1 ■ **A,** Schematic drawing of a lipid bilayer membrane containing a single open K⁺ channel. An outwardly directed K⁺ concentration gradient is present. **B,** The electrical equivalent of the membrane shown in A. The open K channel is modeled as a conductor (or equivalently, a resistor) with a conductance, γ_K, equal to that of the open channel. The resistor is in series with a battery that represents the K⁺ concentration gradient, and it has a voltage equal to E_K. The capacitor represents the ability of the lipid bilayer to separate charge and is parallel to the channel.

"driving force" for the net potential difference exerted on a charge. We use the symbol E to represent theoretical potentials, such as the equilibrium potential of an ion (see Chapter 4), and the symbol V for actual voltages, such as the membrane potential (V_m).

Current

If mobile charges are present in an area of potential difference, positive charges tend to move toward the more negative potential and negative charges tend to move toward the more positive potential. This movement of charge is a *current (I)*. The current at a point in a circuit is defined as the net movement of positive charge past that point per unit time. The movement of 1 coulomb of charge per second is a current of 1 ampere (A). In wires and electronic devices the current is carried by electrons. In biological systems, however, current is carried by mobile ions (e.g., Na^+, K^+, Cl^-, H^+, Ca^{2+}) moving in an aqueous environment.

By convention, when an arrow is used to indicate current flow, it indicates the *net* movement of *positive* charge. The physical reality corresponding to such a representation could be either positive charges moving in the direction of the arrow or negative charges moving in the opposite direction.

Resistance and Conductance

The current that flows through a conductive material is proportional to the voltage across the material. We refer to such a material as either a conductor or a resistor. In electronic circuits resistors are made of carbon or some other low-conductivity material and are characterized by their resistance (R). Intuition tells us that the current through the resistor should increase as the driving force (voltage, or V) across the resistor increases. This relationship is quantitatively given by Ohm's Law, which states that the current through a resistor is directly proportional to the voltage across it:

$$V = I \times R \qquad [1]$$

Resistance is measured in ohms (Ω): a current of 1 ampere will flow through a 1-ohm resistor with a driving force of 1 volt across it. Open ion channels behave electrically like conductors (or resistors): the membrane potential drives ion movement through open channels. The ability of a channel to pass current is characterized as its conductance (g or γ), which is the reciprocal of resistance: $g = 1/R$. The unit of conductance is the siemens (S): $1\ S = 1/\Omega = \Omega^{-1}$.

To understand the relationship expressed by Ohm's Law, we should consider that the flow of electrical current driven by a voltage difference is analogous to many other relationships between flow and driving force. One example is the relationship between bulk water flow and hydrostatic pressure. In Chapter 3 the quantitative relationship for water flow across a membrane was expressed as:

$$J_v = L_p\ \Delta P \qquad [2]$$

where J_v is volume flow, L_p is the hydraulic conductivity of the membrane, and ΔP is the hydrostatic pressure difference. A similar equation could be used to describe water flow through a pipe, where the "conductivity" would be directly proportional to the cross-sectional area of the pipe. Thus electrical current flow through an electrically conductive material driven by a voltage difference is analogous to fluid flow through a fluid-restrictive pathway driven by a hydrostatic pressure difference.

Capacitance

A capacitor is a device that can store, or separate, charges of opposite sign. A parallel plate capacitor has two parallel conducting plates (e.g., made of metal foil) separated by an insulator (e.g., mica, Mylar, glass, air). Biological membranes have capacitive properties because the lipid bilayer is an effective electrical insulator that allows soluble ions to be separated across the membrane. The amount of charge stored on a capacitor is directly proportional to the voltage across the capacitor:

$$Q = C \times V \qquad [3]$$

where Q is the charge in coulombs, V is the voltage in volts, and C is the capacitance of the device in farads. Note that $+Q$ coulombs are stored on one plate and $-Q$ coulombs on the other plate. The capacitance of a given device, or a given area of membrane, is a constant, so Equation [3] shows that if the amount of charge stored on a capacitor (Q) increases, the potential difference (V) across the capacitor must increase.

By taking the time derivative of Equation [3], we obtain

$$\frac{dQ}{dt} = C \times \frac{dV}{dt} \quad \text{or} \quad I_c = C \times \frac{dV}{dt} \qquad [4]$$

The quantity dQ/dt (charge per unit time, or coulombs per second) is by definition a current (I_c, the capacitive current). Thus, in contrast to a resistor, where the current is proportional to the voltage, in a capacitor the current is proportional to the *rate of change* of the voltage. This important relationship shows that if the voltage is changing (i.e., dV/dt is nonzero), capacitive current is flowing. Conversely, $I_c = 0$ when the voltage is constant (i.e., when $dV/dt = 0$).

In the hydrostatic pressure analogy, a large-diameter cylindrical tank that can store water is analogous to the electrical capacitor. The hydrostatic pressure exerted by a column of water is directly proportional to the height of the column. Thus, as water flows into the tank, the height of the water increases (water is stored) and the hydrostatic pressure increases (Box C-1). Similarly, as current flows into a capacitor, charges become separated (or stored) on the capacitor and the voltage across the capacitor changes.

■ CURRENT FLOW IN SIMPLE CIRCUITS

The circuits described in the following sections are analyzed with use of the rules for circuit analysis described in Box C-2.

A Battery and Resistor in Parallel

The circuit in Figure C-2, A, shows a battery with a voltage of V_b volts connected via a switch to a

> **BOX C-1**
>
> ### *Cylindrical Tank of Fluid Is Analogous to an Electrical Capacitor*
>
> A cylindrical tank of cross-sectional area A contains a fluid with a density of ρ at a height of h (Figure C-1). The volume of the tank (V) is:
>
> $$V = A \times h$$
>
> **Figure C-1** ■ **A cylindrical tank with a cross-sectional area A contains a fluid with a density of ρ at a depth of h.**
>
> The mass of fluid contained in the tank is:
>
> $$m = \rho \times V = \rho \times A \times h$$
>
> The weight of the fluid in the tank is:
>
> $$w = m \times g = \rho \times g \times A \times h$$
>
> where g is the acceleration caused by gravity. The pressure, Δp, that the fluid exerts on the bottom of the tank is its weight divided by the cross-sectional area of the tank:
>
> $$\Delta P = \frac{w}{A} = \rho \times g \times h$$
>
> Thus the hydrostatic pressure (ΔP) exerted by a column of water is directly proportional to the height of the column. The storage tank is analogous to a capacitor in electrical circuits. The capacitor equation (Equation [3] in the text) shows that the amount of charge stored on a capacitor is proportional to the potential difference across it. Similarly, the amount of water (charge) stored in the tank is proportional to the hydrostatic pressure (potential) exerted by the water because pressure is proportional to the height of the water.

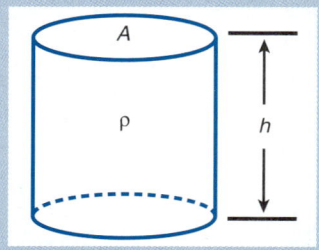

resistance of R ohms. With the switch open no current flows, so the voltage across R is zero. When the switch is closed, a current (I) flows from the positive pole of the battery through the resistor and back to the negative pole of the battery. The current instantaneously takes on a value of V_b/R amperes (from Ohm's Law), as shown in Figure C-2, *B*. When a capacitor is added to this circuit, time delays are introduced (i.e., voltage changes are no longer instantaneous), as shown in a later section.

A hydraulic version of this pure resistive circuit is shown in Figure C-3. A pump that delivers a constant hydrostatic pressure (ΔP) is connected via a valve to a small-diameter, water-filled tube. With the valve closed the hydrostatic pressure difference between the two ends of the tube is zero, so no water flows. When the valve is opened (equivalent to closing a switch in an electrical circuit), water immediately flows out the tube at a constant rate (equivalent to the current flow in an electrical circuit), driven by pressure ΔP (equivalent to the voltage).

A Resistor and Capacitor in Parallel

Next we consider the effect of placing a capacitor in parallel with a resistor (Figure C-4, *A*). Current flow through this circuit is shown with a constant current generator connected to the circuit through a switch. The current generator is designed so that it continuously passes the same, constant amount of current through the circuit. When the switch is closed, a constant current (I_T) is passed through the

BOX C-2

Kirchhoff's Laws Are Used to Analyze Circuits

Two relationships, known as Kirchhoff's Laws, are useful in circuit analysis.

Kirchhoff's Current Law

Current is the movement of charge in a circuit, and when an arrow is used to indicate the direction of current flow, it shows the direction of *net positive charge* movement. Thus, when current flows through a resistor, the end the current enters is at a positive voltage relative to the end the current leaves.

Charge can never accumulate at a point in a circuit. Thus Kirchhoff's First Law states that the sum of the currents flowing into a point in a circuit must equal the sum of the currents flowing out of that point (i.e., there is conservation of charge). Another way to state this law is that the sum of all currents entering and leaving a point in a circuit is zero, if we adopt the arbitrary convention that currents entering are positive and currents leaving are negative. The circuit in Figure C-1 illustrates this law. Using Kirchhoff's Current Law for the point labeled 1 gives the result

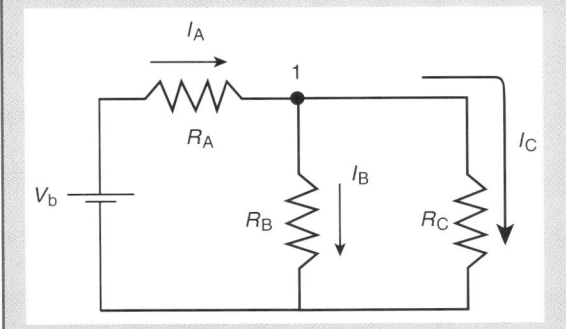

$$I_A = I_B + I_C \qquad [B1]$$

Figure C-1 ■ A battery of voltage V_b is connected to three resistors, R_A, R_B, and R_C, in the manner shown. A current, I_A, flows from the positive terminal of the battery through R_A. At the point labeled 1, some of the current, I_B, flows through R_B and the rest of the current, I_C, flows through R_C.

We will come back to this example later in Box C-3. From Kirchhoff's Current Law we can also deduce that in a series circuit (where elements are connected end to end), the current is the same everywhere.

Kirchhoff's Voltage Law

Elements connected in parallel in a circuit have the same voltage across them. Another way to state this is that the algebraic sum of all voltage drops around a closed loop is zero. When Kirchhoff's Voltage Law is applied, the following sign conventions should be used: (1) the voltage drop across a resistor is positive in the direction of current flow and (2) the voltage drop across a battery is taken as positive if we meet the + pole of the battery going around the loop and negative if we meet the − pole. In the circuit in Figure C-1 the voltage drops across resistors R_A and R_B are $I_A \times R_A$ and $I_B \times R_B$, respectively. If we apply Kirchhoff's Voltage Law to the loop with battery V_b and the resistors R_A and R_B, we would write

$$I_A \times R_A + I_B \times R_B - V_b = 0 \qquad [B2]$$

For the loop with R_B and R_C the voltage law gives

$$I_C \times R_C - I_B \times R_B = 0 \quad \text{or} \quad I_C \times R_C = +I_B \times R_B \qquad [B3]$$

Using Equations [B1], [B2], and [B3], we can solve for $I_A, I_B,$ and I_C as follows.

Rearranging Equation [B2] gives

$$I_A = \frac{V_b - I_B \times R_B}{R_A} \qquad [B4]$$

Substitution of Equations [B3] and [B4] into equation [B1] gives the following equation, which can be solved for I_B:

$$\frac{V_b - I_B \times R_B}{R_A} - I_B - I_B \times \frac{R_A}{R_C} = 0$$

and

$$I_B = \frac{V_b}{R_A + R_B + \frac{R_A \times R_B}{R_C}}$$

If we let $V_b = 10$ volts, $R_A = 10$ ohms, $R_B = 10$ ohms, and $R_C = 20$ ohms, these equations give 0.6, 0.4, and 0.2 ampere for $I_A, I_B,$ and I_C, respectively.

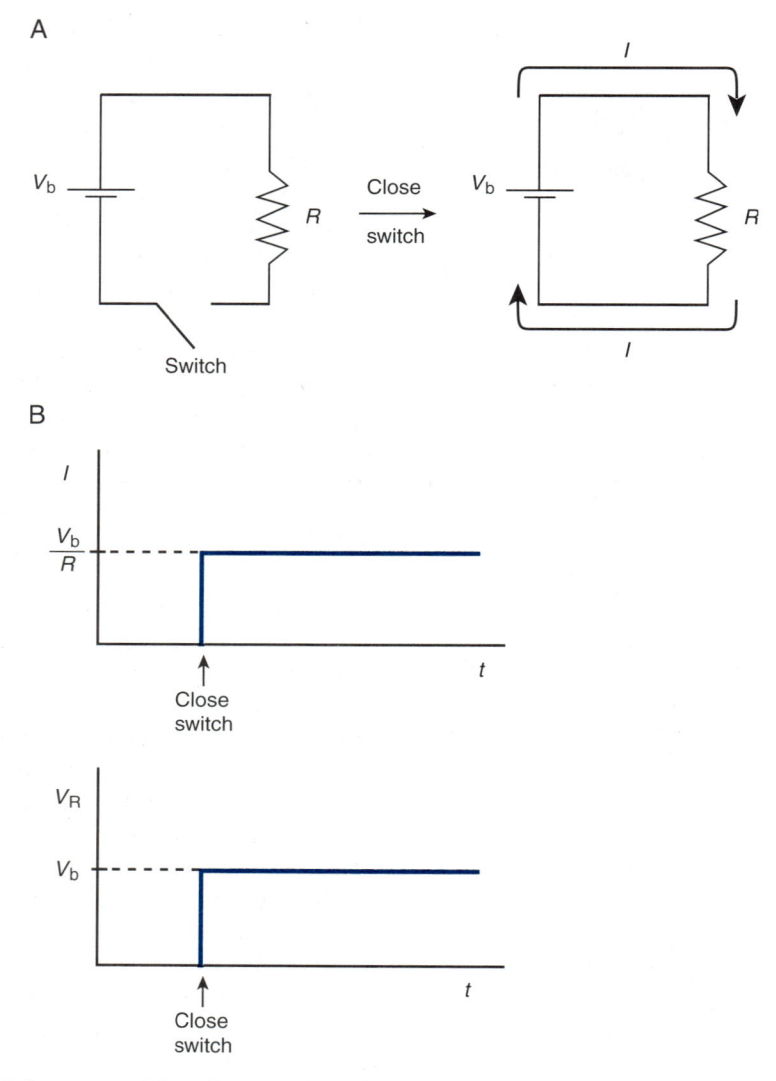

Figure C-2 ■ A, A battery, with voltage V_b, is connected to a resistor of R ohms through a switch. When the switch is closed, a current (I) flows from the positive terminal of the battery, through the resistor, and back to the battery. B, At the instant the switch is closed, the voltage drop across the resistor, V_R, is equal to V_b, and a current of magnitude V_b/R flows through the resistor.

Appendix C

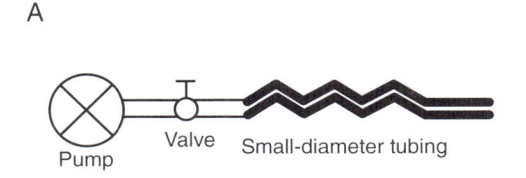

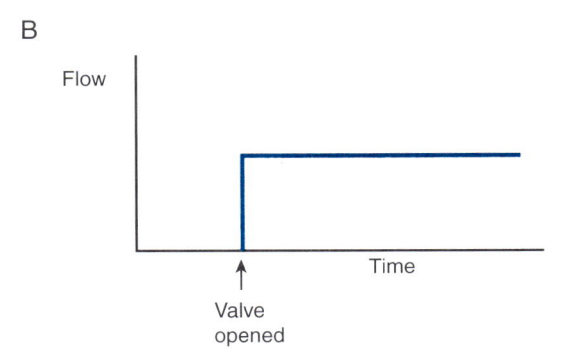

Figure C-3 ■ **A,** A hydraulic analogy of the pure resistive electrical circuit. A constant flow pump is connected through a valve to a length of small-diameter tubing. **B,** At the instant the valve is opened, water flows out of the tube at a rate equal to the flow from the pump.

circuit. At the instant the switch is closed (Figure C-4, *B*), all of this current flows through the capacitor (Box C-3). This capacitive current increases the charge separation across the capacitor, and a potential difference, V_C, develops across the capacitor. Because *R* and *C* are arranged in parallel, the same potential difference develops across *R*: $V_C = V_R$. The voltage across the resistor causes current to flow in the resistor. As the resistive current develops, the capacitive current must decrease because the total current through the circuit, I_T, is constant (Figure C-4, *C*). Eventually the voltage across the circuit will stop changing, a new steady state will be reached, and all of the current will flow through the resistor (Figure C-4, *E*). A mathematical analysis of this circuit shows that I_C, I_R, and V_R all follow exponential time courses (Box C-3), and they are plotted as a function of time in Figure C-5. A comparison of Figure C-2, *B*, and Figure C-5 illustrates that the addition of a capacitor, in parallel with a resistor, causes a delay in the voltage change across the circuit. In a parallel *R-C* circuit the voltage does not change instantaneously in response to an applied current, as it does in a pure resistive circuit. Instead, the voltage changes along an exponential time course.

The time necessary to add, or store, charges on a capacitor may be easier to understand in terms of the hydrostatic pressure analogy. A "hydraulic" version of the parallel *R-C* circuit is shown in Figure C-6. A constant flow pump (the constant current generator) and a length of small-diameter tubing (the resistor) are connected to the base of a large-diameter, cylindrical tank (the capacitor). When the pump is first turned on (with the tank empty), all of the water flows into the tank; none flows out the tube because no driving force, or pressure difference, is present to force water out through the restricted tubing. As the water level in the tank increases, the hydrostatic pressure increases and water begins to flow out the tube, leaving less water available to fill the tank. The hydrostatic pressure in the tank and the outflow increase until the outflow is equal to the flow delivered by the pump and a new stable, steady state is reached. The hydrostatic pressure increases along an exponential time course. The hydrostatic pressure (or voltage) increases slowly because it takes time to fill the tank (or store charge on the capacitor).

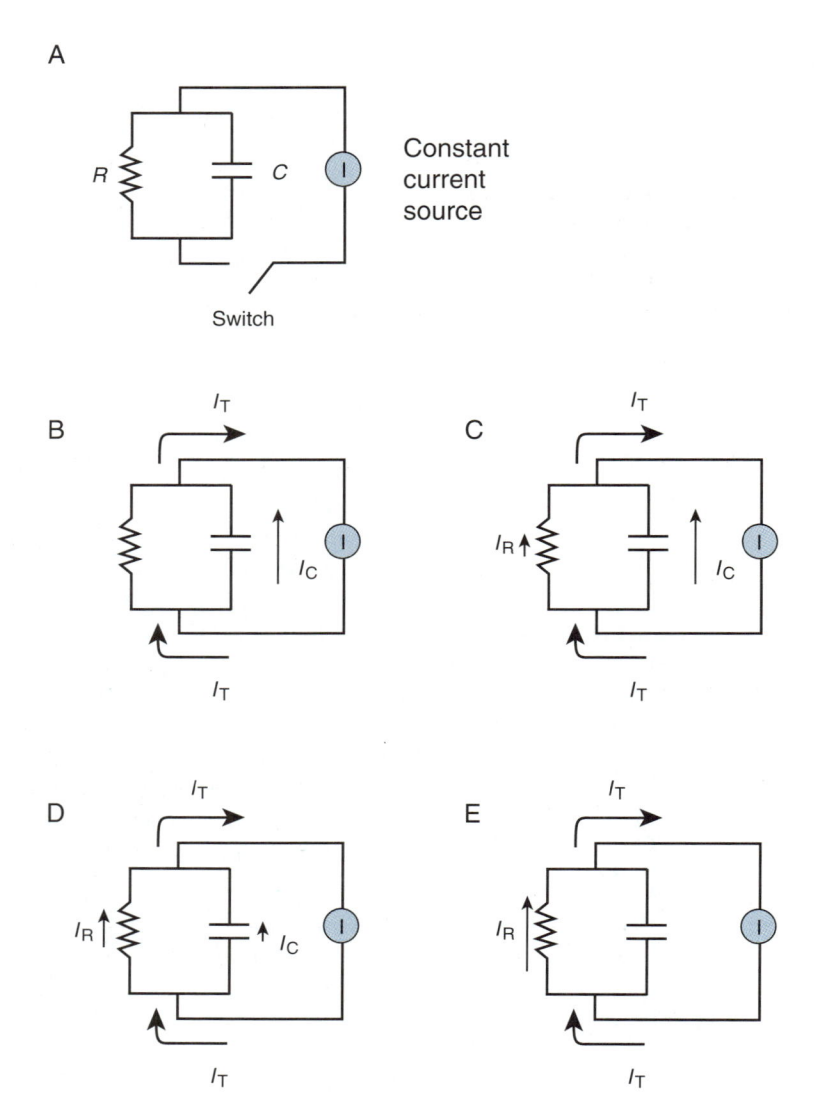

Figure C-4 ■ **A,** A parallel combination of a resistor and capacitor is connected to a constant current source through a switch. **B,** At the instant the switch is closed, all of the current from the source (I_T) flows through the capacitor (I_C). **C,** Shortly after the voltage across the circuit has changed (as a result of I_C), some of the applied current flows through the resistor (I_R). **D,** As the voltage continues to change, more current flows through the resistor and less through the capacitor. **E,** In the final steady state, all of the applied current flows through the resistor.

Appendix C

BOX C-3

A Parallel R-C Circuit Predicts an Exponential Change in Membrane Potential

The predicted time course of the change in membrane potential in response to a step of constant current for a parallel R-C circuit (Figure C-4, A) can be derived as follows. The total membrane current must be the sum of an ionic current and a capacitive current, so we can write

$$I_T = I_R + I_C = \frac{V_R}{R} + C \times \frac{dV_C}{dt} \qquad [B1]$$

where I_R is the current through the resistor and I_C is the capacitive current. The resistor and capacitor are in parallel, so $V_R = V_C$. If we let $V_m = V_R = V_C$, we get

$$I_T = \frac{V_m}{R} + C \times \frac{dV_m}{dt} \qquad [B2]$$

This linear first-order differential equation can be solved with use of the methods described in Appendix A to give the following relationship:

$$V_m(t) = V_{m,\infty}\left[1 - \exp\left(\frac{-t}{\tau_m}\right)\right] \qquad [B3]$$

where $\tau_m = R \times C$ and $V_{m,\infty} = I_T \times R$. We can then readily obtain the following equations for $I_R(t)$ and $I_C(t)$.

For the resistive, or ionic current, we get:

$$I_R(t) = \frac{V_m(t)}{R} = \frac{V_{m,\infty}}{R}\left[1 - \exp\left(\frac{-t}{\tau_m}\right)\right] = I_T\left[1 - \exp\left(\frac{-t}{\tau_m}\right)\right] \qquad [B4]$$

For the capacitive current:

$$I_C(t) = C \times \frac{dV_m(t)}{dt} \qquad [B5]$$

By taking the time derivative of Equation [B3], we get:

$$\frac{dV_m(t)}{dt} = V_{m,\infty} \times \frac{d\left[1 - \exp\left(\frac{-t}{\tau_m}\right)\right]}{dt} = \frac{V_{m,\infty}}{\tau_m} \times \left[\exp\left(\frac{-t}{\tau_m}\right)\right] \qquad [B6]$$

Combining Equations [5] and [6] gives:

$$I_C(t) = \frac{C \times V_{m,\infty}}{\tau_m}\left[\exp\left(\frac{-t}{\tau_m}\right)\right]$$

$$= \frac{C \times I_T \times R}{C \times R}\left[\exp\left(\frac{-t}{\tau_m}\right)\right]$$

$$= I_T \times \exp\left(\frac{-t}{\tau_m}\right)$$

Using these equations, we can show that at $t = 0$, $I_R = 0$ and $I_C = I_T$ and at $t = \infty$, $I_R = I_T$ and $I_C = 0$. Thus, at the instant the current step, I_T, is applied, all of the current is capacitive. The magnitude of I_C then falls to zero along an exponential time course. The resistive (or ionic) current is zero initially, and it increases along an exponential time course. When a new steady state is reached, all of the applied current is ionic current.

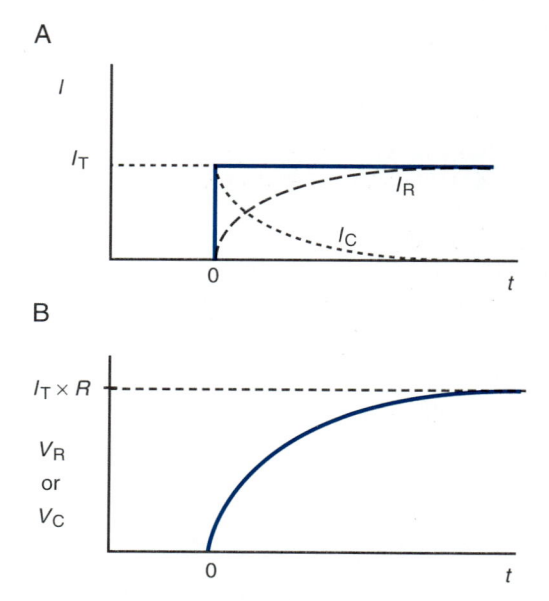

Figure C-5 ■ The voltage, capacitive current, and resistive current in a parallel *R-C* circuit all follow an exponential time course in response to a constant current step.

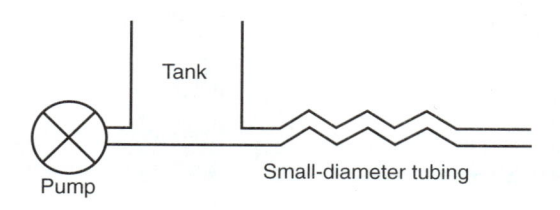

Figure C-6 ■ A hydraulic analogy of the electrical *R-C* circuit. The constant flow pump is analogous to a constant current generator, the storage tank is analogous to a capacitor, and the small-diameter tubing is analogous to a resistor.

APPENDIX D

Answers to Study Problems

■ CHAPTER 2

1. The relationship between the distance and time of diffusion is $d \propto \sqrt{t}$; that is, the distance diffused is proportional to the square root of time (e.g., for three-dimensional diffusion, $d = \sqrt{6Dt}$). One way to solve the problem is to plug numbers in: first, 5 μm = $\sqrt{6 \cdot D \cdot 1 \text{ sec}}$; second, 10 μm = $\sqrt{6 \cdot D \cdot t}$. The first equation allows us to solve for D: squaring the first equation gives 25 μm² = $6D$ sec, which means that $D = 25/6$ μm²/sec. Substituting the value of D into the second equation gives 10 μm = $\sqrt{6 \cdot (25/6 \text{ μm}^2 \text{ sec}^{-1}) \cdot t} = \sqrt{(25 \text{ μm}^2 \text{ sec}^{-1}) \cdot t}$. This can be solved by squaring both sides to give 100 μm² = $(25 \text{ μm}^2 \cdot \text{sec}^{-1}) \cdot t$, which means that $t = 4$ sec. The thing to notice is that, because of the square root dependence on time, to go twice as far by diffusion takes four (2^2) times as long.

2. The expressions should be written as $J_{\text{inward}} = P_K \times [K^+]_o$ and $J_{\text{outward}} = P_K \times [K^+]_i$. A net flux is positive when it brings material *into* the cell. Therefore the correct expression for the net flux of K^+ is $J_K = J_{\text{inward}} - J_{\text{outward}} = P_K ([K^+]_o - [K^+]_i)$.

■ CHAPTER 3

1. In solving all of these problems, "very large volume of plasma" implies the "infinite bath" condition. In other words, the extracellular fluid volume is so large that a bit of solute or water entering or leaving the cell will have essentially *no effect* on either the extracellular volume or the concentrations of solutes in the extracellular fluid.

   a. Answer: Water will move out of the cell. The final cell volume will be one half the initial volume. Explanation: The cell was initially equilibrated, which must mean that the intracellular concentration of permeant solute was $C_P = 300$ mM and the intracellular concentration of impermeant

281

solute was $C_{NP} = 10$ mM. When we consider the situation at equilibrium, we need not worry about the permeant solute because it can cross the cell membrane (and the intracellular and extracellular permeant solute concentrations will always become equal automatically). When the extracellular impermeant solute concentration is increased to 20 mM, an osmotic imbalance occurs, with the inside of the cell having a deficit of impermeant solute. Because the impermeant solute concentration in the cell cannot be changed by solute movement (an impermeant solute cannot cross the cell membrane), the only way the cell can cope with the osmotic imbalance is to *lose water and shrink its volume*. The reduction in cell volume would increase the impermeant solute concentration inside until the intracellular and extracellular impermeant solute concentrations become equal. To calculate the volume change, we note that the initial equilibrium condition is $C_{NP,cell,init} = C_{NP,bath,init}$ (impermeant solutes in the cell and bath are balanced) and the final equilibrium condition is $C_{NP,cell,final} = C_{NP,bath,final}$ (impermeant solutes in the cell and bath are once again balanced). Concentration is just the number of moles per volume of solution; therefore the two equalities may be written as

$$\frac{n_{NP,cell,init}}{V_{cell,init}} = C_{NP,bath,init} = 10 \text{ mM} \quad \text{and}$$

$$\frac{n_{NP,cell,final}}{V_{cell,final}} = C_{NP,bath,final} = 20 \text{ mM}$$

We know that the *number of moles* of impermeant solute inside the cell must remain constant because any impermeant solute originally inside the cell must remain there at all times. In other words, $n_{NP,cell,init} = n_{NP,cell,final} = n_{NP,cell}$. Substituting this back into the two equations above and rearranging gives

$$V_{cell,init} = \frac{n_{NP,cell}}{10 \text{ mM}} \quad \text{and} \quad V_{cell,final} = \frac{n_{NP,cell}}{20 \text{ mM}}$$

Solving these two equations (e.g., by dividing the second equation by the first) gives

$$\frac{V_{cell,final}}{V_{cell,init}} = \frac{1}{2}$$

In other words, the final cell volume will be half the initial volume.

b. Answer: Water will initially move out of the cell (so the cell volume will decrease), but then the volume will gradually return to the initial volume as equilibrium is reestablished (i.e., the final cell volume will be the same as the initial cell volume). Explanation: When the extracellular permeant solute concentration is increased to 400 mM, initially an osmotic imbalance will occur. Because the membrane is more permeable to water than solutes, water will respond to the osmotic imbalance first by leaving the cell, so the cell should start to shrink. Even as water leaves the cell, the permeant solute, being driven by its concentration gradient across the cell membrane, will gradually permeate into the cell. Water will follow osmotically, which will cause the cell volume to grow. Osmotic equilibrium can be reestablished only when the *impermeant* solutes are balanced across the cell membrane. Since the extracellular impermeant solute concentration was always 10 mM, equilibrium requires that the intracellular impermeant solute concentration return to 10 mM, which was its initial value. This can happen only if the cell swells back to its initial volume.

c. Answer: Water will initially enter the cell, causing an increase in cell volume. Then, in response to permeant solute movement, water will leave the cell and cell volume will decrease. The final cell volume will be one half the initial cell volume. Explanation: As soon as the extracellular solute concentrations change, an osmotic imbalance occurs; the total solute concentration inside is greater than the total solute concentration outside. Because water is the most permeant species, it crosses the cell membrane the fastest and will be the first to respond to the osmotic imbalance by moving into the cell. This causes the cell to swell initially. Even as water enters the cell, the permeant solute, being driven by its concentration gradient across the cell membrane, will gradually permeate out of the cell. Water will follow osmotically, which will cause the cell volume to shrink. As before, when a new osmotic equilibrium is established, the final volume of the cell is determined only by the presence of *impermeant* solutes. Since the outside impermeant solute concentration was changed from 10 mM to 20 mM, the situation concerning impermeant solutes is identical to that in part *a* of this problem. Following the solution of part *a*, the final cell volume will be one half the initial cell volume.

■ CHAPTER 4

1. E_{Na} is defined by the Nernst equation:

$$E_{Na} = \frac{RT}{(+1)F} \ln \left(\frac{[Na^+]_o}{[Na^+]_i} \right)$$

After substituting in $RT/F = 26.7$ mV, and $[Na^+]_i = 5$ mM, we can solve for $[Na^+]_o = 10.6$ mM.

2. a. V_m can be calculated through the GHK equation:

$$V_m = 26.7 \ln \frac{0.8(3) + 1.0(145) + 0.5(5)}{0.8(140) + 1.0(15) + 0.5(105)} = -4.8 \text{ mV}$$

b. Use the Nernst equation:

$$E_{Cl} = \frac{RT}{(-1)F} \ln \left(\frac{[Cl^-]_o}{[Cl^-]_i} \right) = \frac{26.7}{-1} \ln \frac{105}{5} = -81.3 \text{ mV}$$

c. If Cl^- is allowed to move, it will move so as to drive the membrane potential toward E_{Cl}. Since $V_m = -4.8$ mV, Cl^- must move *into the cell* to drive V_m toward $E_{Cl} = -81.3$ mV. By definition, an inward flux is a *positive* flux (see Box 4-5).

d. The Cl^- flux is carrying negative charges into the cell, which has the same electrical effect as bringing positive charges out of the cell. A positive current is defined as the flow of positive charges out of the cell. Therefore the Cl^- current is a *positive (or outward) current*.

3. The Na^+ pump normally counteracts the osmotic consequences of the Donnan effect and thus helps maintain cell volume. When the Na^+ pump is inhibited, the osmotic imbalance arising from the Donnan effect would tend to cause the cell to be hyperosmotic relative to the extracellular fluid. This means that water would enter and cause the cell to swell.

■ CHAPTER 5

1. The primary function of gated ion channels is to increase the permeability of the membrane to a specific ion. To increase the membrane K^+ permeability, the β-cell could alter the K^+ channel properties in the following ways:
   - The number of *open* channels could be increased or decreased. The overall permeability of the membrane will be directly related to the number of open channels.
   - The amount of time the channel is opened could be varied: the longer the channels are open, the higher the membrane permeability.
   - The permeability (or conductance) of a single open channel could be increased.

Typically, cellular mechanisms exist to regulate the number of open channels and the amount of time the channel is open. The permeability of a single open channel is usually constant.

2. The most likely location of this amino acid would be in the segment of the P region that forms the selectivity filter of the Na^+ channel. The selectivity filter in an ion channel is a narrow region in the aqueous permeation pathway that determines what ions will be permitted to pass through the channel. The selectivity filter works, in part, by making it energetically more favorable for a specific ion to enter that region of the pore. The structure of the selectivity filter is determined mainly by the specific amino acids that form this part of the channel.

A single amino acid substitution in this region could significantly alter the structure or the chemical properties of the selectivity filter. For example, the amino acid substitution described in this question might make it energetically more favorable for the divalent Ca^{2+} ion to enter the selectivity filter.

CHAPTER 6

1. a. The concentration gradient for Cl^- will cause Cl^- ions to enter the cell through the open channel. Thus the inside of the cell will have a slight excess of negative charges and the membrane potential (V_m) will move in the negative direction. The developing V_m tends to impede the further entry of Cl^- until $V_m = E_{Cl} = -70.5$ mV, at which point the net Cl^- flux goes to zero and V_m stops changing.

   b. The V_m follows a single exponential time course (Figure D-1) with a time constant (τ_m),

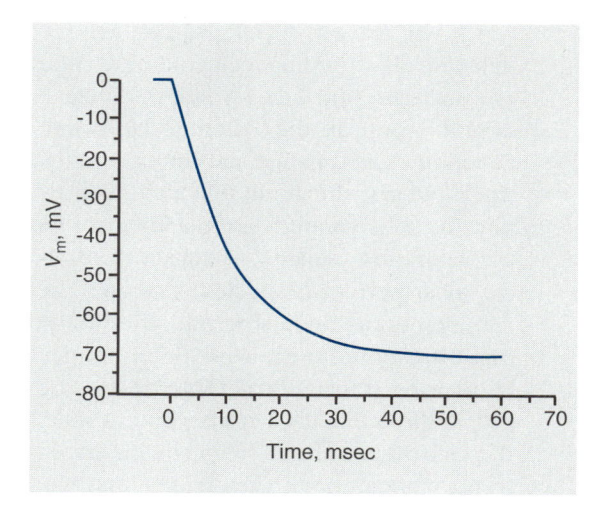

Figure D-1 ■ After the opening of the Cl^- channel (at time = 0 in this graph), the membrane potential, V_m, goes from an initial value of 0 mV to a final value of −70.5 mV along an exponential time course. The time constant of the exponential (the membrane time constant, τ_m) is 10^{-2} sec.

$$\tau_m = R_m \times C_m$$

$$R_m = \frac{1}{\gamma_{Cl}} = \frac{1}{10^{-11} S} = 10^{11} \text{ ohms}$$

$$C_m = 10^{-6} \text{ F/cm}^2 \times 10 \times 10^{-8} \text{ cm}^2 = 10^{-13} \text{ F}$$

$$\tau_m = 10^{11} \text{ ohms} \times 10^{-13} \text{ F} = 10^{-2} \text{ sec}$$

2. a. The change in membrane potential will decrease as a function of distance away from the site of current injection according to the following equation:

$$\Delta V_m(x) = \Delta V_m(x=0) \times \exp\left(\frac{-x}{\lambda}\right)$$

In this problem $\Delta V_m(x=0) = -30$ mV, and the length constant, λ, can be calculated:

$$\lambda = \sqrt{\frac{r_m}{r_i}} = \sqrt{\frac{2.5 \times 10^4 \text{ ohms} \times \text{cm}}{1 \times 10^5 \text{ ohms/cm}}} = \sqrt{0.25 \text{ cm}^2}$$

$$= 0.5 \text{ cm}$$

The change in V_m at $x = 4$ mm (0.4 cm) can then be calculated:

$\Delta V_m (x = 0.4) = (-30 \text{ mV}) \times \exp\left(\frac{-0.4 \text{ cm}}{0.5 \text{ cm}}\right) =$

$-30 \text{ mV} \times 0.45 = -13.5 \text{ mV}$

Thus V_m is −83.5 mV at a distance of 4 mm from the site of current injection.

b. If the Cl⁻ channels are blocked, the membrane resistance (r_m) would increase. This would increase the length constant. With an increase in length constant, the membrane potential would change more slowly as a function of distance away from the site of current injection. Thus the membrane potential would be *more negative* at 4 mm from the site of current injection, since the membrane potential would not have decreased as much because of the longer length constant.

3. a. The membrane time constant, τ_m (= $r_m \times c_m$), provides a quantitative measure of the rate of decay of the EPSP. Given the values in the table, dendrites 1 and 2 have the same value of τ_m (4×10^{-4} sec). Thus the EPSP decay rates would be the same.

b. The length constant,

$$\lambda = \sqrt{\frac{r_m}{r_i}}$$

provides a quantitative measure of the decay of subthreshold signals with distance: with a shorter length constant, a change in membrane potential will decay faster as a function of distance. The length constants of the two dendrites can be determined as follows:

$$\lambda_{\text{Dendrite1}} = \sqrt{\frac{2 \times 10^6 \text{ ohms} \times \text{cm}}{1 \times 10^{10} \text{ ohms/cm}}} = \sqrt{2 \times 10^{-4} \text{ cm}^2}$$

$$= 0.014 \text{ cm}$$

$$\lambda_{\text{Dendrite2}} = \sqrt{\frac{2 \times 10^4 \text{ ohms} \times \text{cm}}{1 \times 10^6 \text{ ohms/cm}}} = \sqrt{2 \times 10^{-2} \text{ cm}^2}$$

$$= 0.14 \text{ cm}$$

Thus the size of the EPSP would decrease more with distance in dendrite 1 because dendrite 1 has a shorter length constant.

A subthreshold EPSP would not be detected in the cell body because at a distance of 2 cm from the synapse the amplitude of the subthreshold EPSP would decline essentially to zero, even in the case of dendrite 2, which has the longer length constant. This is shown by the following calculation:

$$\Delta V_m (x = 2 \text{ cm}) = \Delta V_m (x = 0) \times \exp\frac{-2 \text{ cm}}{0.14 \text{ cm}}$$

$$= \Delta V_m (x = 0) \times 6.2 \times 10^{-7} \approx 0$$

■ CHAPTER 7

1. a. The Na⁺ conductance can be calculated by use of Ohm's Law. The maximum Na⁺ conductance occurs when all of the Na⁺ channels are open. If all of the Na⁺ channels are opened at +20 mV, the use of Ohm's Law at this voltage will give $g_{\text{Na,max}}$.

$$g_{\text{Na}} = \frac{I_{\text{Na}}}{(V_m - E_{\text{Na}})}$$

$$g_{\text{Na,max}} = \frac{-2.0 \times 10^{-3} \text{ A/cm}^2}{(0.02\text{V} - 0.06\text{V})} = 50 \times 10^{-3} \text{ S/cm}^2$$

b. When all of the Na⁺ channels are open, that is, when the channel open probability is "1" ($p_o = 1$), the Na⁺ conductance is maximal, or $g_{\text{Na}} = g_{\text{Na,max}}$.

c. The relationship between g_{Na} and channel open probability is given by $g_{\text{Na}} = N_T \times p_o \times \gamma_{\text{Na}}$, where N_T is the total number of Na⁺ channels, p_o is the probability that a single channel is open, and γ_{Na} is the conductance of a single Na⁺ channel. Because $g_{\text{Na,max}} = N_T \times \gamma_{\text{Na}}$, then $g_{\text{Na}} = p_o \times g_{\text{Na,max}}$ or

$$p_o = \frac{g_{\text{Na}}}{g_{\text{Na,max}}}$$

At −20 mV,

$$g_{\text{Na}} = \frac{-2.0 \times 10^{-3} \text{ A/cm}^2}{(-0.02 \text{ V} - 0.06 \text{ V})} = 25 \times 10^{-3} \text{ S/cm}^2$$

Thus

$$p_o = \frac{25 \times 10^{-3} \text{ S/cm}^2}{50 \times 10^{-3} \text{ S/cm}^2} = 0.5$$

d. These calculations illustrate one of the most important properties of voltage-gated ion channels: the open probability of the channel changes with the membrane potential.

2. a. The depolarization opens voltage-gated Na$^+$ channels. The Na$^+$ electrochemical gradient causes Na$^+$ ions to enter the cell through the open channels, thereby generating an inward I_{Na}. The inward I_{Na} deposits some positive charges on the inside surface of the membrane (i.e., it causes an outward I_C to flow), causing the membrane potential to move in the positive direction. This depolarization opens more voltage-gated Na$^+$ channels, and this positive feedback of membrane potential on the opening of Na$^+$ channels causes V_m to approach E_{Na} rapidly. Next, two processes begin at about the same time. The Na$^+$ channels close as a result of inactivation, and voltage-gated K$^+$ channels start to open. The K$^+$ electrochemical gradient causes K$^+$ to exit the cell. This outward ionic current (I_K) deposits positive charges on the outside surface of the membrane (or, it generates an inward I_C), which makes V_m move in the negative direction.

b. The initial outward current is an outward capacitive current that depolarizes the membrane toward threshold. The inward current that follows is generated by the inward I_{Na} that flows during the upstroke of the action potential. The final phase of outward current is generated by the outward I_K that flows during the repolarization of the action potential.

c. If a neuron is stimulated at a point along the axon, an action potential would propagate away in both directions. Propagation is normally unidirectional in most neurons because they are usually stimulated at only one end, near the cell body in α motor neurons and at distal terminals in sensory neurons. The action potential is then propagated along the axon to the other end of the cell. When stimulated in this manner, the membrane behind the action potential becomes refractory.

3. • *Length constant.* The conduction velocity increases with an increase in the length constant. During a propagated action potential the upstroke of the action potential results from an inward Na$^+$ current. Some of this inward current flows down the axon ahead of the action potential and provides a stimulus to bring the membrane potential from the resting level toward the action potential threshold. In an axon with a longer length constant the membrane would be brought to threshold farther from the point where the action potential upstroke is occurring.

• *Time constant.* The conduction velocity increases with a decrease in the time constant. With a shorter time constant the membrane potential changes more rapidly in response to current flow across the membrane. If the membrane potential changes more rapidly at a point along the axon, the action potential will rise to its peak and decline more rapidly at that point. Thus the action potential can move more quickly from one patch of membrane to the next and consequently increase the conduction velocity.

• *Na$^+$ channel density.* The conduction velocity increases with an increase in the Na$^+$ channel density. If the Na$^+$ channel

Appendix D

density increases, the magnitude of the Na$^+$ current also will increase. The rate of rise of the action potential (dV_m/dt) is directly proportional to the capacitive current, I_C. Because I_C will increase with I_{Na}, the rate of depolarization will increase with an increase in Na$^+$ channel density.

■ CHAPTER 8

1. Even the small influx of Ca^{2+} ions that occurs during an action potential can significantly increase [Ca^{2+}]$_i$. The reason is that the normal [Ca^{2+}]$_i$ is very low, about 100 nM. The following calculation illustrates the point. In cardiac ventricular myocytes an average I_{Ca} of about 20×10^{-12} A flows for 100 msec (which is comparable to the duration of a cardiac action potential). The amount of charge, in coulombs, that enters the cell is equal to the product of the current, in coulombs/sec, and time, in seconds:

$$q_{Ca} = I_{Ca} \times t = 20 \times 10^{-12} \text{ coul/sec} \times 0.1 \text{ sec}$$
$$= 2 \times 10^{-12} \text{ coul}$$

Charge can be converted to moles to obtain the number of moles of Ca^{2+} that entered the cell:

$$n_{Ca} = \frac{q_{Ca}}{zF} = \frac{2 \times 10^{-12} \text{ coul}}{2 \times 96,485 \text{ coul/mole}}$$
$$= 1 \times 10^{-17} \text{ moles}$$

The volume of the spherical cell is

$$\text{Volume} = \frac{4\pi r^3}{3} = \frac{4\pi \times (5 \times 10^{-4} \text{ cm})^3}{3}$$
$$= 5.2 \times 10^{-10} \text{ cm}^3 = 5.2 \times 10^{-13} \text{ liter}$$

This is the average volume of a ventricular myocyte. Neglecting any Ca^{2+} buffering that would occur in the cell, the I_{Ca} would produce a change in [Ca^{2+}]$_i$ of

$$\frac{1 \times 10^{-17} \text{ moles}}{5.2 \times 10^{-13} \text{ liters}} = 19 \times 10^{-6} \text{ M (19 μM)}$$

Such a change in concentration would be relatively insignificant for Na$^+$ or K$^+$ because their concentrations are in the millimolar range. But, because resting [Ca^{2+}]$_i$ is very low (about 100 nM; see Chapter 11), not much Ca^{2+} need enter the cell to raise [Ca^{2+}]$_i$ significantly. In actuality, the rise in [Ca^{2+}]$_i$ is never as large as this calculation indicates because most cells contain large amounts of Ca^{2+} buffering proteins that rapidly bind much of the Ca^{2+} that enters the cells.

2. The depolarization of the resting potential would increase the number of K$_A$ channels that are inactivated. Thus fewer K$_A$ channels would be available to contribute to the cell's electrical activity. When the membrane potential depolarizes after an action potential in the burst, less outward I_A current will be activated to oppose the depolarization. As a result, threshold will be reached faster, resulting in a higher action potential frequency in the burst.

3. Insulin secretion occurs as a result of the Ca^{2+} influx through L-type Ca^{2+} channels that open during the burst of action potentials in the pancreatic β-cells. The Ca^{2+} influx could be enhanced in several ways:
    a. A lengthening of the duration of the burst of action potentials at a constant action potential frequency would be expected to increase Ca^{2+} influx because the L-type Ca^{2+} channels will be open more frequently. The burst duration could be prolonged by blocking BK$_{Ca}$ or K$_{ATP}$ channels.
    b. A change in the number, or open probability, of L-type Ca^{2+} channels could also be used to alter Ca^{2+} influx. The activity of the L-type Ca^{2+} channel in pancreatic β-cells is potentiated by protein kinases A and C. Cellular mechanisms that activate protein kinase A or C in the β-cell therefore enhance Ca^{2+} influx, which, in turn, triggers increased insulin secretion.

CHAPTER 9

1. a. Glucose is electrically neutral, so there is no electrical component for its potential energy. That leaves the chemical component: $\mu_{G,in} = \mu^0_G + RT\ln[G]_i$.

   b. Ca^{2+} is electrically charged, so we expect that the membrane potential will influence its potential energy. For Ca^{2+} inside the cell, $\mu_{Ca,in} = \mu^0_{Ca} + RT\ln[Ca^{2+}]_i + 2FV_m$. Recall that the membrane potential is defined as the inside potential relative to the outside potential, and we define the outside potential to be 0 mV. Therefore, irrespective of charge, the electrical component of the potential energy is 0 for any species. For Ca^{2+} outside the cell, the electrochemical potential energy is thus $\mu_{Ca,out} = \mu^0_{Ca} + RT\ln[Ca^{2+}]_o$.

CHAPTER 10

1. The cotransport systems normally mediate large net movements of solutes into cells. This results in an osmotic burden that should cause cells to swell. Some exceptions are the Na^+-dependent neurotransmitter reuptake mechanisms, but here the extracellular concentrations are very low and only small amounts of solute are involved. Thus even a large (100- to 1000-fold) concentration gradient does not impose a large osmotic burden on the neurons or glia. Epithelial cells avoid osmotic catastrophe by expressing transport mechanisms (ion channels or simple carrier systems) that permit the net transfer of solutes *across* the cells so that normally no net buildup of osmotically active solutes (*osmolytes*) takes place within the cells. In contrast, the exchangers, by exchanging one solute for another, normally have little effect on the total solute concentration within cells. The Na^+ that enters the cells by Na^+-coupled transport is rapidly extruded by the Na^+ pump (see Chapter 11) so that Na^+ does not accumulate within the cells.

2. $[Ca^{2+}]_i$, at equilibrium, would be close to 100 mM $\{[Ca^{2+}]_i = [Ca^{2+}]_o \times \exp(-zV_mF/RT); [Ca^{2+}]_i = 1 \times \exp(-2 \times -60/26.7); [Ca^{2+}]_i = 90$ mM$\}$. This very high level of intracellular Ca^{2+} would form $CaCO_3$ and $Ca_3(PO_4)_2$ precipitates. The high $[Ca^{2+}]_i$ also would contribute to high intracellular osmolarity, which would lead to cell swelling.

3. $[Na^+]_i$ must be higher than in most cells (i.e., much greater than about 6 to 10 mM), or the membrane potential (V_m) must be considerably more positive than in most cells. Indeed, both are true because in these photoreceptor cells there is a large inward (Na^+) depolarizing current in the dark (called the "dark current"). Therefore energy in the Na^+ electrochemical gradient is insufficient to maintain $[Ca^{2+}]_i$ close to 100 nM with a 3 Na^+-for-1 Ca^{2+} exchange. The extra energy necessary to extrude Ca^{2+} from these cells is obtained by coupling of the fourth Na^+ and a K^+. This carrier, which is the product of a different gene than the cardiac Na^+/Ca^{2+} exchanger, also transports only 1 net charge during each cycle.

4. One alternative is an ATP-driven proton pump (see Chapter 11), but the turnover rate of pumps is at least 10-fold slower than that of coupled carriers that mediate countertransport (Table 10-1; the turnover rate of the Na^+/H^+ exchanger may be much greater than that of the Na^+/Ca^{2+} exchanger because only 1 Na^+ needs to bind to the Na^+/H^+ exchanger to initiate the transport cycle). Therefore too many copies of an H^+ pump might be needed to transfer H^+ at a sufficiently rapid rate to keep up with cellular demands. *Note*: Whether the transport system utilizes ATP directly is not a consideration because the same amount of energy must be used, in the long run (see Chapter 11), to extrude H^+.

5. The 1 Na^+-to-1 glucose cotransporter (e.g., SGLT-2) should be able to concentrate glucose about 100-fold across the apical membrane of the proximal tubule epithelial cell. Because glucose can exit the cell by facilitated diffusion across the basolateral membrane, the intracellular glucose concentration will approximate that in the plasma (5 mM). The SGLT-2 Na^+-glucose cotransporter should *theoretically* be able to remove sufficient glucose from the tubular fluid to lower the glucose concentration in the renal tubular fluid to about 0.05 mM. But this assumes that the cotransporter operates at 100% efficiency *and* that it reaches equilibrium, both of which seem unlikely. On these assumptions, in the 60 liters of fluid/day that leaves the proximal tubules, the total amount of glucose remaining in the urine would be a *minimum* of 3 millimoles/day or 540 mg/day (which appears to be negligible). The 1 Na^+-to-1 glucose cotransporter, however, is unlikely to be able to remove virtually all of the glucose in the filtered load because efficiency and transport rate fall off as the glucose concentration in tubular fluid declines below the carrier's K_m for glucose (≈ 2 mM, the concentration at which transport velocity is half-maximal). Under these circumstances the presence of a second cotransporter, with a 2 Na^+-to-1 glucose coupling ratio and higher affinities for glucose ($K_m \approx 0.4$ mM) and for Na^+ ($K_m \approx 3$ versus 100 mM), in the distal part of the proximal tubule, could decrease glucose in the urine to a negligible level.

■ CHAPTER 11

1. By stimulating the Na^+ pump, the α-adrenergic agonists lower $[Na^+]_i$ and transiently hyperpolarize the smooth muscle cells (because the pump is electrogenic). The lower $[Na^+]_i$ (and local $[Na^+]_o/[Na^+]_i$ gradient; see Box 11-3 and Figure 11-4) will tend to drive more Ca^{2+} out of the cells through the Na^+/Ca^{2+} exchanger and thus lower the $[Ca^{2+}]_i$ level and remove Ca^{2+} from the contractile apparatus.
2. The Na^+ electrochemical gradient generated by the Na^+ pump serves as a storage battery with a large capacity. No other ion electrochemical gradient in the cell is comparable in this respect. (This results from the fact that $[Na^+]_o \gg [Na^+]_i$ and the extracellular fluid volume is very large.) Moreover, the secondary active transport systems all have faster turnover rates than ATP-driven pumps. Thus all these systems can rapidly transport the secondarily coupled solutes without rapidly dissipating the Na^+ electrochemical gradient.
3. The same transport systems in different cells, or even in different places in a single cell, may have different functions and may need to be regulated differently. One example, given in Chapter 11, is the different distribution and function of the Na^+ pump catalytic (alpha) subunit isoforms within individual cells. Another example is that the SERCA in cardiac muscle, but not the SERCA in twitch-type skeletal muscle (see Chapter 14), is regulated by a small inhibitory protein phospholamban. When phospholamban is phosphorylated, it can no longer inhibit the cardiac muscle SERCA and cardiac relaxation is accelerated. The main point is that these numerous, functionally different transport systems are needed to maintain exquisite control of the intracellular environment in all cells.

■ CHAPTER 12

1. Contraction of skeletal and cardiac muscles is activated by a "switch" in the thin (actin) filaments. When the cytosolic Ca^{2+} level is elevated, Ca^{2+} binds to troponin C (TnC). This induces a conformational change in the troponin complex so that troponin I rotates out of the way and thereby permits myosin heads to interact with the actin. In smooth

muscles, in contrast, the Ca^{2+} binds to calmodulin (CaM). The Ca·CaM complex then binds to and activates myosin light chain kinase (MLCK). The activated MLCK then phosphorylates the 20-kD myosin regulatory light chain (MLC20). This enables the myosin heads to interact with actin to form cross-bridges. Thus the Ca^{2+}-sensitive "switch" that activates contraction in skeletal and cardiac muscles is located on the thin filaments (TnC), whereas in smooth muscles it is located on the thick filaments (MLC20).

2.
- Skeletal muscle cells are attached to the skeleton by tendons. Most skeletal muscles are under voluntary control. A primary function of many skeletal muscles is to shorten and generate force in order to produce movement of skeletal levers.
- Cardiac muscle cells (myocytes) make up the wall of each heart chamber and must contract synchronously so that the lumen volume is reduced and the chamber can eject its contents. In heart muscle the action potential spreads rapidly from cell to cell through gap junctions between the cells. This is important in the heart, where the muscle cells must contract synchronously to reduce the lumen volume.
- Smooth muscle cells are the types of muscle cells contained within the walls of hollow organs such as the gastrointestinal tract, arteries and veins, urinary bladder, bronchi, and ureters. The contractile fiber bundles in smooth muscle cells are oriented obliquely to the long axis of the cell, so that some contractile force is transmitted laterally. Thus in a cylindrical organ, such as an artery or the intestine, smooth muscle cells that are oriented nearly end to end (with some overlap) around the lumen constrict the lumen when they contract. In contrast, contraction of longitudinally oriented smooth muscle cells, as in the longitudinal muscle layer of the intestine, causes the organ to shorten. In saccular organs such as the urinary bladder, lateral as well as longitudinal forces cause the wall of the organ to contract relatively uniformly, leading to a reduction in organ (and lumen) volume.

3. Many smooth muscles must remain contracted for long periods. To maintain the $[Ca^{2+}]_i$ level substantially above the contraction threshold for a long time, the transport systems that move Ca^{2+} into and out of the cytosol would have to be reset to minimize large Ca^{2+} fluxes and a large energy expenditure that is normally required to resequester or extrude the Ca^{2+}. An alternative is to reset (increase in this case) the sensitivity of the contractile machinery to Ca^{2+}. In this way the contraction can be maintained at a relatively low $[Ca^{2+}]_i$ level. This is important because sustained elevation of $[Ca^{2+}]_i$ may turn on too many other, extraneous Ca^{2+}-dependent processes.

■ CHAPTER 13

1. In both skeletal and cardiac muscle, excitation-contraction (E-C) coupling is initiated by a depolarization of the surface membrane that propagates into the T-tubules and activates L-type Ca^{2+} channels (DHPRs). In both types of muscle the L-type Ca^{2+} channels are functionally coupled to elements of the sarcoplasmic reticulum (SR). These functional couplings occur at triads in skeletal muscle and at dyads and peripheral couplings in cardiac muscle. At these functional couplings, DHPRs in the surface membrane lie opposite Ca^{2+} release channels (ryanodine receptors, or RyRs) in the SR. Activation of the DHPRs causes Ca^{2+} release channels in the SR to open, allowing Ca^{2+} to be released from the SR.

   In spite of the similarities in E-C coupling between skeletal and cardiac muscle, there are several important differences. In skeletal muscle a Ca^{2+} release channel in the SR is opened as a result of a mechanical link between the voltage sensor (DHPR) and the Ca^{2+} release channel (RyR); Ca^{2+} entry is unnecessary. In cardiac muscle the RyRs/Ca^{2+}-release channels are opened by Ca^{2+}-induced Ca^{2+} release (CICR): Ca^{2+} enters the cell through L-type Ca^{2+} channels, binds to the RyRs/Ca^{2+} release channels, and opens them. Thus extracellular Ca^{2+} is essential for E-C coupling in cardiac muscle but is not required in skeletal muscle. All of the Ca^{2+} required for contraction in skeletal muscle comes from the SR. Another important difference involves the recycling of Ca^{2+}. In skeletal muscle virtually all of the Ca^{2+} released during a contraction is returned to the SR by SERCA pumps. In cardiac muscle a significant amount of Ca^{2+} enters during each action potential. Therefore, to maintain Ca^{2+} in the steady state, Na^+/Ca^{2+} exchangers (primarily) and plasma membrane Ca^{2+}-ATPase (PMCA) pumps must pump some Ca^{2+} out of the cell after each contraction.

2. Perhaps the Ca^{2+} release channels that are not opened by a mechanical link to a DHPR are opened by CICR. That is, when the RyRs that are mechanically coupled to the voltage-sensitive DHPRs open and release Ca^{2+} from the SR, the released Ca^{2+} may, in turn, activate adjacent RyRs that are *not* situated opposite the DHPRs.

3. a. Mechanisms that influence the availability of Ca^{2+} for smooth muscle contraction include (1) those that mediate or regulate Ca^{2+} entry (e.g., voltage-gated Ca^{2+} channels, Ca^{2+}-activated K^+ channels, receptor-operated channels, store-operated channels, the Na^+ pump, and the Na^+/Ca^{2+} exchanger); (2) those that mediate or regulate Ca^{2+} extrusion from the myocytes (plasma membrane Ca^{2+} pump, the Na^+ pump, and the Na^+/Ca^{2+} exchanger); and (3) those that mediate or regulate Ca^{2+} sequestration in the SR (SERCA, the Na^+ pump, and the Na^+/Ca^{2+} exchanger).

b. Mechanisms that influence smooth muscle contraction by altering the sensitivity of the contractile apparatus to Ca^{2+} (see Chapter 12) include phosphorylation of myosin light chain kinase (MLCK) and myosin light chain phosphatase (MLCP).

c. The numerous mechanisms that contribute to the regulation of smooth muscle contraction are apparently needed to vary contraction in a graded fashion, to maintain tonic contraction, and to respond to the multiple types of neuronal and hormonal signals that influence smooth muscle contraction in different smooth muscles (e.g., in circular and longitudinal smooth muscles in the intestinal wall).

d. The numerous mechanisms involved in the regulation of smooth muscle contraction provide many opportunities for therapeutic intervention with a variety of different agents that can act selectively on the different mechanisms.

■ CHAPTER 14

1. Upon stimulation, the muscle first develops force (tension) at constant length (Figure E-2, *A*) between points *a* and *b*. This is a period of isometric force development. When the muscle force exceeds the attached load, the muscle begins to shorten isotonically (i.e., at constant force; from *b* to *c*). At point *c* the muscle begins to relax (lengthen) at constant force. This isotonic relaxation ends at *d* when the muscle returns to its initial length. Muscle force continues to decline at constant length until the muscle is fully relaxed (at *e*). These phases of the contraction (isometric contraction [*a-b*], isotonic shortening [*b-c*], isotonic relaxation [*c-d*], and isometric relaxa-

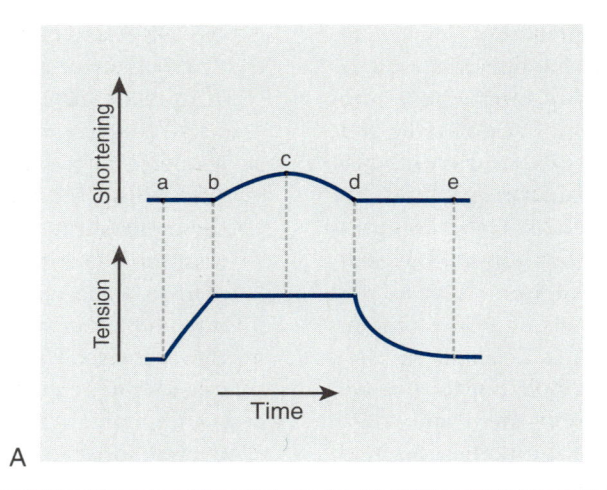

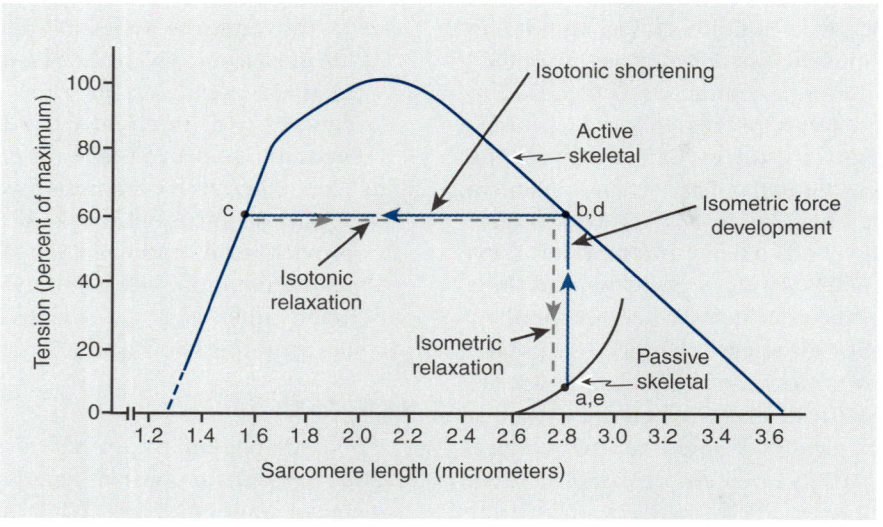

Figure D-2 ■ **A,** During this partly isometric, partly isotonic contraction, the muscle first undergoes isometric force development (between *a* and *b*). This is followed by isotonic shortening (*b* to *c*), isotonic relaxation (*c* to *d*), and, finally, isometric relaxation (*d* to *e*). **B,** The four phases of the contraction are illustrated on the length-tension curve. The muscle begins at rest, at an initial sarcomere length of 2.8 μm (point *a*). After stimulation the muscle develops force at constant length (isometric force). When the muscle force exceeds the attached load (at *b*), the muscle begins to shorten (isotonic shortening). At point *c*, the muscle begins to relax (lengthen) at constant force (isotonic relaxation), until the muscle returns to its initial length (at *d*). Muscle force then declines at constant length (isometric relaxation) until the muscle is fully relaxed (at *e*).

tion [*d-e*]) are also illustrated on the length-tension curve in Figure D-2, *B*.
2. The increase in contractility would result in more isotonic shortening and thus a greater length change in individual ventricular myocytes. Because the ventricular myocytes are interconnected to form a sac (the ventricle), the larger length change (i.e., increased shortening) in the individual ventricular myocytes would produce a smaller final ventricular volume.
3. The force generated by whole skeletal muscle is altered physiologically in two ways. First, the number and type of motor units activated at the same time can be varied. Second, the frequency of stimulation of the motor unit can be varied. As a result the force can vary from as little as that of a single twitch to as much as that of a fused tetanus.

    In ventricular muscle the primary physiological mechanism for altering force involves regulating the level of $[Ca^{2+}]_i$: mechanisms that raise peak $[Ca^{2+}]_i$ or increase the duration of the elevated $[Ca^{2+}]_i$ will increase force. Conversely, mechanisms that lower peak $[Ca^{2+}]_i$ or reduce the duration of the elevated $[Ca^{2+}]_i$ will decrease force. For example, stimulation of β-adrenergic receptors with norepinephrine increases contractility in cardiac muscle by increasing Ca^{2+} influx through voltage-gated Ca^{2+} channels. As in skeletal muscle, the force developed by cardiac muscle depends on the initial length of the muscle fiber. In ventricular muscle the initial fiber length will be determined by the ventricular end-diastolic volume.
4. When the dephosphorylation of myosin light chain (MLC) is slow, more cross-bridges can remain attached simultaneously. Moreover, if MLC becomes dephosphorylated while the cross-bridges are still attached, detachment will be slowed. These factors contribute to the tonic contractions that are maintained with very little hydrolysis of ATP by the myosin ATPase. In contrast, skeletal and cardiac muscles could not perform their normal functions if they were unable to relax rapidly.

APPENDIX E

Review Examination

1. Which of the following statements about diffusion is **FALSE**?
   A. Molecules diffuse from regions of high concentration to regions of low concentration.
   B. Diffusion flux (J) is directly proportional to the concentration gradient ($\Delta C/\Delta x$).
   C. Diffusion tends to even out concentration differences.
   D. Diffusion is the result of the random motion of molecules
   E. The distance molecules diffuse is directly proportional to time (i.e., $d \propto t$).

2. If a collection of molecules is found to diffuse a distance d in 9 seconds, how long will it take the same molecules to diffuse twice as far?
   A. 9 seconds.
   B. 18 seconds.
   C. 36 seconds.
   D. 81 seconds.
   E. None of the above.

3. Which of the following statements about membrane permeability is **FALSE**?
   A. The cell membrane is more permeable to small, nonpolar solutes than to polar solutes because nonpolar solutes dissolve better in the membrane.
   B. A difference in solute concentration on the two sides of the membrane can drive a diffusive flux of molecules through the membrane.
   C. Increasing the thickness of a membrane reduces the diffusive flux through the membrane.
   D. The net solute flux through a cell membrane is the result of balancing influx and efflux.
   E. Increasing the diffusion coefficient of a solute molecule in the membrane does not change the permeability of the membrane to that solute.

4. If the intracellular and extracellular Na⁺ and K⁺ concentrations are symbolized as $[Na^+]_o$, $[Na^+]_i$, $[K^+]_o$, and $[K^+]_i$, and the respective membrane permeabilities are symbolized as P_{Na} and P_K, which of the following statements about unidirectional fluxes is correct?
   A. $J_{Na, in \to out} = P_{Na}[Na^+]_i$
   B. $J_{K, out \to in} = P_K[K^+]_o$
   C. $J_{K, in \to out} = P_K[K^+]_i$
   D. All of the above are correct.
   E. All of the above are incorrect.

5. A cell containing 300 mM nonpermeant solute is initially equilibrated with an extremely large volume of plasma that also contains 300 mM nonpermeant solute. The initial cell volume is 1 picoliter. The solute concentration of the plasma is then suddenly increased by the addition of 100 mM of a *permeant* solute. Which of the following is **FALSE**?
   A. After new osmotic equilibrium is reached, the cell volume will be 1 picoliter.
   B. The final concentration of permeant solute in the cell will be 100 mM.
   C. After new osmotic equilibrium is reached, the cell volume will be 0.75 picoliter.
   D. The final concentration of nonpermeant solute inside the cell will be 300 mM.
   E. The cell will initially shrink slightly and then recover to its original volume.

6. Which of the following statements is **FALSE**?
   A. Injecting, into the circulation, a substance that cannot cross the blood-brain barrier tends to reduce brain edema.
   B. Adding a permeant solute to the plasma will cause red blood cells to shrink permanently.
   C. Inflammatory mediators released by mast cells increase the permeability of capillary walls, thus leading to edema.
   D. Capillary hydrostatic pressure drives fluid filtration, whereas capillary colloid osmotic pressure drives fluid reabsorption.
   E. Proteins that cannot readily permeate the capillary wall are the principal cause of the osmotic pressure difference between the plasma and the interstitial tissue fluid.

7. The membrane potential of a cell is $V_m = -60$ mV, and the intracellular and extracellular Cl⁻ concentrations are $[Cl^-]_i = 7$ mM and $[Cl^-]_o = 105$ mM, respectively. Which of the following statements is **FALSE**?
   A. The Cl⁻ *current* is inward.
   B. The Cl⁻ *flux* is inward.
   C. The Cl⁻ equilibrium potential is $E_{Cl} = -72$ mV.
   D. There is an outward *driving force* on Cl⁻.
   E. If $V_m = E_{Cl}$, there will be no net flux of Cl⁻ ions across the cell membrane.

8. Which of the following is (are) essential for generating a stable, nonzero membrane potential?
   A. The cell membrane must be permeable to at least one type of ion.
   B. The net current through the plasma membrane must be zero.
   C. The net flux of ions through the plasma membrane must be zero.
   D. A and B are correct.
   E. A, B, and C are correct.

9. If the cell's sodium pumps are inhibited by ouabain, all of the following will happen **EXCEPT**:
   A. The Donnan effect will cause osmotic imbalance.
   B. [K⁺] will fall in the cell.
   C. The membrane potential will hyperpolarize.
   D. The cell volume will increase.
   E. [Na⁺] will rise in the cell.

10. For a neuron, the equilibrium potentials for several common ions were found to be

$E_H = -12$ mV, $E_{Na} = +50$ mV, $E_K = -90$ mV, $E_{Ca} = +135$ mV, and $E_{Cl} = -50$ mV. If the membrane potential of the neuron is at $V_m = -60$ mV, which of the following statements about ion fluxes is **FALSE**?
   A. Cl^- flux is inward and H^+ flux is inward.
   B. The K^+ and Na^+ fluxes flow in opposite directions.
   C. Ca^{2+} flux is inward and Na^+ flux is inward.
   D. There is net H^+ influx, which would tend to make the inside of the cell more acidic.
   E. If more Cl^- channels are opened, the resulting change in Cl^- flux will tend to depolarize the cell.

11. Intracellular and extracellular concentrations for the three common monovalent ions are given below for a cell.

Ion	In (mM)	Out (mM)
K^+	140	5
Na^+	5	145
Cl^-	5	105

If the relative permeabilities for the three ions are 1:10:0.2 (K^+:Na^+:Cl^-), what is the expected membrane potential of the cell (rounding to two significant digits)? (**Note:** At 37° C, $RT/F = 26.7$ mV and $2.303RT/F = 61.5$ mV.)
   A. -89 mV.
   B. -53 mV.
   C. -33 mV.
   D. +52 mV.
   E. +90 mV.

12. Which of the following statements is **FALSE**?
   A. Chemical potential energy is stored in concentration gradients.
   B. The electrochemical potential for an ion is zero if the membrane potential is at $V_m = 0$ mV.
   C. If the electrochemical potential of an ion is the same on the inside and outside of the cell membrane, that ion is at equilibrium.
   D. Diffusion is an example of a transport process driven by a gradient in electrochemical potential.
   E. A gradient in electrochemical potential drives the transport of ionic substances.

13. After demyelination, the axonal membrane in the region between two nodes of Ranvier:
   A. Depolarizes at approximately the same rate during a propagated action potential as it did before demyelination.
   B. Has a smaller membrane time constant (τ_m) because the membrane resistance is lower and the membrane capacitance is unchanged.
   C. Has a lower membrane resistance and more charge separation across the membrane at the resting potential (-70 mV).
   D. Has a larger membrane time constant (τ_m) because the membrane capacitance is larger and the membrane resistance is unchanged.
   E. None of the above.

14. Two nonmyelinated axons have the same resistance and capacitance *per unit area* of membrane but are different in diameter. The passive cable properties of these axons were investigated, and the following values of resistance and capacitance per unit length of axon were determined (assume that $r_o = 0$):

	r_m	r_i	c_m
Axon 1	3×10^4 $\Omega \times$ cm	1.5×10^6 Ω/cm	3×10^{-8} F/cm
Axon 2	3×10^6 $\Omega \times$ cm	1.5×10^{10} Ω/cm	3×10^{-10} F/cm

Which of the following is **TRUE**?
   A. The membrane time constant in axon 1 is smaller than in axon 2.
   B. Axon 2 is larger in diameter than axon 1.
   C. The effect of a subthreshold stimulus can

be seen over a longer distance in axon 2 than in axon 1.
D. The action potential would propagate faster in axon 1.
E. The length constant is the same in both axons.

15. All of the following contribute to the muscle paralysis found in hyperkalemic periodic paralysis **EXCEPT**:
    A. Some Na$^+$ channels are open in the steady state, causing membrane depolarization.
    B. Some Na$^+$ channels do not inactivate completely.
    C. An increase in extracellular K$^+$ produces membrane depolarization.
    D. Membrane depolarization increases Na$^+$ efflux through the Na$^+$ pump, resulting in a reduction in the amount of Ca^{2+} stored in the sarcoplasmic reticulum.
    E. Membrane depolarization causes skeletal muscle to become mechanically inactivated.

16. All of the following are true of voltage-gated L-type Ca^{2+} channels **EXCEPT**:
    A. Their open probability increases as the membrane potential moves in the positive direction.
    B. They can be opened by phosphorylation.
    C. During an action potential generated by voltage-gated Ca^{2+} channels, the amount of Ca^{2+} entering the cell can significantly increase the concentration of Ca^{2+} in the cytoplasm.
    D. The number of functional Ca^{2+} channels in cardiac cell membranes can be altered by increasing the concentration of intracellular cyclic AMP (cAMP).
    E. They are blocked by dihydropyridines (e.g., nifedipine).

17. Which of the following statements about current flow across an "isolated patch" of membrane (e.g., a small spherical cell) is **FALSE?**
    A. An inward ionic current will produce a depolarization only if it causes an outward capacitive current.
    B. Outward capacitive current always causes the membrane potential to become more positive.
    C. Inward capacitive current never causes the membrane potential to become more positive.
    D. An outward ionic current can never cause the membrane potential to become more positive.
    E. While current is being passed across the membrane through an external current source, the capacitive current is equal in magnitude, and opposite in direction, to the ionic current.

18. Assume that an Na$^+$ channel stays open and allows Na$^+$ ions to flow through at all times. Which of the following statements about the current through this single *open* Na$^+$ channel is **FALSE?**
    A. The current has a constant amplitude if the membrane potential is held at a constant level.
    B. The current would decrease in amplitude as the membrane potential changed from the resting potential to the peak of the action potential.
    C. The current would increase and then decrease while the membrane potential was voltage clamped at 0 mV.
    D. The current amplitude can be calculated from Ohm's Law.
    E. The net current through the channel is zero if the membrane potential is at the Na$^+$ equilibrium potential.

19. Which of the following would be the Cl$^-$ current flowing through 100 open Cl$^-$ channels if the membrane potential is -70 mV, E_{Cl} is -45 mV, and the conductance of a single open chloride channel is 20 pS (pS = 10^{-12} S; 1 S = 1 A/V).

A. 50 pA. B. −50 pA.
C. 0.5 pA. D. −0.5 pA.
E. −250 pA.

20. Which of the following statements about Ca^{2+}-activated potassium (BK_{Ca}) channels is **FALSE**?
    A. In neurons that generate a burst of action potentials, outward current through BK_{Ca} channels helps to terminate the burst.
    B. BK_{Ca} channels could contribute outward current to help repolarize individual action potentials.
    C. BK_{Ca} channels always carry outward current under physiological conditions.
    D. At negative membrane potentials (about −80 mV), with $[Ca^{2+}]_i$ <100 nM, BK_{Ca} channels are mostly closed.
    E. Ca^{2+} ions bind to a site on the extracellular side of the BK_{Ca} channel to activate the channel.

21. When the plasma glucose concentration rises above about 5 mM, pancreatic β-cells secrete insulin in response to a rise in $[Ca^{2+}]_i$. $[Ca^{2+}]_i$ increases because:
    A. Glucose blocks K_{ATP} channels, leading to membrane depolarization and the opening of voltage-gated Ca^{2+} channels.
    B. Glucose binds to a receptor on the voltage-gated Ca^{2+} channel and increases the channel open probability.
    C. Glucose metabolism increases $[ATP]_i$ and ATP directly opens voltage-gated Ca^{2+} channels.
    D. Glucose metabolism increases $[ATP]_i$ and ATP blocks K_{ATP} channels, leading to membrane depolarization and the opening of voltage-gated Ca^{2+} channels.
    E. None of the above.

22. All of the following events are involved in the increase in cardiac contractility caused by epinephrine **EXCEPT**:
    A. The cytosolic cyclic AMP (cAMP) concentration increases.
    B. Ca^{2+} entry through voltage-gated L-type Ca^{2+} channels is enhanced.
    C. Na/Ca exchangers in the plasma membrane are inhibited.
    D. cAMP-dependent protein kinase phosphorylates L-type Ca^{2+} channels.
    E. Epinephrine activates adenylate cyclase by binding to β-adrenergic receptors.

23. Which of the following statements is **FALSE**?
    A. Voltage-gated K^+ channels in squid axons and A-type K^+ channels are opened by membrane depolarization, but the open probability of Ca^{2+}-activated K^+ channels decreases with depolarization.
    B. Under physiological conditions a current flowing through any type of K^+ channel tends to oppose membrane depolarization.
    C. A-type K^+ channels inactivate during maintained depolarization.
    D. Ca^{2+}-activated K^+ channels can be opened by an increase in $[Ca^{2+}]_i$.
    E. All K^+ channels normally pass outward current under physiological conditions.

24. Which of the following statements concerning the voltage-gated macroscopic sodium (g_{Na}) and potassium (g_K) conductances of the squid giant axon is **FALSE**?
    A. In a voltage clamp experiment, if the membrane potential is stepped to 0 mV, g_{Na} would activate faster than g_K.
    B. Both g_{Na} and g_K are voltage dependent and time dependent.
    C. Both g_{Na} and g_K have an activation and an inactivation phase during a depolarizing voltage clamp step.
    D. g_{Na} is proportional to the number of open sodium channels.
    E. g_K is proportional to the probability that a potassium channel is open.

25. Which of the following events does **NOT** occur during a propagated action potential along a myelinated nerve axon?

A. Propagation occurs by local circuit current flow.
B. Inward sodium current at one node of Ranvier causes inward current to flow at an adjacent node, which depolarizes that node toward threshold.
C. Na$^+$ channels become inactivated.
D. The action potential rapidly propagates from one node of Ranvier to the next.
E. If E_{Cl} is always more negative than the membrane potential, an inward Cl$^-$ flux is flowing.

26. All of the following statements are true of membrane capacitance (C_m) **EXCEPT**:
    A. The decrease in C_m that results from demyelination is one of the factors contributing to slowing or blocking of action potential propagation.
    B. Biological membranes typically have a membrane capacitance of about 1×10^{-6} F/cm^2.
    C. The rate of change of V_m in a small spherical cell, in response to a constant current stimulus, would decrease if C_m increased while R_m did not change.
    D. C_m is equal to the amount of charge separated across the membrane, in coulombs, per volt of membrane potential.
    E. If the membrane potential is changing, the amount of charge separated across the membrane is changing and a capacitive current is flowing.

27. All of the following statements about voltage-gated Na$^+$ channels are true **EXCEPT**:
    A. They pass only inward current under normal physiological conditions.
    B. Potassium ions interfere with Na$^+$ channel inactivation in skeletal muscle cells from patients with hyperkalemic periodic paralysis.
    C. They have an open probability that depends on time and membrane potential.
    D. They inactivate during the action potential, causing the membrane to be refractory to additional stimuli for a short period of time.
    E. Inward current through Na$^+$ channels in axons generates the upstroke of the action potential.

28. Which or the following is **NOT** a property of *all* ion channels?
    A. Ion channels increase the permeability of the membrane to ions.
    B. Ion channels are integral membrane proteins that extend across the lipid bilayer.
    C. An ion channel is a pore that is not open at all times.
    D. Ion channels exhibit selectivity by allowing only certain ions to flow through the channel.
    E. All of the above are properties of all ion channels.

29. Which of the following statements about ion channel structure is **FALSE?**
    A. Voltage-gated Na$^+$, K$^+$, and Ca^{2+} channels contain structural similarities indicating that they are members of a gene superfamily.
    B. Voltage-gated Na$^+$, K$^+$, and Ca^{2+} channels contain a P region, or loop, that lines the pore of the channel.
    C. Inward rectifier K$^+$ channels and voltage-gated K$^+$ channels are composed of subunits with six membrane-spanning helical segments.
    D. The selectivity filter in the bacterial KcsA K$^+$ channel is formed by several main-chain carbonyl oxygen atoms from amino acids in the P region.
    E. Voltage-gated Na$^+$, K$^+$, and Ca^{2+} channels all contain a membrane-spanning segment (S4) having several positive charges that act as a voltage sensor.

30. All of the following are true of membrane transport **EXCEPT**:

A. Special water channels (aquaporins) are responsible for high water permeability across some cell membranes.
B. Single carrier molecules, such as the simple glucose carrier (GLUT), can transport substrate at a rate of 1000 to 5000 molecules/sec.
C. Insulin modulates the glucose carriers (GLUTs) in skeletal muscle and thereby speeds the rate of glucose uptake into these cells, but it does not affect the intracellular glucose concentration in the cells under steady-state conditions.
D. The diffusion of nonpolar compounds across cell membranes is directly proportional to their solubility in water.
E. Ions normally cross the plasma membrane at a very slow rate unless they are transported by special integral membrane proteins (e.g., carriers, channels, or pumps).

31. All of the following are characteristic of transport across cell membranes **EXCEPT:**
    A. Carriers behave like channels that are open to only one side of the membrane at a time.
    B. Carriers that mediate facilitated diffusion of a single solute species cannot maintain a concentration gradient for that solute in the steady state.
    C. Carriers that mediate facilitated diffusion of a single solute species can "cycle" only when the solute is bound.
    D. Carrier-mediated transport can be modulated by phosphorylation.
    E. Carrier-mediated transport can be regulated by cycling carriers into and out of the plasma membrane.

32. Glucose absorption in the intestinal tract and reabsorption in the renal tubules are dependent on sodium-glucose cotransporters (SGLTs) in the brush border membranes of intestinal and renal epithelial cells. Assume that:

    The glucose concentration in the blood plasma = 4 mM.
    The Na^+ concentrations are 145 mM in blood plasma, 10 mM in the cytoplasm, and 135 mM in kidney tubular fluid.
    The membrane potentials (V_m) are –62 mV (cytosol with respect to tubule lumen) and –58 mV (cytosol with respect to blood plasma).
    $RT/F = 26.7$ mV.
    What is the theoretical limit to which an Na^+-glucose cotransporter, with a 1 Na^+:1 glucose coupling ratio (SGLT-2), could reduce the glucose concentration in the tubule lumen?
    A. 0.4 mM.
    B. 0.3 mM.
    C. 0.2 mM.
    D. 0.04 mM.
    E. 0.03 mM.

33. All of the following are true of glucose transport in human cells **EXCEPT:**
    A. All cells express an Na^+-glucose cotransporter (SGLT).
    B. Some cells express an Na^+-glucose cotransporter with a coupling ratio of 1 Na^+:1 glucose.
    C. Some cells express an Na^+-glucose cotransporter with a coupling ratio of 2 Na^+:1 glucose.
    D. All cells that express an Na^+-glucose cotransporter (SGLT) must also express a (simple) glucose carrier (GLUT).
    E. The simple glucose carrier (GLUT) activity in some cell types is modulated by insulin.

34. The "sodium/calcium exchanger" in vertebrate photoreceptors (rod and cone cells in the retina) mediates the exchange of 4 Na^+ for 1 Ca^{2+} plus 1 K^+. A rise in the extracellular K^+ concentration can be expected to:
    A. Decrease the exchanger-mediated transport of Ca^{2+} from the cytoplasm to the extracellular fluid.

B. Increase the exchanger-mediated transport of Ca^{2+} from the cytoplasm to the extracellular fluid because of a reduction in the K^+ concentration gradient.
C. Increase the exchanger-mediated transport of Ca^{2+} from the cytoplasm to the extracellular fluid because of a membrane depolarization.
D. Increase the exchanger-mediated entry of Na^+ into the cells.
E. B, C, and D are all correct.

35. The following are all characteristics of sodium pumps **EXCEPT:**
    A. Sodium pumps in the kidney and in the brain consume more than half of the ATP hydrolyzed in those organs.
    B. The hormone aldosterone regulates sodium pumps by promoting the synthesis and insertion of new sodium pumps into the plasma membrane of certain epithelial cells.
    C. Sodium pumps can be regulated by phosphorylation at a site other than the catalytic site.
    D. Sodium pumps are electrogenic: they generate a current and normally contribute a few (e.g., 1 to 3) millivolts to the resting membrane potential.
    E. Most cells have two different sodium pumps that are the products of different genes: one is located in the plasma membrane, and the other in the endoplasmic reticulum.

36. All of the following are true of transport ATPases **EXCEPT:**
    A. The Na^+ pump (Na^+,K^+-ATPase) ultimately provides the energy for most secondary active transport mechanisms.
    B. The Na^+,K^+-ATPase normally generates an inward electric current.
    C. The gastric H^+,K^+-ATPase can extrude protons from an intracellular environment with pH of 7.2 to a very acidic extracellular environment (pH 2 to 3).
    D. Wilson disease and Menkes disease are associated with genetic defects in two different copper-transporting ATPases.
    E. The multidrug resistance (MDR) transport proteins are ATPases that actively transport anticancer agents such as doxorubicin (Adriamycin) out of cells.

37. Inhibition of the Na^+ pump by ouabain (with no change in plasma Na^+ concentration) will lead to all of the following **EXCEPT:**
    A. Swelling of skeletal muscle cells.
    B. Reduction of neurotransmitter (e.g., dopamine) reuptake at nerve terminals.
    C. Augmentation of Ca^{2+}-dependent secretion of catecholamine by adrenal medullary cells.
    D. Augmentation of glucose and amino acid (e.g., alanine) absorption from the intestinal lumen.
    E. Cell acidification.

38. The sodium pump does all of the following **EXCEPT:**
    A. Helps regulate the glucose concentration in skeletal muscle.
    B. Contributes directly to the resting membrane potential.
    C. Contributes indirectly to the resting membrane potential by regulating $[K^+]_i$.
    D. Helps regulate Ca^{2+} stores in the sarcoplasmic and endoplasmic reticulum and Ca^{2+} signaling.
    E. Helps regulate cell volume.

39. The multidrug resistance (MDR) proteins include all of the following **EXCEPT**:
    A. P-type transport ATPases.
    B. Transport proteins that may be up-regulated in the presence of their substrates.
    C. Primary active transporters.
    D. Transport proteins that actively concentrate many types of drugs in cells.

E. Transport proteins that underlie drug resistance to many anticancer agents.

40. Which *one* of the following statements about regulation of solute transport is **TRUE**:
    A. Insulin stimulates glucose uptake into skeletal muscle cells by increasing the number of Na$^+$-glucose cotransporter molecules in the plasma membrane.
    B. Histamine stimulates the secretion of acid into the stomach lumen by increasing the number of H$^+$,K$^+$-ATPase molecules in the parietal cell basolateral membrane.
    C. Histamine stimulates the secretion of acid into the stomach lumen by increasing the number of Na$^+$/proton exchanger molecules in the oxyntic cell apical membrane.
    D. Dopamine can modulate the activity of some sodium pumps by promoting phosphorylation of the pump at a site *different* from the phosphorylation site required for activation of Na$^+$ extrusion and pump cycling.
    E. The Na$^+$/proton exchanger requires a 2 Na$^+$:1 H$^+$ coupling ratio to lower intracellular pH to 7.4 when extracellular pH = 7.4.

41. All of the following statements about Ca^{2+} homeostasis are true **EXCEPT**:
    A. The free Ca^{2+} concentration in the endoplasmic reticulum and sarcoplasmic reticulum, ER/SR ([Ca^{2+}]$_{ER/SR}$), of quiescent (resting) cells is normally greater than 10^{-4} M.
    B. Most of the Ca^{2+} in the lumen of the ER or SR is free Ca^{2+} (i.e., not bound to proteins).
    C. The free Ca^{2+} concentration in the cytosol ([Ca^{2+}]$_i$) of quiescent cells is normally about 10^{-7} M.
    D. Partial Na$^+$ pump inhibition can induce a large increase in [Ca^{2+}]$_{ER/SR}$ despite a very small increase in [Na$^+$]$_i$.
    E. The plasma membrane Ca^{2+} pump (PMCA) plays an important role in maintaining [Ca^{2+}]$_i$ in quiescent (resting) cells.

42. A 25-year-old man comes to your office with a chief complaint that his muscles are stiff after he exercises. On physical examination you find nothing remarkable. However, when you ask him to flex and extend his arms rapidly and repeatedly, you notice that he soon slows down and his muscles seem to remain tense and contracted longer and longer. He reports that his older brother has a similar problem. The impaired skeletal muscle relaxation could be explained by a defect causing *reduced activity* of which one of the following skeletal muscle channels/transporters?
    A. Ryanodine receptors (sarcoplasmic reticulum [SR] Ca^{2+}/channels).
    B. Dihydropyridine receptors (L-type Ca^{2+} channels).
    C. Plasma membrane Ca^{2+} pump (PMCA).
    D. SR Ca^{2+} pump (SERCA).
    E. Na$^+$/Ca^{2+} exchanger.

43. All of the following statements about transepithelial cell transport are true **EXCEPT**:
    A. The main driving force for Cl$^-$ reabsorption in the small intestine and the renal proximal tubule cells is the −3 to −5 mV (lumen negative) transepithelial electrical potential gradient.
    B. Most of the Cl$^-$ reabsorbed in the small intestine and the renal proximal tubules is transported through the cells (i.e., by the transcellular pathway).
    C. Pancreatic acinar cell secretions are a major source of the Na$^+$ that is used to drive Na$^+$-coupled solute transport across intestinal cell apical membranes.
    D. Net transport of many solutes across epithelia is ultimately driven by the Na$^+$ pump in the basolateral membrane.

E. Net solute transport across epithelia depends on the presence of different transporters (carriers, pumps, or channels) in the apical and basolateral membranes.

44. All of the following statements about water (re)absorption across epithelia are true **EXCEPT:**
    A. Net water transport may occur by active transport of water molecules.
    B. Net water transport is always coupled to solute transport
    C. Net water transport across leaky epithelia is always driven by an osmotic gradient.
    D. Water absorbed across tight epithelia normally passes through the epithelial cells (i.e., it occurs through the transcellular route).
    E. Antidiuretic hormone (ADH) promotes water transport across some tight epithelia by promoting the insertion of aquaporins (water channels) into the apical membrane of the epithelial cells.

45. Secretory diarrhea is dependent on which one of the following cyclic AMP (cAMP)-mediated mechanisms:
    A. Increased activation of Cl⁻ channels in the apical membrane of intestinal epithelial cells.
    B. Increased activation of Cl⁻ channels in the basolateral membrane of intestinal epithelial cells.
    C. Increased insertion of aquaporins (water channels) into the apical membrane of intestinal epithelial cells.
    D. Increased insertion of aquaporins into the basolateral membrane of intestinal epithelial cells.
    E. Inhibition of the Na⁺ pump in the basolateral membrane of intestinal epithelial cells.

46. Which of the following statements about the structure of skeletal muscle is **FALSE?**
    A. Thick filaments interdigitate with thin filaments, so that each thick filament is surrounded by a hexagonal array of thin filaments.
    B. Bundles of thick and thin filaments run obliquely across the cell.
    C. Thick filaments are composed mostly of myosin.
    D. Thin filaments are composed of actin, tropomyosin, troponin, and nebulin.
    E. Surrounding each myofibril is an extensive membrane-enclosed intracellular compartment, the sarcoplasmic reticulum.

47. In the presence of high $[Ca^{2+}]_i$ all of the following steps occur in the cross-bridge cycle in skeletal muscle **EXCEPT:**
    A. ATP binds to myosin, causing the cross-bridge to detach.
    B. With ADP and P_i bound to the myosin head, myosin binds to actin with low affinity.
    C. When ATP is hydrolyzed to ADP and P_i, the angle between the myosin head and the thin filament changes from 45 degrees to 90 degrees.
    D. The release of ADP, P_i, and Ca^{2+} results in a strong attachment between myosin and actin.
    E. Force is generated when the angle between the myosin head and the thin filament changes from 45 degrees to 90 degrees.

48. All of the following are features of both skeletal and cardiac muscle **EXCEPT:**
    A. Individual muscle cells are electrically connected through gap junction channels.
    B. Ca^{2+} ions initiate contraction by binding to troponin C.
    C. The contractile elements are organized in sarcomeres.
    D. Force is generated by a sliding filament mechanism.
    E. In resting muscle cells, cross-bridges

cannot form because tropomyosin covers the myosin binding sites on actin.

49. In skeletal muscle the activation of contraction by Ca^{2+} involves the regulatory proteins tropomyosin and troponin in which of the following ways?
   A. When $[Ca^{2+}]_i$ rises into the micromolar range, it binds to troponin C and weakens the affinity of troponin I for actin.
   B. Troponin T binds to troponin I, troponin C, and tropomyosin and is responsible for linking the troponin complex to tropomyosin.
   C. Tropomyosin moves on the thin filament to either cover or expose myosin binding sites on actin.
   D. A, B, and C are all true.
   E. Only B and C are true.

50. All of the following are true of both skeletal and cardiac muscle contraction **EXCEPT:**
   A. Contraction is initiated by a depolarization of the surface membrane.
   B. Almost all of the Ca^{2+} that activates the contraction is pumped back into the sarcoplasmic reticulum (SR) by SR Ca^{2+} (SERCA) pumps.
   C. L-type Ca^{2+} channels (dihydropyridine receptors, or DHPRs) in the surface membrane are activated by depolarization.
   D. Ca^{2+} is released from the SR into the cytoplasm through open Ca^{2+}-release channels (ryanodine receptors) in the SR.
   E. Ca^{2+} release channels in the SR are opened at specialized junctions between SR and T-tubule membranes.

51. The activation of Ca^{2+} release from the sarcoplasmic reticulum (SR) during a contraction in skeletal muscle:
   A. Occurs by the same mechanism as in cardiac muscle.
   B. Is caused by Ca^{2+} entering the cell through L-type Ca^{2+} channels in the surface membrane.
   C. Occurs through Ca^{2+}-release channels opened by IP_3 binding.
   D. Is independent of the membrane potential.
   E. None of the above.

52. Which of the following is **FALSE?**
   A. The opening of sarcoplasmic reticulum (SR) Ca^{2+}-release channels in cardiac muscle involves Ca^{2+}-induced Ca^{2+} release.
   B. The activity of both the Na^+/Ca^{2+} exchanger and SR Ca^{2+} pump (SERCA) decreases $[Ca^{2+}]_i$ and causes the relaxation of cardiac muscle.
   C. Extracellular Ca^{2+} is required for E-C coupling in cardiac muscle.
   D. All of the Ca^{2+} that activates cardiac muscle contraction comes from the SR.
   E. The Ca^{2+} release through Ca^{2+} release channels can be visualized as Ca^{2+} "sparks."

53. Which of the following statements about FF (fast, fatigable), FR (fast, fatigue-resistant), and S (slow) motor units in skeletal muscle is **FALSE?**
   A. S motor units generate the smallest forces and do not fatigue.
   B. Whole muscle often contains mixtures of FF, FR, and S motor units.
   C. A motor unit is a single skeletal muscle cell and the α motor neuron that innervates it.
   D. FR motor units are more resistant to fatigue than FF motor units.
   E. FF motor units generate the largest tetanic forces and are usually recruited after S and FR motor units.

54. The force generated by cardiac muscle can be increased by all of the following **EXCEPT:**
   A. Increasing the duration of the cardiac action potential.
   B. Inhibiting Na^+/Ca^{2+} exchangers in the plasma membrane.

C. Activating β-adrenergic receptors in cardiac muscle.
D. Increasing the end-diastolic volume of the heart.
E. Increasing the frequency of stimulation of the heart.

55. In a pure isometric contraction the force generated by whole skeletal muscle can be increased by all of the following **EXCEPT**:
    A. Increasing the number of motor units that are activated.
    B. Increasing the frequency of stimulation of the muscle.
    C. Increasing the sarcomere length from 1.4 μm to 1.6 μm.
    D. Increasing the sarcomere length from 2.4 μm to 3.0 μm.
    E. Decreasing the rate of Ca^{2+} uptake by the sarcoplasmic reticulum (SR) Ca^{2+} pump (SERCA) into the SR.

56. All of the following are true of the relationship between isotonic force and velocity of shortening in skeletal muscle **EXCEPT**:
    A. As the isotonic force generated by the muscle increases, the velocity of shortening decreases.
    B. The maximum velocity of shortening (V_0) occurs when the muscle shortens with no attached load.
    C. The maximum velocity of shortening is a reflection of the maximum rate of cross-bridge cycling.
    D. The maximum velocity of shortening is inversely proportional to myosin ATPase activity.
    E. If the load attached to the muscle is greater than the maximum force the muscle can generate, the velocity of shortening is zero.

57. The maximum force in a twitch contraction in skeletal muscle is smaller than the maximum tetanic force because:
    A. The amount of Ca^{2+} released during a twitch is not enough to saturate all the troponin C binding sites.
    B. During a twitch there is not enough time to fully stretch series elastic elements in the muscle.
    C. $[Ca^{2+}]_i$ remains elevated for a longer time during a tetanus.
    D. A, B, and C are all true.
    E. Only B and C are true.

58. All of the following statements about malignant hyperthermia (MH) are true **EXCEPT**:
    A. MH is triggered by exposure to volatile, halogenated anesthetics.
    B. Dihydropyridines (e.g., nifedipine) are used to prevent attacks of MH.
    C. An episode of MH is characterized by a sustained increase in $[Ca^{2+}]_i$ in skeletal muscle.
    D. Most cases of MH are associated with a point mutation in the gene that encodes the skeletal muscle sarcoplasmic reticulum (SR) Ca^{2+} release channel.
    E. In an episode of MH, continuous cross-bridge cycling and SR Ca^{2+} pump (SERCA) activity produce an increase in body temperature that can be fatal.

59. Which one of the following statements is **FALSE**?
    A. In an isotonic contraction the velocity of shortening is constant.
    B. In an isometric contraction the muscle generates force and then relaxes at constant length.
    C. In an isotonic contraction the muscle shortens against a constant load.
    D. Under physiological conditions most skeletal muscle contractions are partly isotonic and partly isometric.
    E. When skeletal muscle is activated with an attached load, the first phase of the contraction is isometric force development.

60. All of the following are true **EXCEPT**:

A. Smooth muscles do not exhibit the striation patterns observed in skeletal muscle because the thick and thin filament bundles are not in register.
B. Smooth muscle, like skeletal muscle, requires troponin C (TnC) for contractile activation.
C. The "dense bodies" of smooth muscles are analogous to the Z lines of skeletal muscle because both are composed primarily of α-actinin.
D. The "dense bodies" of smooth muscles are analogous to the Z lines of skeletal muscle because the thin filaments are inserted into the dense bodies.
E. In saccular organs such as the urinary bladder, smooth muscle contraction exerts both longitudinal and lateral forces so that the volume contracts uniformly.

61. Smooth muscle contraction can be activated by all of the following **EXCEPT**:
   A. Ca^{2+} binding to calmodulin.
   B. Ca^{2+} binding to sarcoplasmic reticulum (SR) Ca^{2+} pump (SERCA).
   C. Phosphorylation of myosin light chain.
   D. Inositol-1,4,5-trisphosphate (IP_3).
   E. Ca^{2+} binding to the ryanodine receptor (RyR).

62. Smooth muscle relaxation is promoted by all of the following **EXCEPT**:
   A. Dephosphorylation of myosin light chain.
   B. Elevating the concentration of cyclic AMP (cAMP) in the smooth muscle cytoplasm.
   C. Decreasing the activity of myosin light chain phosphatase.
   D. Phosphorylation of myosin light chain kinase.
   E. Opening Ca^{2+}-dependent K^+ channels.

63. Mechanisms involved in the activation of smooth muscles may include all of the following **EXCEPT**:
   A. Depolarization initiated by some neurotransmitters such as acetylcholine.
   B. Acetylcholine-induced release of nitric oxide (NO).
   C. Release of Ca^{2+} from the sarcoplasmic reticulum (SR).
   D. Pharmacomechanical coupling that involves little or no change in membrane potential.
   E. Ca^{2+}-independent changes in the sensitivity of the contractile apparatus to Ca^{2+}.

64. Activation of smooth muscle differs from that of skeletal muscles in that:
   A. Smooth muscles are never activated by membrane depolarization.
   B. Smooth muscles are not dependent on sarcoplasmic reticulum (SR) Ca^{2+} release.
   C. Smooth muscles are activated by a troponin-tropomyosin–regulated mechanism.
   D. Smooth muscles generate much less force per unit cross-sectional area (= "stress").
   E. Smooth muscle contraction velocity is slower.

65. All of the following are true of tonic smooth muscles **EXCEPT**:
   A. The unitary actin-myosin cross-bridge force is much smaller than in skeletal muscle.
   B. Smooth muscle cross-bridge attachments last several times longer than skeletal muscle cross-bridge attachment.
   C. Compared with skeletal muscle, a much larger fraction of the smooth muscle actin-myosin cross-bridges are attached at any time.
   D. Tonic smooth muscles can maintain contraction with little consumption of ATP.
   E. The rate of ADP dissociation from myosin in smooth muscles is very slow when the cross-bridges are attached.

Answers to Review Examination

1. E	18. C	34. A	50. B
2. C	19. B	35. E	51. E
3. E	20. E	36. B	52. D
4. D	21. D	37. D	53. C
5. C	22. C	38. A	54. E
6. B	23. A	39. D	55. D
7. A	24. C	40. D	56. D
8. D	25. B	41. B	57. E
9. C	26. A	42. D	58. B
10. A	27. B	43. B	59. A
11. D	28. E	44. A	60. B
12. B	29. C	45. A	61. B
13. C	30. D	46. B	62. C
14. D	31. C	47. D	63. B
15. D	32. E	48. A	64. E
16. B	33. A	49. E	65. A
17. E			

Index

A

A bands
  in muscle contraction
    of cardiac muscle, 189f
    of skeletal muscle, 182, 184, 185f, 186f
  structure of, 180, 180n, 181, 183f
ABC (ATP-binding cassette) transporters, 163-165, 164f, 165b
Absolute refractory period, 77, 79f
Acetylcholine (ACh)
  and skeletal muscles, 225
  and smooth muscles, 217
Acetylcholine (ACh)-gated ion channels, 112-113, 114b
Actin, 177
  in thin filaments, 182, 185f
Actin filaments, in smooth muscle, 191, 192f
Action potential(s)
  agents that block Na^+ or K^+ channels and, 89, 91b, 92f
  in cardiac muscle cell, 101f
  conduction velocity of, 91-93, 93b
    myelination and, 93-95, 94f, 94t, 95f
  as cyclical process of channel opening and closing, 87, 91f
  defined, 53, 75
  firing patterns of, 105-109, 106f
  frequency of, 108-109, 109f
  generation by voltage-gated Na^+ and K^+ channels of, 86-89, 90f-92f, 91b
  in pancreatic beta (β)-cells, 110, 111f
  propagation of, 54, 89-95
    in myelinated axons, 93-95, 95f
    in nonmyelinated axons, 89-91, 93b, 93f
    unidirectional, 91
  properties of, 75-77, 76f, 79f

Page numbers followed by f indicate figures; those followed by t indicate tables; those followed by b indicate boxed material; those followed by n indicate footnotes.

Activation, 81, 82
  declining phase of, 81
Activation gate, 83, 84f, 85, 87f
Active tension, 230-231, 231f
Active transport, 149-175
  across epithelial cells, 165-174
    absorption of Cl^- in, 169-170, 170f
    functional diversity and, 167-168
    net water flow and net solute flow in, 172-174
    secretion of substances by epithelia in, 170-171, 171b, 172f, 173b
    sources of Na^+ for apical membrane Na^+-solute cotransport in, 168-169, 169f
    structure and, 165, 166f, 167f
  ATPases in, 150
    copper-transporting, 162-163, 162b, 163b
    H^+,K^+-, 160-161, 161f, 162b
  ATP-driven Ca^{2+} pump in, 158-159, 160b
  by ATP-binding cassette transporters, 163-165, 164f, 165b
  Ca^{2+} storage in sarcoplasmic/endoplasmic reticulum in, 157-158, 158b, 159b
  coupling in parallel or in series for, 160
  interconversion of chemical energy and electrochemical potential energy in, 149-150
  intracellular Ca^{2+} signaling in, 154-157
  plasma membrane Na^+ pump in, 150-154, 151f, 153f, 154f, 155b, 156f
  primary, 150
  secondary, 134-135, 135b, 138
  tertiary, 145-146, 145f
A-currents (I_A), 107
Adenosine triphosphatase(s) (ATPases)
  in active transport, 150
  Ca^{2+}-dependent, 157-158, 158b, 159b
  copper-transporting, 162-163, 162b, 163b
  F-type, 150
  H^+,K^+-, 160-161, 161f, 162b

311

Adenosine triphosphatase(s) (ATPases) (cont'd)
  multidrug resistance, 163
  Na^+,K^+-. See Na^+,K^+-ATPase
  P-type, 150
  sarcoplasmic/endoplasmic reticulum Ca^{2+}-dependent. See Sarcoplasmic/endoplasmic reticulum Ca^{2+}-dependent ATPase (SERCA)
  V-type, 150
Adenosine triphosphate (ATP)
  hydrolysis of, 178
  in smooth muscle contraction, 243-244, 246b, 247f
Adenosine triphosphate (ATP)-binding cassette (ABC) transporters, 163-165, 164f, 165b
Adenosine triphosphate (ATP)-driven Ca^{2+} pump, 158-159, 160b
Adenosine triphosphate (ATP)-sensitive K^+ channel, 100t, 106b, 109-110, 111b, 111f, 112b
ADH (antidiuretic hormone), in water transport across tight epithelia, 173-174
AE1 (anion exchanger type 1), 145
Aganglionic colon, 214, 214b
Agonist receptors, 217
Agre, Peter, 129n
Albumin
  and colloid osmotic pressure, 28b
  and edema, 29b
Allergic response, and edema, 29b
"All-or-none" response, 77
Alpha (α)-actinin
  in skeletal muscle, 181
  in smooth muscle, 191
Alpha (α)-ketoglutarate (αKG^{2-}), coupling to countertransport of organic anions of, 145, 145f
Alpha (α) motor neuron
  in motor unit, 225
  structure of, 53-54, 54f
Amphipathic helices, 132f
Amphipathic phospholipids, 3
Amphiphilic helices, 131
Amphiphilic phospholipids, 3
Angina pectoris, nitroglycerin for, 217, 217b
Angiogenesis, and tumor growth, 13b
Anion exchanger type 1 (AE1), 145
Antidiuretic hormone (ADH), in water transport across tight epithelia, 173-174
Antiport, 134
Apical membrane
  Cl^- uptake at, 170, 170f
  of epithelial cells, 165, 166f, 167f
  ion gradients across, 168
  sources of Na^+ for Na^+-solute cotransport across, 168-169, 169f
Apical surface, of epithelial cells, 165, 166f

Aquaporins, 129, 172
Aqueous pore, ion movement through, 54-55, 55f, 56b
Arterial smooth muscle, 243, 244, 245f
ATP. See Adenosine triphosphate (ATP)
ATPases. See Adenosine triphosphatase(s) (ATPases)
Autonomic nervous system, 190, 211
Avogadro's number, 56b
Axon, 53, 54f
  equivalent circuit of, 72, 72f
Axon diameter, and conduction velocity, 94, 94f
Axon hillock, 53, 54f
Axoplasmic resistance, and passive spread of electrical subthreshold signals, 69-73, 70f, 71b, 71t, 72f

B

Bartter's syndrome, 171, 171b
Basolateral membrane
  of epithelial cells, 165, 166f, 167f
  ion gradients across, 168
  K^+ secretion across, 170f
Basolateral surface, of epithelial cells, 165, 166f
Becker's myotonia, 201b
Benign prostatic hypertrophy (BPH), 243b
Bernard, Claude, 2n
Beta (β)-adrenergic agonists, inhibition of glucose uptake by, 134
Beta (β)-adrenergic receptor activation, modulation of L-type Ca^{2+} channels in cardiac muscle by, 113
Beta (β)-cells, glucose-induced insulin secretion from, 109-110, 111b, 111f, 112b
Bicarbonate (HCO_3^-), exchange with chloride of, 122, 123b, 124b-125b, 125f
Bilayer membranes, 3-4, 4f
Biochemical signals, 2, 4
Biological membranes, 3-4, 4f
  transport across
    carrier-mediated, 130-134, 131b, 132b, 132f, 133f
    channel, carrier, and pump proteins in, 128-130, 128f, 129t
    lipid solubility and, 127-128
Biomembranes. See Biological membranes
BK_{Ca} channel, 109, 110f
Bladder, tight epithelium of, 174
Blood pressure
  high, salt retention and, 171b
  low, salt wasting and, 171, 171b
Blood-brain barrier, 29b
Body, organization of, 2-4, 2f
BPH (benign prostatic hypertrophy), 243b
Brain edema, 29b
Brody disease, 159b
Bulk flow, 173
Bursts, of action potentials, 106, 106f

Index

C

Cable equation, 72
   resistance units used in, 71b
Calcium (Ca^{2+})
   in excitation-contraction coupling, 202-205, 203f, 204b, 205f, 206f
   in malignant hyperthermia, 204, 204b
   in muscle contraction
      cardiac, 211
         Ca^{2+} in, 188, 190, 210-211, 226f, 235
      skeletal, 188
         binding with troponin C of, 188, 227
         Ca^{2+}-induced release of, 208-211, 210f, 212b, 213b, 213f
         concentration of, 226, 226f, 227-228
         extracellular, 202-203, 203f
         storage in sarcoplasmic reticulum of, 203-205, 204b, 205f, 206f
      smooth
         elevation of cytosolic, 191-195, 193f, 194f, 195b
         maintaining balance of, 218, 220f
         relation with myosin, phosphorylation and mechanical force in, 242-243, 244f, 245f
   intracellular, physiological roles of, 143-144
Calcium (Ca^{2+})-activated K^+ channels, 100t, 106b, 109, 110f
Calcium (Ca^{2+}) antagonist drugs, 104, 104f, 105b
Calcium (Ca^{2+}) channel(s)
   beta (β)-adrenergic receptor activation of, 113
   in cardiac muscle, 210-211, 210f, 212b, 213b, 213f
   location and functions of, 100t
   structure of, 58
   voltage-gated, 99-104
      contribution to action potentials by, 100, 101f
      structure of, 58
      types of, 100, 102b, 203t
Calcium (Ca^{2+}) channel blockers, as therapeutic agents, 104, 104f, 105b
Calcium (Ca^{2+}) concentration
   depolarization and, 202
   free, 157
   total intracellular, 157
Calcium (Ca^{2+}) currents, recording of, 101-104, 103f
Calcium (Ca^{2+})-dependent ATPase, 157-158, 158b, 159b
Calcium (Ca^{2+}) homeostasis, 154-157, 159
Calcium (Ca^{2+})-independent regulatory mechanisms, modulation of smooth muscle contraction by, 195, 195b
Calcium (Ca^{2+})-induced calcium (Ca^{2+}) release (CICR), 208-211, 212f
Calcium (Ca^{2+}) overload, 157
Calcium (Ca^{2+}) pump
   plasma membrane, 156f, 158-159, 160b
      ATP-driven, 158-159, 160b
   in cardiac muscle, 210f
   in smooth muscle, 218
   SERCA as. See Sarcoplasmic/endoplasmic reticulum Ca^{2+}-dependent ATPase (SERCA)
   turnover number for, 129t
Calcium (Ca^{2+}) release, in cardiac muscle contraction, 208-211, 210f, 212b, 213b, 213f
Calcium (Ca^{2+}) release channels, 203, 204, 205-206, 206f, 208f
Calcium (Ca^{2+}) signaling, intracellular, 154-157
Calcium (Ca^{2+}) sparks, 211, 213b
Calcium (Ca^{2+}) storage, in sarcoplasmic/endoplasmic reticulum
   mediation by Ca^{2+}-ATPase of, 157-158, 158b, 159b
   for skeletal muscle contraction, 203-205, 204b, 205f, 206f
Calcium (Ca^{2+}) transport, 158-159
Calcium (Ca^{2+}) transporters
   in Ca^{2+} homeostasis, 159
   localization of, 159
Calmodulin (CaM), 219b
Calreticulin (CR), 220f
Calsequestrin (CS), 203, 220f
cAMP (cyclic adenosine monophosphate) system, 113
Cannon, Walter B., 2n
Capacitance, 43b, 65, 66b
Capacitive currents
   with open ion channel, 65-67, 68f
   with voltage clamps, 80, 80f
Capacitor, 65
Capillary density, and metabolic rate of tissue, 12, 13b
Capillary hydrostatic pressure, 26-29, 26f, 27f
Capillary oncotic pressure, 26-27, 26f, 27f
Capillary wall, direction of fluid flow through, 26-29, 26f, 27f, 28b, 29b
Carbamino compounds, 125f
Carbon dioxide (CO_2)
   metabolism of, 124b
   transport of, 124b, 125f
Carbonic anhydrase, 124b
Cardiac muscle
   beta (β)-adrenergic receptor activation of Ca^{2+} channels in, 113
   contraction of, 188-190, 208-211, 234-238
      Ca^{2+} in, 188, 190, 210-211, 226f, 235
      Ca^{2+} release in, 208-211, 210f, 212b, 213b, 213f
      end-diastolic volume and, 237-239, 237f
      energy supply for, 190
      excitation-contraction coupling in, 208-211
      force development in, 226f, 234-235
      force-velocity relationship in, 238, 238f
      length-tension relationships in, 231f, 235-237
      long duration of, 234-235
      sarcolemma and sarcoplasmic reticulum in, 209-210

Cardiac muscle (cont'd)
    synchronous, 190
    twitch, 234
    striation of, 188-190, 189f
    structure and function of, 188-190, 189f
Cardiac muscle cell, 188, 189f
Cardiotonic steroids
    and Ca^{2+} signaling, 160b
    Na^+ pump as receptor for, 152-154, 155b
Carrier(s)
    model of, 128f
    simple, 130
Carrier molecule, ion transport via, 54, 55
Carrier proteins, 17-20
    in transport across biological membranes, 130-134, 131b, 132b, 132f, 133f
Carrier-mediated transport, 130-134, 131b, 132b, 132f, 133f
Cations, flux of, 39b-40b, 39f
Cell(s), biological membranes of, 3-4, 4f
Cell body, 53, 54, 54f
Cell volume changes
    persistent, 31-32, 32f, 33b-34b
    transient, 30, 30f, 31b
Cellular physiology, 5
Cerebral edema, 29b
Ceruloplasmin, 162
CFTR (cystic fibrosis transmembrane conductance regulator), 165, 165b, 173
Changes in volume, 30
Channel(s). *See also* Ion channel(s)
    gated, 128f
    model of, 128f
    permeability through, 129-130
    stretch-activated, cation-permeable, 214-215
    transport through
        "gating" and, 130
    speed of, 129-130, 129t
Channel proteins, in transport across biological membranes, 128-130, 128f, 129t
Charge movement, in excitation-contraction coupling, 205-206, 207b, 208f
Chemical energy, interconversion of electrochemical potential energy and, 149-150, 178
"Chemical force," 118, 119b, 119f
Chemical potential energy
    gradient of, 118, 119b-120b
    of ion, 118-120, 121b
Chloride (Cl^-)
    absorption by transcellular route of, 169f
    equilibrium potential for, 47
    intracellular and extracellular concentrations of, 38t
    mutations in, 201b

reabsorption of, 168, 169-170, 170f
    in resting membrane potential, 45
Chloride (Cl^-) channels, in secretory diarrhea, 171, 173b
Chloride (Cl^-) conductance, in cystic fibrosis, 165b
Chloride (Cl^-) permeability, of skeletal muscle, 200-201, 201b
Chloride (Cl^-)-selective channels, in basolateral membrane, 170f
Chloride (Cl^-) transporters, 170, 170f
Chloride-bicarbonate (Cl^-/HCO_3^-) exchange, 122, 123b, 124b-125b, 125f, 144-145
    in gastric acid secretion, 161
Chloride-bicarbonate (Cl^-/HCO_3^-) exchanger, 170
    in chloride absorption by transcellular route, 169f
Cholesterol
    in biomembranes, 3
    in lipid bilayers, 128
Chronotropic effect, 235n
CICR (Ca^{2+}-induced Ca^{2+} release), 208-211, 212f
Circulatory system, in homeostasis, 2
Cl^-. *See* Chloride (Cl^-)
CMS (congenital myasthenic syndromes), 114b, 114f
CO_2 (carbon dioxide)
    metabolism of, 124b
    transport of, 124b, 125f
Cognate, 217
Colloid osmotic pressure, 26-27, 26f, 27f, 28b
Colon, aganglionic, 214, 214b
Compartmentation, 2-3
Competitive inhibition, of carrier-mediated transport, 133
Concentration difference, diffusion and, 18b-19b, 19f
Concentration gradient(s), 8, 9f, 12
    of cotransported solute, 137-139, 137f, 138b
    and diffusion of solute across membrane, 12-13, 14f-15f
    membrane permeability and, 18b-19b, 19f
Conductance(s)
    calculation of, 81
    defined, 81
    macroscopic, 82
    rising phase of, 80-81
    unit of, 81
    voltage-dependent, 81-83, 83f, 84f, 85b
Conductance levels, of ion channels, 83-84, 86f
Conduction velocity, 91-93, 93b
    and axon diameter, 94, 94f
    myelination and, 93-95, 94f, 94t, 95f
Conductor, resistance of, 71b
Congenital myasthenic syndromes (CMS), 114b, 114f
Congenital stationary night blindness (CSNB), X-linked, 100, 103b
Contractures, 200, 200f
Copper (Cu^+)-requiring metalloenzymes, 162, 162b
Copper (Cu^{2+})-transporting ATPases, 162-163, 162b, 163b

Index

Cotransport, 134
  energetic consequences of, 137-139, 138b
  physiology and pathophysiology of, 136b
Cotransported solute, concentration or electrochemical gradient of, 137-139, 137f, 138b
Cotransporters
  sodium-glucose, 136-139, 136f, 137f, 138b, 139b
  sodium-iodine, 136, 136b
Countertransport, 134-135
  coupled, 141-143, 142f, 143f, 144b
  exchange of sodium for calcium and protons by, 141-143, 142f, 143f, 144b
  by simple carriers, 133-134
Coupled cotransport, energetics of, 137-139, 138b
Coupled countertransport, 141-143, 142f, 143f, 144b
Coupled transport, 134-135, 135b
  for multiple systems, 144-146, 145f
CR (calreticulin), 220f
Cross-bridge(s), 182, 184, 184f
  force and displacement generated by single, 230, 232b
  in smooth muscle, 242, 242b, 244, 246b, 247f
Cross-bridge cycling
  in skeletal muscle, 184-188, 187f, 232
  in smooth muscle, 191-195, 194f, 242, 242b
"Cross-linkase," 162b
CS (calsequestrin), 203, 220f
CSNB (congenital stationary night blindness), X-linked, 100, 103b
Cu^{2+} (copper)-requiring metalloenzymes, 162, 162b
Cu^{2+} (copper)-transporting ATPases, 162-163, 162b, 163b
Current(s), sign conventions for, 46b, 46t
Current-voltage relationships, passive membrane properties and, 65, 66b, 67f
Cyclic adenosine monophosphate (cAMP) system, 113
Cyclic guanosine monophosphate-dependent protein kinase (G-kinase), vasodilation caused by, 217b
Cystic fibrosis, 165b
Cystic fibrosis transmembrane conductance regulator (CFTR), 165, 165b, 173
Cytochrome c oxidase, 162b
Cytotoxic agents, and multidrug resistance proteins, 164-165

D

D600, calcium channel block by, 104, 104f
Deactivation, 82
Defective glucose transporter protein syndrome, 132b
Demyelinating diseases, 95, 95b
Dendrites, 53, 54, 54f
Dense bodies, plasma membrane–associated, 191, 192f
Dephosphorylation of myosin regulatory light chain, 193f, 194-195, 194f
Depolarization, 87, 91f

Ca^{2+} entry during, 202-203, 203f
  inactivation of Na^+ channels during maintained, 84-86, 87f, 88b-89b
  initiation of muscle contraction by, 199-202, 200f, 201b, 201f
  of T-tubule membrane, 202, 203f
Desmin, 191
DHPRs (dihydropyridine receptors)
  in cardiac muscle, 211, 213f
  in skeletal muscle, 202-203, 205-206, 206f, 207b, 208f
Diabetes insipidus, 129
Diabetes mellitus, 130
  non–insulin-dependent, 110, 111b
Diarrhea, secretory, 171, 173b
Diffusing capacity of the lung (D_L), 16b
Diffusion, 7-17
  across membrane barrier, 12-17, 14f-15f, 16b
    and concentration difference, 18b-19b, 19f
    lipid solubility and, 127-128
  and capillary density, 12, 13b
  constraint of cell biology and physiology by, 11-12, 13b
  defined, 7, 8f
  facilitated, 130, 131b
  Fick's First Law of, 7-9, 9f
    and diffusion across membrane barrier, 12-17, 14f-15f, 16b
    and gas transport in lung, 16b, 16f
  ion transport via, 54-55, 55f, 56b
  quantitative examination of random, microscopic movements of molecules in, 9-10, 10f, 11f
  root-mean-squared displacement as measure of, 10-11
  square-root-of-time dependence of, 11, 12f
Diffusion barrier, 16b, 16f
Diffusion coefficient, 8
Diffusion constant, 8
Digoxin, Na^+ pump as receptor for, 152-154, 155b
Dihydropyridine receptors (DHPRs)
  in cardiac muscle, 211, 213f
  in skeletal muscle, 202-203, 205-206, 206f, 207b, 208f
Diltiazem, as calcium channel blocker, 104
D_L (diffusing capacity of the lung), 16b
Donnan effect, 48-49, 48f, 50b-51b
Dopamine beta (β)-hydroxylase, 162b
Driving force, 64
  and rate of transport through open channels, 130
Duty cycle ratio, 241
Dyads, 209, 210f
Dynein motors, 177-178

E

E-C coupling. *See* Excitation-contraction (E-C) coupling
Economy, of muscle contraction, 244
Edema, 29, 29b

EDN3 (endothelin 3) gene, 214b
EDNRB (endothelin B receptor) gene, 214b
Efficiency, of muscle contraction, 244
Efflux, 15
Elastic elements, in skeletal muscle, 226-227, 226f, 227b
Electric field, 44b
Electrical potential energy, of ion, 118-120, 121b
Electrical potential gradient
  defined, 39b
  movement of ions driven by, 39b-41b
Electrical signals, 4-5
Electrical syncytium, 190, 190n
Electrochemical equilibrium, 38
Electrochemical gradient
  of cotransported solute, 137-139, 137f, 138b
  steady-state, 130
Electrochemical potential, 120
Electrochemical potential energy, 120, 121b
  interconversion of chemical energy and, 149-150, 178
  Nernst equation for, 120-121, 122f, 123b
  and transport processes, 117-126, 123b-125b
Electroneutral exchange, 122
Electroneutrality principle, 44b
Electrotonic conduction, 70
Electrotonic potentials, 64
End-diastolic volume, and cardiac muscle contraction, 237-238, 237f
Endocytosis, 20
Endofacial configuration, of carrier, 128f, 130
Endoplasmic reticulum (ER), Ca^{2+} storage in, 157-158, 158b, 159b
Endoplasmic reticulum Ca^{2+}-dependent ATPase. *See* Sarcoplasmic/endoplasmic reticulum Ca^{2+}-dependent ATPase (SERCA)
Endothelin 3 (EDN3) gene, 214b
Endothelin B receptor (EDNRB) gene, 214b
Enteric nervous system, 214
Enterotoxins, and secretory diarrhea, 173b
Environment, internal, 1, 2n
Epithelial cell(s), active transport across, 165-174
  absorption of Cl^- in, 169-170, 170f
  functional diversity and, 167-168
  net water flow and net solute flow in, 172-174
  secretion of substances by epithelia in, 170-171, 171b, 172f, 173b
  sources of Na^+ for apical membrane Na^+-solute cotransport in, 168-169, 169f
  structure and, 165, 166f, 167f
Epithelial cell monolayer, 165, 166f
Epithelial membrane potentials, 166f
Epithelium(ia)
  functional diversity of, 167-168
  structure of, 165, 166f, 167f

substances secreted by, 170-171, 171b, 172f, 173b
  water transport across, 172-174
Equilibrium potential, 38, 41-42
  for Cl^-, 47
Equivalent electrical circuit(s), 64
  of axon, 72, 72f
  of excitable membrane, 64-65, 64f, 65f, 66b
  parameters used in, 71t
  of passive, resting membrane, 67, 69f
  of patch of axon membrane, and action potential generation, 86-87, 90f
ER (endoplasmic reticulum), Ca^{2+} storage in, 157-158, 158b, 159b
Escherichia coli, secretory diarrhea caused by, 173b
Exchange, 134
Excitation-contraction (E-C) coupling, 199-223
  in cardiac muscle, 208-211
  charge movement in, 205-206, 207b, 208f
  defined, 200
  depolarization of T-tubule membrane in, 202, 203f
  direct mechanical interaction between sarcolemmal and sarcoplasmic reticulum membrane proteins in, 202-207
  extracellular Ca^{2+} not required for, 202-203, 203f
  mechanical nature of, 205-206, 207b, 208f, 209f
  in skeletal muscle, 199-208
  in smooth muscle, 211-218
  voltage sensors for, 200, 205, 206, 207b, 208f
Exocytosis, 20
Exofacial configuration, of carrier, 128f, 130
Extracellular environment, 3
Extracellular fluid, osmotic pressure of, 24b

F

Facilitated diffusion, 130, 131b
Familial persistent hyperinsulinemic hypoglycemia of infancy, 110, 112b
Fanconi-Bickel syndrome, 141
Faraday, 118
"Fast channel syndrome," 114b
Fast twitch
  fatigable (FF) motor units, 232, 233, 234, 235f, 236b
  fatigue resistant (FR) motor units, 232, 233, 234, 235f, 236b
Fatigue, 233
Fatigue index, 233
FF (fast twitch, fatigable) motor units, 232, 233, 234, 235f, 236b
Fick's First Law of Diffusion, 7-9, 9f
  and diffusion across membrane barrier, 12-17, 14f-15f, 16b
  and gas transport in lung, 16b, 16f
Filtration constant, 25

Index

Finite bath condition, 33b-34b
Fluid flow, through capillary wall, direction of, 26-29, 26f, 27f, 28b, 29b
Fluid mosaic, 3
Flux(es), 8, 9f
  driven by chemical force, 119b
  ionic, 42-44, 45
  net, through membrane, 15-17
  of positive ions being driven by an electric field, 39b-40b, 39f
  sign conventions for, 46b, 46t
Folkman, Judah, 13b
Force, 229
  chemical, 118, 119b, 119f
  measurement of, 229f
  muscle length and, 230-231, 231f
Force development
  in cardiac muscle, 226f, 234-235
  in skeletal muscle, 226-228, 226f
  in smooth muscle, 242-243, 244f, 245f
Force transient, duration of, 226f
Force-velocity relationship
  in cardiac muscle, 238, 238f
  in skeletal muscle, 229-232, 229f, 231f, 233f
  in smooth muscle, 239-241, 240f
FR (fast twitch, fatigue resistant) motor units, 232, 233, 234, 235f, 236b
Frank-Starling relationship, 237
F-type ATPases, 150
Fused contractions, 228-229, 228f
FXYD family, 154

G

G-actin, 182
Gamma (γ)-aminobutyric acid (GABA)-gated ion channels, 112
Gamma (γ)-aminobutyric acid (GABA) receptor channel, 100t
Gamma (γ)-glutamyl-cysteinyl-glycine (GSH), cotransport with glutathione of, 163
Gap junctions, 190, 215
Gas transport, in lung, Fick's First Law of Diffusion and, 16b, 16f
Gastric acid secretion
  history of physiology of, 251-252
  mediation by H^+,K^+-ATPase of, 160-161, 161f, 162b
Gastric glands, 161
Gastric hyperacidity, 161, 162b
Gastric parietal cell, 161
  HCl secretion by, 161, 161f
Gastrin, 161, 161f
Gastrointestinal system, in homeostasis, 2
Gated channel, model of, 128f

Gating
  of ion channels, 55
  and transport through channels, 130
Gating currents, 83, 85b, 85f
Gene superfamily, 58
GHK (Goldman-Hodgkin-Katz) equation, 45, 46b, 46t
G-kinase (cyclic guanosine monophosphate–dependent protein kinase), vasodilation caused by, 217b
Globulins, and colloid osmotic pressure, 28b
Glucose transport
  defects in, 140-141, 141b
  with sodium, 136-139, 136b, 136f, 137f, 138b, 139b
  two-step sequential, 139-140, 140f
Glucose transporter 1 (GLUT-1)
  carrier-mediated transport by, 131b
  competitive and noncompetitive inhibition of, 133
  defects in, 131-132, 132b
  glucose uptake mediated by, 133f
  structure of, 131-132, 132f
  turnover number for, 129t
Glucose transporter 2 (GLUT-2), in two-step sequential transport, 140, 140f
Glucose transporter 4 (GLUT-4), regulation of, 134
Glucose uptake
  inhibition by beta (β)-adrenergic agonists of, 134
  Na^+-glucose coupling ratio and, 139, 139b
Glucose-galactose malabsorption, 141b
Glucose-induced insulin secretion, ATP-sensitive K^+ channels in, 109-110, 111b, 111f, 112b
GLUT-1. *See* Glucose transporter 1 (GLUT-1)
GLUT-2 (glucose transporter 2), in two-step sequential transport, 140, 140f
GLUT-4 (glucose transporter 4), regulation of, 134
Glutamate receptor channels, 100t
Glutamate-gated ion channels, 112
Glutathione, cotransport of neutral solutes with, 163, 164f
Glutathione-S (GS)-coupled solute, 164f
Glycine-gated ion channels, 112
Glycosuria, 140
Goldman, David E., 45n
Goldman-Hodgkin-Katz (GHK) equation, 45, 46b, 46t
Gonyaulax, 91b
G-proteins (GTP-binding proteins), 219b
Gradient(s)
  of chemical potential energy, 118, 119b-120b
  concentration, 8, 9f, 12
    of cotransported solute, 137-139, 137f, 138b
    and diffusion of solute across membrane, 12-13, 14f-15f
    ion, 37, 168
    membrane permeability and, 18b-19b, 19f
  electrical potential
    defined, 39b
    movement of ions driven by, 39b-41b

Gradient(s) (cont'd)
  electrochemical
    of cotransported solute, 137-139, 137f, 138b
    steady-state, 130
  of potential energy, 118, 119b-120b
Gravitational force, and potential energy, 117-118
GS (glutathione-S)-coupled solute, 164f
GSH (gamma [γ]-glutamyl-cysteinyl-glycine), cotransport with glutathione of, 163, 164f
Guanosine triphosphate (GTP)-binding proteins (G-proteins), 219b

H

H^+ (protons)
  extrusion of, 135, 135b
  in kidneys, 169
H^+ (proton) pump, mediation of gastric acid secretion by, 160-161, 161f, 162b
H zone
  in muscle contraction, 182-184, 185f, 186f
  structure of, 180, 180n
H_2 receptor blockers, 252
H_2O. *See* Water
HCl (hydrochloric acid) secretion, by gastric parietal cell, 161, 161f
HCO_3^- (bicarbonate), exchange with chloride of, 122, 123b, 124b-125b, 125f
Heartburn, 161, 162b
hERG (human ether-a-go-go), 106b
Hirschsprung's disease, 214, 214b
Histamine
  and edema, 29b
  in gastric acid secretion, 161, 161f
H^+,K^+-ATPase, mediation of gastric acid secretion by, 160-161, 161f, 162b
H^+,K^+-ATPase inhibitor, 162b
Hodgkin, Alan L., 45n, 77n
"Holding" potential, 79
Homeostasis, 1-2, 2n
  Ca^{2+}, 154-157, 159
HPP (hyperkalemic periodic paralysis), 86, 88b-89b, 88f
Human ether-a-go-go (hERG), 106b
Huxley
  A.F., 77n, 182, 202, 230
  H.E., 182, 184
Hydraulic conductivity, 25
Hydrochloric acid (HCl) secretion, by gastric parietal cell, 161, 161f
Hydrophilic head group, 3
Hydrophilic solutes, diffusion across lipid bilayers of, 127-128
Hydrophobic fatty acid chains, 3
Hydrophobic substances, diffusion across lipid bilayers of, 127

Hydrostatic pressure, 22
  and direction of fluid flow through capillary wall, 26-29, 26f, 27f, 28b, 29b
  and osmotic pressure, in water movement through membrane, 25-29, 26f, 27f, 28b, 29b
Hyperacidity, gastric, 161, 162b
Hyperinsulinism, familial, 110, 112b
Hyperkalemic periodic paralysis (HPP), 86, 88b-89b, 88f
Hyperosmolar solution, 25b
Hyperpolarization, 65
Hypertension, salt retention and, 171b
Hyperthermia, malignant, 204, 204b
Hypertonic solution, 25b
Hypoglycorrhachia, 132b
Hypotension, salt wasting and, 171, 171b
Hypothyroidism, congenital, caused by defects in Na^+/I^- cotransporter, 136b
Hypotonic solution, 25b

I

I band(s)
  in muscle contraction
    cardiac, 189f
    skeletal, 182-184, 185f, 186f
  structure of, 180
I_A (A-currents), 107
Impermeant solute(s), 23
  imbalance of, 48-49, 48f, 50b-51b
  permanent osmotic effects of, 31-32, 32f, 33b-34b
Inactivation, 81, 82
Inactivation gate, 83, 84f, 85, 87f
Infinite bath condition, 31, 33b
Influx, 15
Inositol trisphosphate (IP_3), in smooth muscle contraction, 218, 219b
Inositol trisphosphate (IP_3) receptors, 156f
Inotropic effect, positive, 113, 235, 235n
Insect venom, and edema, 29b
Insulin, regulation of GLUT-4 by, 134
Insulin secretion, ATP-sensitive K^+ channels in, 109-110, 111b, 111f, 112b
Intercalated disks, in cardiac muscle, 189f, 190
Intermediate(s), phosphorylated, 150
Intermediate filaments, 191
Internal environment, 1, 2n
Internode distance, 94
Interstitial hydrostatic pressure, 26-27, 26f, 27f
Interstitial oncotic pressure, 26-27, 26f, 27f
Intestinal smooth muscle, 214
Intracellular fluid, osmotic pressure of, 24b
Intracellular microelectrodes, study of properties of action potential with, 75-77, 76f, 79f
Intracellular space, 3

Index

Inward ionic current, 89-90
Inward rectifier K^+ channel, 100t, 106b
Iodothyronines, 136b
Iodotyrosines, 136b
Ion(s)
    electrical and chemical potential energy of, 118-120, 121b
    intracellular and extracellular concentrations of, 37, 38t
Ion channel(s), 4f, 53-61
    ACh-gated, 112-113, 114b
    diversity of, 99-116
    electrical behavior of membranes and, 53-54, 54f
    flow of ionic and capacitive currents with open, 65-67, 68f
    function of, 77-83
    GABA-gated, 112
    gated, 55
        glutamate-gated, 112
        glycine-gated, 112
    ion selectivity of, 55-56, 57b
        ligand-gated, 55, 100t, 111-113, 114b
    in membrane conductance, 64-65, 64f
    membrane permeability and, 54-55, 55f, 56b
    regulation by second-messenger pathways of, 113
    structure of, 56-59, 57f, 58f, 60f
    turnover numbers for, 129, 129t
    two conductance levels of, 83-84, 86f
        voltage-gated, 55
            examples of, 100t
            voltage sensor in, 85b, 85f
            voltage-dependent conductances of, 81-83, 83f, 84f, 85b
Ion channel conductance, 64-65, 64f
Ion concentration gradients, 37, 168
Ion currents. *See* Ionic currents
Ion movement
    driven by electrical potential gradient, 39b-41b
    needed to establish physiologic membrane potential, 42, 43b
    through aqueous pore, 54-55, 55f, 56b
Ion pump, 4f
Ionic currents
    dependence on voltage and time of, 79-81, 80f, 81f, 82b
    ionic fluxes and, 45, 46b, 46t
    measurement of, 77, 78b, 78f
    with open ion channel, 65-67, 68f
Ionic flux(es), 42-44, 45
    and ionic currents, 45, 46b, 46t
Ionic permeability(ies), through membranes, 37-42, 38f, 39b-41b, 43b, 44b, 45
Ionic substitutions, for separating current components, 82b, 82f
IP_3 (inositol trisphosphate), in smooth muscle contraction, 218, 219b
IP_3 (inositol trisphosphate) receptors, 156f

Isometric contraction, 229-230, 230f, 233f
Isotonic contraction, 230, 231-232, 233f, 234f
Isotonic solution, 25b

K

K^+. *See* Potassium (K^+)
K_A channels, 107-108, 107f-109f
Katz, Bernard, 45n
KCNQ channels, 106b
KCSA channel protein, 59, 60f
Kinesin, conventional, 179b, 179f, 180f
Kinesin motors, 177-178, 179b-180b, 179f, 180f

L

Lansoprazole (Prevacid), 162b, 252
Lateral intercellular space, of epithelial cells, 166f, 167f
Leaflet, of phospholipids, 3
Leakage channels, 86, 90f
Leakage conductance, 90f
"Leakiness," 165
Leaky epithelia, 172
Length constant, 72, 73, 91-92, 93b
Length-tension curve
    in cardiac muscle, 231f, 235-237
    in skeletal muscle, 229-232, 229f, 231f
    in smooth muscle, 238-239, 239f
Ligand-gated ion channels, 55, 100t, 111-113, 114b
Linear current-voltage relationships, passive membrane properties and, 65, 66b, 67f
Lipid bilayer membranes, 3-4, 4f
    diffusion across, 127-128
Lipid solubility, and diffusion across biological membranes, 127-128
Local anesthetics, blocking of Na^+ channels by, 89, 91b
Local circuit current, in propagation of action potential, 89, 93f
Localization, of Ca^{2+} transporters, 159
Loewi, Otto, 144n
Low blood pressure, salt wasting and, 171, 171b
L-type Ca^{2+} channel, 102b, 102t, 103b
    beta (β)-adrenergic receptor activation of, 113
L-type voltage-gated channels (LVGCC), in smooth muscle, 220f
Lung
    diffusing capacity of, 16b
    gas transport in, Fick's First Law of Diffusion and, 16b, 16f
Lymph production, 29
Lysyl oxidase, 162b

M

M line
    of cardiac muscle, 189f
    of skeletal muscle, 180

MacKinnon, Roderick, 59n
Macromolecules, impermeant, 48-49, 48f, 50b-51b
Malignant hyperthermia (MH), 204, 204b
Meandering, random movements and, 9-10, 10f
Mechanical threshold, 200
Megacolon, congenital aganglionic, 214, 214b
Membrane(s)
    equivalent circuits of an excitable, 64-65, 64f, 65f, 66b
    lipid bilayer, 3-4, 4f
    net flux through, 15-17
    passive electrical properties of, 63-74
        and time course and spread of membrane potential changes, 63-64
    water movement through, osmotic pressure and hydrostatic pressure in, 25-29, 26f, 27f, 28b, 29b
Membrane barrier, diffusion across, 12-17, 14f-15f, 16b
Membrane capacitance, 43b, 65, 66b
    specific, 66b
    and time course of voltage changes, 65-69, 68f-70f
Membrane conductance, ion channels in, 64-65, 64f
Membrane length constant, 72, 73, 91-92, 93b
Membrane microdomains, 4
Membrane permeability, 13-15
    ion channels and, 54-55, 55f, 56b
    to ions, 37-42, 38f, 39b-41b, 43b, 44b
    and transport of solute, 17-20, 17t, 18b-19b, 19f
Membrane permeability coefficients, 17, 17t
Membrane potential, 40b-41b, 41
    depolarization of, 199-202, 200f, 201b, 201f
    during action potential, 76
    electrical subthreshold changes in, passive spread of, 69-73, 70f, 71b, 71t, 72f
    exponential time course of, 67-69, 69f, 70f
    ion movement needed to establish, 42, 43b
    ionic and capacitive current flow and, 65-67, 68f
    magnitude of, 42, 44b
    measuring and manipulating, 66b
    and Na^+/Ca^{2+} exchange, 143
    resting, 42-47
        estimation of, 45, 46b, 46t
        in hyperkalemic periodic paralysis, 88f
        of skeletal muscle, 200-201, 201b
    selective membrane permeability and, 48
    steady-state, 63
    time course and spread of changes in, passive electrical properties of membranes and, 63-64
Membrane resistance, 64, 64f
    equation for, 71b
    and passive spread of electrical subthreshold signals, 69-73, 70f, 71b, 71t, 72f
Membrane time constant, 17, 19b, 68-69, 92
Membrane-mediated processes, 5
Menkes disease, 162, 163b

Metalloenzymes, Cu^{2+}-requiring, 162, 162b
MH (malignant hyperthermia), 204, 204b
MHC (myosin heavy chain) isoform, 242, 242b
Microdomains, membrane, 4
Microtubules, 177
Mitochondria, in cardiac muscle, 189f, 190
Mixing, 21
MLC (myosin light chain) isoform, 242, 242b
MLC phosphorylation. *See* Myosin light chain (MLC) phosphorylation
MLCK (myosin light chain kinase), 191-195, 193f, 194f, 195b
MLCP (myosin light chain phosphatase), 193f, 194, 195b
Mobility coefficient, 119b
Molecular motors, 177-178, 179b-180b, 179f, 180f
Motor units, 225-226, 232-234, 235f, 236b
Multidrug resistance proteins (MRPs), 163-165, 164f
Multidrug resistance transport ATPases, 163
Multiple sclerosis, 95, 95b
Muscle cells, composition of, 178, 181f, 182f
Muscle contraction
    cardiac, 188-190, 208-211, 234-238
        Ca^{2+} in, 188, 190, 210-211, 226f, 235
        Ca^{2+} release in, 208-211, 210f, 212b, 213b, 213f
        end-diastolic volume and, 237-239, 237f
        energy supply for, 190
        excitation-contraction coupling in, 208-211
        force development in, 226f, 234-235
        force-velocity relationship in, 238, 238f
        length-tension curve in, 231f, 235-237
        long duration of, 234-235
        sarcolemma and sarcoplasmic reticulum in, 209-210
        structural basis for, 188-190, 189f
        synchronous, 190
        twitch, 234
    skeletal, 177-188, 199-207, 225-234
        Ca^{2+} in
            binding with troponin C of, 188, 227
            Ca^{2+}-induced release of, 208-211, 210f, 212b, 213b, 213f
            concentration of, 226, 226f, 227-228
            extracellular, 202-203, 203f
            storage in sarcoplasmic reticulum of, 203-205
        Ca^{2+} release channels in, 203, 204, 205-206, 206f, 208f
        cross-bridge cycling in, 184-188, 187f, 232
        depolarization of surface membrane in, 199-202, 200f, 201b, 201f
        efficiency of, 244
        force development in, 226-228, 226f
        force-velocity relationship in, 229-232, 229f, 231f, 233f
        fused, 228-229, 228f
        isometric and isotonic, 229-230, 230f, 231-232, 233f, 234f
        length-tension curve in, 229-232, 229f, 231f

Muscle contraction (cont'd)
  skeletal (cont'd)
    mechanisms that vary total force of, 225-229
    molecular motors in, 177-178, 179b-180b
    motor units in, 225-226, 232-234, 235f, 236b
    myofibrils in, 178, 181f, 182f
    sarcolemma and sarcoplasmic reticulum in, 202-207
    sarcomere in, 178-182, 183f-185f
    sliding filament mechanism of, 182-184, 185f, 186f, 230-231
    T-tubules in, 202, 203f, 205, 205f
    twitch, 201-202, 201f, 226-228, 226f, 227b
    voltage sensor in, 200, 205, 206, 207b, 208f
  smooth, 190-195, 211-218, 238-246
    ATP in, 243-244, 246b, 247f
    Ca^{2+} in
      elevation of cytosolic, 191-195, 193f, 194f, 195b
      maintaining balance of, 218, 220f
      relation with myosin, phosphorylation and mechanical force in, 242-243, 244f, 245f
    cross-bridges in, 242, 242b, 244, 246b, 247f
    depolarization in, 215
    diversification and, 211-214, 246
    force-velocity relationship in, 239-241, 240f
    innervation density and, 214-215, 214b, 215f
    length-tension curve in, 238-239, 239f
    myosin light chain phosphorylation in, 242
    myosin motors in, 177, 242, 242b, 243b
    phasic, 215, 242, 242b
    second messenger in, 218, 219b
    single-unit, 215
    sliding filament mechanism in, 238-239
    structural basis for, 190-191, 192f
    tonic, 215
      ATP in, 243-244, 246b, 247f
      Ca^{2+} channels in, 215-216, 216f
      Ca^{2+} concentration in, 243, 245f
      inositol-1,4,5-trisphosphate in, 218, 219b
      muscle shortening velocity in, 241
      myosin isoforms in, 241, 242b
      myosin light chain phosphorylation in, 242-243, 244f
      pharmacomechanical coupling in, 216-218
Muscle economy, 244
Muscle efficiency, 244
Muscle fibers, composition of, 178, 181f, 182f
Muscle length
  and force, 230-231, 231f
  measurement of, 229f
Muscle shortening velocity
  in cardiac muscle, 238, 238f
  in skeletal muscle, 231-232, 233f, 234f
  in smooth muscle, 239-241, 240f, 242

Myasthenic syndromes, congenital, 114b, 114f
Myelin, 54f
Myelinated neuron, structure of, 53-54, 54f
Myelination, and action potential conduction velocity, 93-95, 94f, 94t, 95f
Myocytes, cardiac, 188, 189f
Myofibrils, 178-182, 181f, 183f
  in cardiac myocyte, 189f
Myogenic tone, 215, 215f
Myosin, 182, 184f
Myosin head rotation, 232, 234f
Myosin heavy chain (MHC) isoform, 242, 242b
Myosin isoforms
  and cross-bridge cycling, 242, 242b
  prostate gland hypertrophy and, 243b
Myosin light chain (MLC) isoform, 242, 242b
Myosin light chain kinase (MLCK), 191-195, 193f, 194f, 195b
Myosin light chain phosphatase (MLCP), 193f, 194, 195b
Myosin light chain (MLC) phosphorylation
  Ca^{2+} activation of, 191-194, 193f
  with Ca^{2+}-independent mechanisms, 195, 195b
  and cross-bridge cycling, 194-195, 194f
  and force development, 244f
  and force-velocity relationship, 240f
  and length-tension relationship, 239
  and velocity of shortening, 242
Myosin motors, 177, 242, 242b, 243b
Myosin regulatory light chain, phosphorylation and dephosphorylation of, 191-195, 193f, 194f
Myotonia, defined, 201n
Myotonia congenita, 201b

N

Na^+. See Sodium (Na^+)
Na^+-K^+-2 Cl^- cotransporter, 170, 170f
Na^+,K^+-ATPase
  cycle of, 150, 153f
  "electrogenic" nature of, 152
  hydrolysis of ATP by, 150-152
  isoforms of alpha (α) subunit of, 154, 155b, 156f
  maintenance of low Na^+ and high K^+ concentrations in cytosol by, 150-154, 155b, 156f
  net reaction mediated by, 152, 154f
  as receptor for cardiotonic steroids, 152-154, 155b
  structure of, 151, 151f
NCX. See Sodium/calcium (Na^+/ Ca^{2+}) exchanger (NCX)
NE (norepinephrine), and smooth muscles, 217
Nebulin, in thin filaments, 182
Negative feedback, 218
Negative "holding" potential, 79
Neher, Erwin, 84n
Nernst, Hermann Walther, 38n

Nernst equation, 38-42, 39b-41b
   for electrochemical potential energy, 120-121, 122f, 123b
   as special case of GHK equation, 47
Nernst potential, 38, 38n, 41-42
Net flux, through membrane, 15-17
Neuromuscular junction, ACh-gated ion channels at, 112-113, 114b
Neuron(s)
   alpha (α) motor
      in motor unit, 225
      structure of, 53-54, 54f
   myelinated, structure of, 53-54, 54f
   sympathetic and parasympathetic, 190, 211
NHE (Na^+/H^+ exchanger), 134-135, 135b, 141
NIC (Na^+-I^- cotransporter), 136, 136b
Nicotinic ACh-receptor channel, 100t
NIDDM (non–insulin-dependent diabetes mellitus), 110, 111b
Nifedipine, as calcium channel blocker, 104
Night blindness, X-linked congenital stationary, 100, 103b
NIS (Na^+-I^- symporter), 136, 136b
Nitrates, organic, vasodilation caused by, 217b
Nitric oxide (NO), and smooth muscles, 217, 217b
Nitroglycerin, vasodilation caused by, 217, 217b
Nodes of Ranvier, 54f, 94
Noncompetitive inhibition, of carrier-mediated transport, 133
Noninfinite bath condition, 33b-34b
Non–insulin-dependent diabetes mellitus (NIDDM), 110, 111b
Nonmyelinated axons, propagation of action potential in, 89-91, 93b, 93f
Nonpolar fatty acid chains, 3, 4f
Nonpolar substances, diffusion across lipid bilayers of, 127
Nonstriated muscle. *See* Smooth muscle(s)
Norepinephrine (NE), and smooth muscles, 217
N-type Ca^{2+} channel, 102b, 102t

O

OA⁻ (organic anions), coupling of alpha (α)-ketoglutarate to countertransport of, 145, 145f
OAT-1 (organic anion transporter-1), 145, 145f
Occluded state, 130
Ohmic current-voltage relationships, passive membrane properties and, 65, 66b, 67f
Ohm's Law, 64
Omeprazole (Prilosec), 162b, 252
Oncotic pressure, 26-27, 26f, 27f, 28b
Optical "trap," 232b
Optimal length, 230, 231f
Organic anion transporter-1 (OAT-1), 145, 145f
Organic anions (OA⁻), coupling of alpha (α)-ketoglutarate to countertransport of, 145, 145f

Organic nitrates, vasodilation caused by, 217b
Osmolality, 23b
Osmolar solution, 23b
Osmolarity, 23b
   vs. tonicity, 25, 25b
Osmole, 23b
Osmosis
   defined, 21-22, 22f
   osmotic pressure drives net transport of water during, 22-25, 23b, 24b, 25b
   reverse, 25n
   units of measurement for, 23b
   water transport during, and changes in volume, 22
Osmotic imbalance, caused by Donnan effect, 48-49, 48f, 50b-51b
Osmotic pressure(s)
   colloid, 26-27, 26f, 27f
   defined, 23
   and direction of fluid flow through capillary wall, 26-29, 26f, 27f, 28b, 29b
   and hydrostatic pressure, in water movement through membrane, 25-29, 26f, 27f, 28b, 29b
   and net transport of water during osmosis, 22-25, 23b, 24b, 25b
   physiologically relevant, 23, 24b
Ouabain, Na^+ pump as receptor for, 152-154, 155b
Outward current, 90-91
Oxygen diffusion, and capillary density, 12, 13b

P

Paracellular pathway, 165, 166f
Parallel elastic element, 226, 227f
Parietal cell, 161
   HCl secretion by, 161, 161f
Partial pressures, 16b
Partition coefficient, 12-13, 14f-15f
Passive electrical properties, of membranes, 63-74
   defined, 63-64
   and linear current-voltage relationships, 65, 66b, 67f
   and time course and spread of membrane potential changes, 63-64
Passive solute transport, 127-147
Passive tension
   in cardiac muscle, 238
   in skeletal muscle, 230, 231f
Patch clamp, 84, 86f
Pathophysiology, 5
Peripheral couplings, 209, 210f
Peristalsis, 214
Permeability(ies)
   membrane, 13-15
      ionic, 37-42, 38f, 39b-41b, 43b, 44b, 45
      and transport of solute, 17-20, 17t, 18b-19b, 19f

Index

Permeability(ies) (cont'd)
  selective, 37-42
    and concentration gradient, 38f
    and membrane potential, 43b, 44b, 48
    and Nernst equation, 37-42, 39b-41b
  through channels, 129-130
Permeability coefficients, 54
Permeant ion, equilibrium potential for, 47
Permeant solute(s), transient changes in cell volume with, 30, 31b, 31f
Persistent hyperinsulinemic hypoglycemia of infancy (PHHI), 110, 112b
Pharmacomechanical coupling, 216-218
Phospholipid(s)
  amphiphilic (amphipathic), 3
  in biomembranes, 3
Phospholipid bilayers, permeability of, 128
Phosphorylated intermediates, 150
Phosphorylation, myosin light chain
  Ca^{2+} activation of, 191-194, 193f
  with Ca^{2+}-independent mechanisms, 195, 195b
  and cross-bridge cycling, 194-195, 194f
  and force development, 244f
  and force-velocity relationship, 240f
  and length-tension relationship, 239
  and velocity of shortening, 242
Plasma membrane, 3-4, 4f
  electrical forces between ions separated by, 42, 44b
  ion concentration gradients across, 37
Plasma membrane Ca^{2+} pump (PMCA), 156f, 158-159, 160b
  ATP-driven, 158-159, 160b
  in cardiac muscle, 210f
  in smooth muscle, 218
Plasma membrane–associated dense bodies, 191, 192f
Polar head groups, 3, 4f
Polar solutes, diffusion across lipid bilayers of, 127-128
Pore, model of, 128f
Positive inotropic effect, 113, 235, 235n
Postsynaptic potentials, 63
Potassium (K^+)
  in depolarization of membrane potential, 200f
  equilibrium potential for, 43b, 44
  Na^+ pump and transport into cells of, 169
  in resting membrane potential, 45
  secretion across epithelium of, 170, 170f, 171
  selective permeability to, 37-38, 38f
  transport of, 120-121, 122f, 123b
Potassium (K^+) channel(s)
  agents that block, and shape of action potential, 89, 91b, 92f
  ATP-sensitive, 100t, 106b, 109-110, 111b, 111f, 112b
  Ca-activated, 100t, 106b, 109, 110f
  inward rectifier, 100t, 106b
  location and functions of, 100t
  membrane conductance for, 65, 65f
  Ohm's Law for, 64
  regulation of action potential firing patterns by, 105-107, 106f
  structure of, 58-59, 58f, 60f
  turnover number for, 129t
  two-pore, 100t, 106b
  voltage-gated
    current flow through, 80, 81f
    generation of action potential by, 86-89, 90f-92f, 91b
    open, and refractory period, 87-89
    rapidly inactivating, 107-109, 107f-109f
    structure of, 58, 58f, 106b
Potassium (K^+) concentration(s)
  extracellular, 38t
  intracellular, 38t, 150
Potassium (K^+) current, macroscopic, 81, 81f
Potassium (K^+) homeostasis, pump-leak model of, 150
Potassium (K^+)-selective channels, 104-110
  in apical membrane, 170f
  and associated heritable diseases, 105t
  ionic selectivity of, 55
  regulation of action potential firing patterns by, 105-107, 106f
  structural and functional diversity of, 104-105, 106b
Potassium-chloride (K^+-Cl^-) cotransporter, 169f, 170, 170f
Potential energy
  chemical
    gradient of, 118, 119b-120b
    of ion, 118-120, 121b
  defined, 118
  electrochemical, 120, 121b
    in analysis of transport processes, 121-126, 123b-125b
    Nernst equation for, 120-121, 122f, 123b
  and force, 117-118
  and transport processes, 117-126
Prevacid (lansoprazole), 162b, 252
Prilosec (omeprazole), 162b, 252
Propagation time constant, 92
Proportionality constant, in Starling equation, 25
Prostate gland hypertrophy, 243b
Protein(s)
  carrier, 17-20
  dissolved, and colloid osmotic pressure, 28b
  signaling, 3
  transmembrane, 3
  transport, 3
Proton(s) (H^+)
  extrusion of, 135, 135b
  in kidneys, 169
Proton (H^+) pump, mediation of gastric acid secretion by, 160-161, 161f, 162b

P-type ATPases, 150
P-type Ca^{2+} channel, 102b, 102t
Puffer fish, 91b
Pump proteins, in transport across biological membranes, 128-130, 128f, 129t
"Pump-leak model," of Na^+ and K^+ homeostasis, 150

Q

Q-type Ca^{2+} channel, 102b, 102t

R

Random movements, 7
   and meandering, 9-10, 10f
   spreading of molecules in space by, 10, 11f
"Random walk," of single molecule, 9-10, 10f
Rate constant, in membrane permeability, 18b
Receptor-operated channels (ROCs), 218, 220f
"Red tide," 91b
Reflection coefficient, 24
Refractory period(s), 87-89
   absolute and relative, 77, 79f
Relative refractory period, 77, 79f
Relaxation, of skeletal muscle, 207
Renal proximal tubule, net reabsorption of NaCl and H_2O by, 167f
Renal tubular acidosis, 145
Repolarization, 87, 91f
Resistance equation, 71b
Resistance units, used in cable equation, 71b
Resistivity, 71b
Respiratory system, in homeostasis, 2
Resting length, of smooth muscle, 238-239
Resting membrane potential, 42-47
   estimation of, 45, 46b, 46t
   in hyperkalemic periodic paralysis, 88f
   of skeletal muscle, 200-201, 201b
RET gene, 214b
Reverse osmosis, 25n
Reversibility, of simple carriers, 133
Rho-associated protein kinase (ROK), 193f, 195b
ROCs (receptor-operated channels), 218, 220f
Root-mean-squared (RMS) displacement, as measure of diffusion, 10-11
R-type Ca^{2+} channel, 102t
Ryanodine receptors (RyRs), 156f
   in cardiac muscle, 210f, 211, 213f
   in skeletal muscle, 203, 204, 204b, 205
   in smooth muscle, 220f

S

S (slow twitch, fatigue resistant) motor units, 232, 233, 234, 235f, 236b
Sakmann, Bert, 84n
Salt retention, 171, 171b
Salt wasting, 171, 171b
Saltatory conduction, 94
Sarcolemma
   in cardiac muscle, 189f, 209-210
   voltage sensor in, 200
Sarcolemmal membrane proteins, interaction between sarcoplasmic reticulum and, 202-207
Sarcomere
   in muscle contraction
     of cardiac muscle, 189f
     of skeletal muscle, 185f
   structure of, 178-182, 183f-185f
Sarcoplasmic reticulum (SR), 178, 181f
   Ca^{2+} storage in
     mediation by Ca^{2+}-ATPase of, 157-158, 158b, 159b
     for skeletal muscle contraction, 203-205, 204b, 205f, 206f
   in cardiac muscle, 209-210, 210f
   and T-tubules, 205, 205f, 206f
Sarcoplasmic reticulum (SR) membrane proteins, interaction between sarcolemmal membrane proteins and, 202-207
Sarcoplasmic/endoplasmic reticulum Ca^{2+}-dependent ATPase (SERCA), 156f, 157
   in Ca^{2+} homeostasis, 159
   in cardiac muscle, 210f, 211
   in coupled transport, 160
   crystal structure of, 158b
   isoforms of, 158, 159b
   in muscle contraction, 203, 204
   in muscle relaxation, 207
   in smooth muscle, 220f
   turnover number for, 129t
Saxitoxin (STX), 89, 91b
Sea anemone toxin, 89, 91b
Second messenger(s)
   and ion channel activity, 113
   communication between departments via, 4
   in pharmacomechanical coupling, 218, 219b
Secondary active transport, 134-135, 135b, 138
Secretory diarrhea, 171, 173b
Selective permeability, 37-42
   and concentration gradient, 38f
   and membrane potential, 43b, 44b, 48
   and Nernst equation, 37-42, 39b-41b
Selectivity filter, 55, 57b, 129
Semifused tetanus, 229
SERCA. *See* Sarcoplasmic/endoplasmic reticulum Ca^{2+}-dependent ATPase (SERCA)
Series elastic element, 226, 227f
SGLTs. *See* Sodium and glucose cotransporters (SGLTs)
Shortening, measurement of, 229f

Signaling mechanisms, 5
Signaling proteins, 3
Sildenafil (Viagra), 217, 217b
Simple carriers
  glucose, 131-132, 132f
  reversibility and countertransport by, 133-134
Single-channel currents, measurement of, 84, 86f
"Size principle," 234
Size-ordered recruitment, of motor units, 234, 236b, 236f
Skeletal muscle
  contraction of, 177-188, 199-207, 225-234
    Ca^{2+} in
      binding with troponin C of, 188, 227
      Ca^{2+}-induced release of, 208-211, 210f, 212b, 213b, 213f
      concentration of, 226, 226f, 227-228
      extracellular, 202-203, 203f
      storage in sarcoplasmic reticulum of, 203-205
    Ca^{2+} release channels in, 203, 204, 205-206, 206f, 208f
    cross-bridge cycling in, 184-188, 187f, 232
    depolarization of surface membrane in, 199-202, 200f, 201b, 201f
    efficiency of, 244
    force development in, 226-228, 226f
    force-velocity relationship in, 229-232, 229f, 231f, 233f
    fused, 228-229, 228f
    isometric and isotonic, 229-230, 230f, 231-232, 233f, 234f
    length-tension curve in, 229-232, 229f, 231f
    mechanisms that vary total force of, 225-229
    molecular motors in, 177-178, 179b-180b
    motor units in, 225-226, 232-234, 235f, 236b
    myofibrils in, 178, 181f, 182f
    sarcolemma and sarcoplasmic reticulum in, 202-207
    sarcomere in, 178-182, 183f-185f
    sliding filament mechanism of, 182-184, 185f, 186f, 230-231
    T-tubules in, 202, 203f, 205, 205f
    twitch, 201-202, 201f, 226-228, 226f, 227b
    voltage sensor in, 200, 205, 206, 207b, 208f
  excitation-contraction coupling in, 199-208
  high resting Cl⁻ permeability of, 200-201, 201b
  relaxation of, 207
Skeletal muscle cells, composition of, 178, 181f, 182f
Skou, Jens, 151n
Sliding filament mechanism
  in skeletal muscle, 182-184, 185f, 186f, 230-231
  in smooth muscle, 238-239
Slow twitch, fatigue resistant (S) motor units, 232, 233, 234, 235f, 236b
Smooth muscle(s)
  activation of, 215-218
  contraction of, 190-195, 211-218, 238-246
    ATP in, 243-244, 246b, 247f
    Ca^{2+} in
      elevation of cytosolic, 191-195, 193f, 194f, 195b
      maintaining balance of, 218, 220f
      relation with myosin, phosphorylation and mechanical force in, 242-243, 244f, 245f
    cross-bridges in, 242, 242b, 244, 246b, 247f
    depolarization in, 215
    diversification and, 211-214, 246
    force-velocity relationship in, 239-241, 240f
    innervation density and, 214-215, 214b, 215f
    length-tension relationship in, 238-239, 239f
    myosin light chain phosphorylation in, 239, 240f, 242
    myosin motors in, 177, 242, 242b, 243b
    phasic, 215, 242, 242b
    second messenger in, 218, 219b
    single-unit, 215
    sliding filament mechanism in, 238-239
    structural basis for, 190-191, 192f
    tonic, 215
      ATP in, 243-244, 246b, 247f
      Ca^{2+} channels in, 215-216, 216f
      Ca^{2+} concentration in, 243, 245f
      inositol-1,4,5-trisphosphate in, 218, 219b
      muscle shortening velocity in, 242
      myosin isoforms in, 241, 242b
      myosin light chain phosphorylation in, 242-243, 244f
      pharmacomechanical coupling in, 216-218
  diversification of, 211-214
  excitation-contraction coupling in, 211-218
  locations of, 190
  multiunit, 215
  phasic, 215, 242, 242b
  single-unit, 215
  structure and function of, 190-195, 192f-194f, 195b
  tonic, 215-218, 216f, 242, 242b
  variations in density of innervation of, 214-215, 214b, 215f
  vascular, 215-218, 216f
  vs. skeletal and cardiac muscle, 190-191
SOCs (store-operated channels), 218, 220f
Sodium (Na^+)
  cotransport of, 136-139, 136b, 136f, 137f, 138b, 139b
  equilibrium potential for, 42
  reabsorption of, 168-169
  in resting membrane potential, 45
Sodium and glucose cotransporters (SGLTs), 136-139
  coupling in series of, 139-140, 140f
  energetic consequences of cotransport by, 137-139, 138b
  inherited defects in, 140-141, 141b
  mechanism of, 136, 136f
  transport reactions mediated by, 137, 137f
Sodium bicarbonate ($NaHCO_3$), secretion by exocrine pancreas of, 168

Sodium (Na⁺) channel(s)
　activation and inactivation gates of, 83, 84f
　agents that block, and shape of action potential, 89, 91b, 92f
　deactivation of, and refractory period, 87-89
　in hyperkalemic periodic paralysis, 86, 88b-89b, 88f
　inactivation during maintained depolarization of, 84-86, 87f, 88b-89b
　location and functions of, 100t
　membrane conductance for, 65, 65f
　structure of, 56-57, 57f
　voltage-gated
　　activation gate and inactivation gate of, 85, 87f
　　current flow through, 80, 81f
　　generation of action potential by, 86-89, 90f-92f, 91b
　　structure of, 57, 57f
Sodium chloride (NaCl)
　net reabsorption of, 167f
　secretion across epithelium of, 171, 172f
Sodium (Na⁺) concentration
　extracellular, 38t
　intracellular, 38t, 150
Sodium (Na⁺) currents
　gating, 85b, 85f
　in hyperkalemic periodic paralysis, 88f
　macroscopic, 80-81, 81f
　recording of, 103f
Sodium (Na⁺) homeostasis, pump-leak model of, 150
Sodium (Na⁺) pump
　in Ca²⁺ homeostasis, 159
　in coupled transport, 134, 160
　cycle of, 150, 153f
　"electrogenic" nature of, 152
　hydrolysis of ATP by, 150-152
　isoforms of alpha (α) subunit of, 154, 155b, 156f
　and K⁺ transport into cells, 169, 170f
　in kidneys, 169
　maintenance of low Na⁺ and high K⁺ concentrations in cytosol by, 150-154, 155b, 156f
　net reaction mediated by, 152, 154f
　as receptor for cardiotonic steroids, 152-154, 155b, 160b
　reversibility of, 152b
　structure of, 151, 151f
　turnover number for, 129t
Sodium (Na⁺)-solute cotransport, across apical membrane, 168-169, 169f
Sodium (Na⁺) transporters, in Ca²⁺ homeostasis, 159
Sodium/calcium (Na⁺/Ca²⁺) exchange, 141-143, 142f, 143f, 144b
Sodium/calcium (Na⁺/Ca²⁺) exchanger (NCX), 141, 142f, 143, 143f, 156f
　in Ca²⁺ homeostasis, 159
　in cardiac muscle, 210f, 211
　in coupled transport, 160

　in smooth muscle, 218, 220f
　turnover number for, 129t
Sodium-glucose (Na⁺-glucose) coupling ratio, and glucose uptake, 139, 139b
Sodium-iodine (Na⁺-I⁻) cotransporter (NIC), 136, 136b
Sodium-iodine (Na⁺-I⁻) symporter (NIS), 136, 136b
Sodium/proton (Na⁺/H⁺) exchange, 134-135, 135b, 141
　across apical membrane, 168
　in reabsorption of Na⁺, 169
Sodium/proton (Na⁺/H⁺) exchanger (NHE), 134-135, 135b, 141
Solvent drag, 173
Soma, 53, 54, 54f
Specific membrane capacitance, 66b
Sphincters, 246
"Spike," 77
Square-root-of-time dependence, of diffusion, 11, 12f
SR. *See* Sarcoplasmic reticulum (SR)
Starling, Ernest, 25n
Starling equation, 25
　and direction of fluid flow through capillary wall, 26-29, 26f, 27f, 28b, 29b
Steady-state electrochemical gradient, 130
Steroids, cardiotonic
　and Ca²⁺ signaling, 160b
　Na⁺ pump as receptor for, 152-154, 155b
Store-operated channels (SOCs), 218, 220f
Stress, 239
Stretch-activated, cation-permeable channels, 214-215
Striated muscle, 178, 182f
STX (saxitoxin), 89, 91b
Subcellular compartments, 3
Subcellular organelles, biological membranes of, 3-4, 4f
Substrate specificity, of carrier-mediated transport, 133
Subthreshold potentials, electrical, passive spread of, 69-73, 70f, 71b, 71t, 72f
Sugar transporters, 130-132, 131b, 132b, 132f
Sulfonylurea drugs, for non–insulin-dependent diabetes mellitus, 110, 111b
Surface-to-volume ratio, in membrane permeability, 18b
Sympathetic neurons, 190, 211
Synapses, 53, 54f
Syncytium, 215
　electrical, 190, 190n

T

Taylor, R., 202
Tension, 229
Terminal branches, 54f
Terminal cisterns, 205, 205f, 206f
Tertiary active transport, 145-146, 145f
Tetanus, 201b, 228f, 229
Tetanus toxin, 229n

Tetraethylammonium ions, 89, 91b
Tetrodotoxin (TTX), 56, 56n, 89, 91b, 92f
Thick filaments
    in sliding filament mechanism, 182-184, 185f, 186f
    in smooth muscle, 192f
    structure of, 178-182, 181f, 183f, 184f
Thin filaments
    in sliding filament mechanism, 182-184, 185f, 186f
    in smooth muscle, 192f
    structure of, 178-182, 181f, 183f, 185f
Thomsen's disease, 201b
Threshold, 76
Thyroxine, synthesis of, 136b
Tight epithelia, water transport across, 173-174
"Tight" junctions, 165, 166f, 167f
Time constant
    membrane, 17, 19b, 68, 92
    propagation, 92
Titin, 181
Tone
    myogenic, 215, 215f
    in smooth muscle, 195
Tonic block, 104
Tonic force, in smooth muscle, 195
Tonicity, *vs.* osmolarity, 25, 25b
Transcellular pathway, 165, 166f
Transition state, 130
Transmembrane proteins, 3
Transport
    across biological membranes
        carrier-mediated, 130-134, 131b, 132b, 132f, 133f
        channel, carrier, and pump proteins in, 128-130, 128f, 129t
    across epithelial cells, 165-174
    active. *See* Active transport
    cotransport, 134
        energetic consequences of, 137-139, 138b
        physiology and pathophysiology of, 136b
    countertransport, 133-135
        coupled, 141-143, 142f, 143f, 144b
        exchange of sodium for calcium and protons by, 141-143, 142f, 143f, 144b
        by simple carriers, 133-134
    coupled, 134-135, 135b
        for multiple systems, 144-146, 145f
    passive solute, 127-147
    through channels
        "gating" and, 130
        speed of, 129-130, 129t
Transport processes, 4-5
    coupling in series of, 139-141, 140f, 141b
    electrical potential energy in analysis of, 121-126, 123f-125f
    electrochemical potential energy and, 117-126

Transport proteins, 3
Transport systems, functional coupling in parallel or in series of, 160
Transporters, turnover numbers for, 129t
Transverse tubules. *See* T-tubule(s)
Triads, 205, 205f, 206f
Triiodothyronine, synthesis of, 136b
Tropomyosin, in thin filaments, 182, 185f
Troponin, in thin filaments, 182, 185f
Troponin C, 182
    Ca^{2+} binding to, 188, 227
Troponin I, 182
    binding to, 188
Troponin T, 182
    binding to, 188
T-tubule(s), 178, 181f
    of cardiac muscle, 189f
    and sarcoplasmic reticulum, 205, 205f, 206f
T-tubule membrane, depolarization of, 202, 203f
TTX (tetrodotoxin), 56, 56n, 89, 91b, 92f
T-type Ca^{2+} channel, 102b, 102t
Tubovesicles, 161
Tumor growth, angiogenesis and, 13b
Turnover numbers, 129, 129t
Twitch contraction
    of cardiac muscle, 234
    of skeletal muscle, 201-202, 201f, 226-228, 226f, 227b
Two-pore K^+ channel, 100t, 106b
Tyrosinase, 162b

U

Ultrafiltrate, 168
Unitary displacement step, 241
Unitary force, 241
Urinary bladder, tight epithelium of, 174
Use-dependent block, 104
Uterine smooth muscle, 214

V

Valinomycin, turnover number for, 129t
van't Hoff, Jacobus Henricus, 23n
van't Hoff's Law, 23
Varicosities, 211-213
Vasodilation, 217b
Vasopressin, and water permeability, 129
Vectorial movement, 133
Viagra (sildenafil), 217, 217b
Vibrio cholerae, secretory diarrhea caused by, 173b
Vimentin, 191
Voltage clamps
    recording of calcium currents with, 101-104, 103f
    for study of ion channel function, 77, 78b, 78f
Voltage gating, and transport through channels, 130

Voltage sensor, 200, 205, 206, 207b, 208f
Voltage-dependent conductances, of voltage-gated ion channels, 81-83, 83f, 84f, 85b
Voltage-gated Ca^{2+} channels, 99-104
   contribution to action potentials by, 100, 101f
   structure of, 58
   types of, 100, 102b, 203t
Voltage-gated ion channels, 55
   examples of, 100t
   voltage sensor in, 85b, 85f
   voltage-dependent conductances of, 81-83, 83f, 84f, 85b
Voltage-gated K^+ channels
   current flow through, 80, 81f
   generation of action potential by, 86-89, 90f-92f, 91b
   open, and refractory period, 87-89
   rapidly inactivating, 107-109, 107f-109f
   structure of, 58, 58f, 106b
Voltage-gated Na^+ channels
   activation gate and inactivation gate of, 85, 87f
   current flow through, 80, 81f
   generation of action potential by, 86-89, 90f-92f, 91b
   structure of, 57, 57f
Volume changes, 30

Volume flow, 25
V-type ATPases, 150

W

Water, reabsorption of, 167f, 168
Water movement, through membrane, osmotic pressure and hydrostatic pressure in, 25-29, 26f, 27f, 28b, 29b
Water transport
   across epithelia, 172-174
   during osmosis
      and changes in volume, 22
      osmotic pressure and, 22-25, 23b, 24b, 25b
Wilson disease, 162-163, 163b

X

Xenobiotics, clearance of, 145-146
X-linked congenital stationary night blindness, 100, 103b
X-ray crystallography, of K^+ channel, 58-59, 60f

Z

Z line
   of cardiac muscle, 189f
   of skeletal muscle, 180, 180n, 181, 183f